HEARING AID ASSESSMENT AND USE IN AUDIOLOGIC HABILITATION

HEARING AID ASSESSMENT
AND USE IN
AUDIOLOGIC HABILITATION

Edited By

William R. Hodgson, Ph.D.
Professor of Audiology
Department of Speech and Hearing Sciences
University of Arizona
Tucson, Arizona

AND

Paul H. Skinner, Ph.D.
Professor and Chairman
Department of Speech and Hearing Sciences
University of Arizona
Tucson, Arizona

THE WILLIAMS & WILKINS COMPANY
BALTIMORE

Made in the United States of America

Library of Congress Cataloging in Publication Data

Main entry under title:

Hearing aid assessment and use in audiologic habilitation.

  Bibliography: p.
  Includes indexes.
  1. Hearing aids. 2. Hearing aids—Testing. I. Hodgson, William R. II. Skinner, Paul H. [DNLM: 1. Hearing aids. 2. Hearing disorders—Rehabilitation. WV274 H32]
RF300.H38   617.8'9   76–49041
ISBN 0-683-04090-1

Composed and printed at the
Waverly Press, Inc.
Mt. Royal and Guilford Aves.
Baltimore, Md. 21202, U.S.A.

contributors

(CHAPTER 2)

William F. Carver, Ph.D.
Director,
Division of Audiology and Assistant Professor of Audiology in Otolaryngology
Department of Otolaryngology
Washington University School of Medicine
St. Louis, Missouri

(CHAPTERS 14 and 15)

Theodore J. Glattke, Ph.D.
Associate Professor of Audiology
Department of Speech and Hearing Sciences
University of Arizona
Tucson, Arizona

(CHAPTERS 1, 6, 8, 10, and 12)

William R. Hodgson, Ph.D.
Professor of Audiology
Department of Speech and Hearing Sciences
University of Arizona
Tucson, Arizona

(CHAPTERS 5 and 11)

Roger N. Kasten, Ph.D.
Associate Professor of Audiology
Department of Logopedics
Wichita State University
Wichita, Kansas

(CHAPTER 9)

Noel D. Matkin, Ph.D.
Director of Preschool Language and Learning Center
Boys Town Institute for
Communicative Disorders in Children
Omaha, Nebraska

(CHAPTER 3)

Wayne O. Olsen, Ph.D.
Associate Professor
Department of Otorhinolaryngology, Section of Audiology
Mayo Clinic
Rochester, Minnesota

(CHAPTER 12)

Herbert J. Oyer, Ph.D.
Professor of Audiology and Speech Sciences, and
Dean, the Graduate School
Michigan State University
East Lansing, Michigan

(CHAPTER 13)

Mark Ross, Ph.D.
Professor, Department of Speech
University of Connecticut
Storrs, Connecticut

(CHAPTERS 1 and 7)

Paul H. Skinner, Ph.D.
Professor and Chairman
Department of Speech and Hearing Sciences
University of Arizona
Tucson, Arizona

(CHAPTER 4)

Kenneth E. Smith, Ph.D.
Hearing Associates, Inc.
Prairie Village, Kansas

(CHAPTER 11)

Marilyn P. Warren, Ph.D.
Instructor in Audiology
Department of Logopedics
Wichita State University
Wichita, Kansas

table of contents

Contributors v

CHAPTER 1.
Role of Audiology 1
  Introduction 1
  Principles and Assumptions 2
  Recommended Practice in Hearing Aid Assessment 3

CHAPTER 2.
Development of the Hearing Aid and the
  Hearing Aid Industry 5
  Introduction 5
  Pre-Electric Hearing Aids 5
  Electric Hearing Aids 7
  Vacuum Tube Hearing Aids 10
  Transistor Hearing Aids 12
  The Hearing Aid Industry 14

CHAPTER 3.
Physical Characteristics of Hearing Aids 17
  Introduction 17
  Mode of Operation 18
  Electricity and Electronics 19
  Summary 40
  Recommended Readings 40

CHAPTER 4.
Earmolds and Hearing Aid Accessories 42
  Introduction 42
  Earmolds 42
  Earmold Materials and Impression Techniques 43
  Types of Earmolds 46
  Earmold Connectors 46
  Earmold Modification: Canal Length, Tubing, Bore, and
    Filters 49
  Venting 54

Limitations Associated with the Use of Earmolds 58
Clinical Assessment of Earmold Performance 60
Hearing Aid Accessories 60
Batteries 61
Summary 66

CHAPTER 5.
Electroacoustic Characteristics 67
Introduction 67
Instrumentation for Measuring Electroacoustic Character-
istics of Hearing Aids 68
Common Electroacoustic Characteristics 72
Standards 73
From Yesterday to Today 74
Tomorrow and Beyond 76
Electroacoustics 77
Environmental Tests 86
Other Considerations 89

CHAPTER 6.
Speech Acoustics and Intelligibility 90
Introduction 90
Intensity 90
Long-Term Spectrum 94
Individual Speech Sounds 96
Coarticulation and Suprasegmental Factors 103
Conclusion 104

CHAPTER 7.
Relationship of Electro- and Psychoacoustic
Measures 106
Introduction 106
Gain and Comfort Level, Saturation Sound Pressure Level
and Discomfort Level 107
Electroacoustic Distortion: Speech Quality and Perception 112
Frequency Response and Speech Perception 113
Monaural and Binaural Hearing and Monaural Versus
Binaural Hearing Aid Use 115
Body Baffle and Speech Perception 121
Directional Microphones and Speech Perception 123
Telecoils and Speech Perception 125
Conclusion 126

CHAPTER 8.
Clinical Measures of Hearing Aid Performance 127
Introduction 127
Factors That Determine Need for Amplification 128
Factors That Determine Benefits of Amplification 130
Type of Aid 132
Choice of Aided Ear 132
Hearing Aid Selection Procedures and Philosophies 133
Electroacoustic Characteristics and Hearing Aid Evalua-
tion 139
Conclusions 140

CHAPTER 9.
Hearing Aids for Children 145
Introduction 145
Essential Steps in Procuring an Aid 147
Audiologic Re-Evaluation 163
Parent Management 165
Recommended Readings 168

CHAPTER 10.
Special Cases of Hearing Aid Assessment: CROS Aids 170
Introduction 170
The Head Shadow 171
Hearing Aids That Reduce the Effect of the Head Shadow 172
Effect of the Open Earmold 178
Hearing Aids That Utilize the Head Shadow 181
Clinical Evaluation of CROS-Type Hearing Aids 183
Variations of CROS-Type Aids 185
Conclusion 187

CHAPTER 11.
Learning to Use the Hearing Aid 188
Introduction 188
Step One: Examining the Audiologist's Role 190
Step Two: Introducing the Client to the Hearing Aid 191
Step Three: Introducing the Client to Amplified Sound ... 200
Summary 205

CHAPTER 12.
Aural Rehabilitation through Amplification . . .206
Introduction 206
Conceptualization of the Aural Rehabilitation Process ... 207
Amplification and Aural Rehabilitation 208
Research Needs 220

CHAPTER 13.
Classroom Amplification 221
Introduction 221
General Principles 223
Types of Classroom Amplification Systems 229
The "Optimum" Unit 241
Overview 243

CHAPTER 14.
Hearing Aid Facilities and Delivery Systems ..244
Introduction 244
Physical Facilities 244
Delivery Systems 252
Recommended Readings 259

CHAPTER 15.
Some Implications for Research 260
Introduction 260
Wearable and Group Amplification Systems 260
Surgical Modification of the Ear 264
Implantation Techniques 267
Electrical Stimulation 268
Stimulation of Alternate Sensory Systems 271

BIBLIOGRAPHY 273
AUTHOR INDEX 283
SUBJECT INDEX 287

role of audiology

William R. Hodgson, Ph.D.

Paul H. Skinner, Ph.D.

INTRODUCTION

In 1973, a position paper delineating the responsibilities of the audiologist in habilitation of the hearing-impaired was adopted by the American Speech and Hearing Association. This paper defined audiologic habilitation as a comprehensive process including developmental and restorative procedures in auditory language processing as well as the traditional aural rehabilitative programs of auditory training and speechreading instruction. It was emphasized that audiologic habilitation is a professional nonmedical service that is coordinated with medical treatment. Amplification is critically important in audiologic habilitation. The paper states:

> Providing more efficient speech reception for the individual with a peripheral sensorineural impairment is a fundamental responsibility of audiologists. The *hearing aid* is a critical tool in habilitation. Indeed the capability of the recommended hearing aid to provide the optimal acoustic signals needed determines and limits other aspects of the habilitative process.

> . . . .

> Other aspects of the habilitative process, such as counseling, speechreading, auditory training, and speech and language training are often rendered ineffective when professional responsibilities concerning hearing aids are relinquished. Moreover, the selection and effective use of group amplification systems for children in classrooms require audiologic knowledge and supervision, which should be considered primary duties of the audiologist.

The importance of optimal amplification to the audiologic habilitative process requires that audiologists assume the major responsibility for the selection of their client's hearing aids. The selection of an appropriate aid requires extensive knowledge of the performance characteristics of hearing aids, combined with information about the particular auditory parameters necessary for maximum utilization of each client's residual hearing. In addition, professional skills are needed to effect positive changes in human attitudes and behavior. Clearly such knowledge and skill should lie within the expertise of the professional audiologist. Once an amplification device has been provided for a client, it must be maintained in an optimally functioning condition. The audiologist's responsibility must include regular follow-up evaluation of the amplification unit and the client's adjustment to it (ASHA Committee on Rehabilitative Audiology, 1974. Quoted by permission).

Professional practices as outlined in the above statement, which serve the best interests of consumers, are incumbent upon the profession of audiology. Therefore, an objective examination of principles and assumptions associated with effective use of amplification is warranted. We have attempted such examination in this chapter, stating principles and assumptions as axioms.

PRINCIPLES AND ASSUMPTIONS

First, it is assumed that all persons who choose to consider amplification should receive professional evaluation. The audiologic as well as the otologic examination should be done under adequate conditions and by qualified personnel.

A second assumption is that the procurement and use of a hearing aid should be integral aspects of a program in audiologic habilitation. This assumption implies that selection, use, and care of a hearing aid require special testing, evaluation, and counseling. Trial use of amplification may be necessary to determine the adaptability of a client to amplification, and the suitability of a particular hearing aid.

A third assumption is that persons who choose amplification should be assured of objective advice in hearing aid selection. Hearing aids, if misused, can cause physical damage and mental anguish. In principle, determination of the provision of prosthetics or services in health care should be independent of a profit motive. These decisions rather should be determined solely on the basis of the needs of the client. This principle is not in conflict with provision of products or services for profit. Rather, the distinction is that the client should receive treatment or prosthetic devices based upon an objective evaluation of need.

Fourth, we assume that prosthetic devices and related services should be provided to the consumer at a reasonable cost. Often reasonable cost can be evaluated only by arbitrary criteria, and such costs are expected to differ depending upon the method in delivery of services and even the location at which services and prosthetic devices are delivered.

A final assumption pertains specifically to the use of prosthetic devices. Adequate service should be available for repair and replacement just as follow-up evaluation and treatment should be provided for other health needs.

The desirability of incorporating the hearing aid as a component in audiologic habilitation makes it important to consider current practices in dispensing hearing aids. Various dispensing systems are discussed in Chapter Fourteen, where traditional and alternative delivery systems are detailed, and their merits and problems are considered. We take the position that audiologic services are vital regardless of the dispensing system via which hearing aids are provided. Audiologic services provide the client with information about the extent to which he needs and can benefit from amplification, the kind of aid needed, and how to use it effectively. These problems are considered in detail in Chapters Eight through Twelve.

RECOMMENDED PRACTICE IN HEARING AID ASSESSMENT

In view of the stated principles and assumptions, we believe that certain criteria can be developed regarding audiologic recommendations for amplification. Underlying these criteria is the need for thorough understanding by the audiologist of the physical, electro-, and psychoacoustic characteristics related to hearing aids and their use. These considerations are covered in Chapters Two through Seven. Our concept of hearing aid assessment is based on the criteria given below.

First, otologic examination and audiologic evaluation should precede recommendation and selection of a hearing aid. Otologic examination should be conducted to determine the general status or health of the auditory system, possible treatment, and clearance for hearing aid use relating to such matters as placement of an earmold in the ear canal. An audiologic evaluation should be conducted to ascertain auditory sensitivity, discrimination ability, and any special auditory problems. Additionally, monaural versus binaural capabilities or right versus left ear superiority for hearing aid use should be determined, based upon sensitivity, discrimination ability, and dynamic range. These preliminary measures are the primary determinants for successful hearing aid use and audiologic habilitation, and also may provide the basis for special otologic follow-up evaluation.

Second, a hearing aid evaluation should be conducted by an audiologist and a recommendation for a hearing aid should be determined. Recommendations should include maximum gain, saturation sound pressure level, and frequency response characteristics. Decisions should be made regarding the aided ear or ears, ear level or body-worn aid, air or bone conduction, type of earmold, or for any special fittings, such as a CROS (contralateral routing of signals) aid. If successful use of a hearing aid is questionable, recommendation for a trial period should be made.

Third, clinical testing with a wearable hearing aid is recommended for determination of aided speech reception threshold, aided discrimination ability, and aided tolerance level. Additionally, such testing permits assessment of the client's initial reaction to amplification and provides opportunity for explanation of hearing aid use and counseling regarding the advantages and limitations of a hearing aid.

Finally, counseling and training relevent to hearing aid selection and use should include information on hearing aid function and care, training in listening skills for routine and difficult situations, as well as training as warranted in speechreading and language and speech development or conservation.

In summary, we believe that, regardless of the manner in which hearing aids are dispensed, hearing-impaired clients should receive all aspects of the hearing aid assessment. Hearing aid sales should be based upon prior professional evaluations and objective recommendations. Hearing aids should be provided at a reasonable cost, with provision for maintenance and repair. Trial use of aids should be available to clients who demonstrate special hearing problems. Training in the effective use of amplification is essential. The audiologist must assume a fundamental responsibility in the provision of these services. The material in the following chapters constitutes a foundation for hearing aid assessment and use in audiologic habilitation.

chapter *2*

development of the hearing aid and the hearing aid industry

William F. Carver, Ph.D.

INTRODUCTION

When one observes many animals, one notes that their outer ears are rather specialized, especially when compared to man's. Animals' ears are often elongated and much more cupped than man's. Also, many animals can rotate their auricles to maximize the sound-collecting function of the outer ear. One can imagine early man observing this behavior among animals, and putting his hand, cup-shaped, behind his ear for the same purpose. One can also imagine early man, perhaps playing with an animal horn or a conch shell, and, holding the small end to his ear, noting that the sounds were louder.

One would tend to guess that these early "hearing aids" were probably employed more for hunting and survival than for aiding a hearing handicap, although certainly, they must have been used by those with hearing losses too.

PRE-ELECTRIC HEARING AIDS

Pre-electronic prefabricated "hearing aids" were not called hearing aids, but speaking tubes, deaf aids or instruments, and ear trumpets (Berger, 1970). Probably the largest and most complete collection of these early ear trumpets (as well as electronic aids) is at Kent State University in Kent, Ohio. This large and quite complete collection was obviously assembled with a great deal of patience and effort by Dr. Kenneth Berger.

There is also a smaller collection at Central Institute for the Deaf in St.

Louis. What is interesting when one observes these exhibits, is the extreme variety — indeed, inventiveness — which early manufacturers employed to make these old aids more attractive, less cumbersome, and less obvious. Yes, even in the early history of pre-electric hearing aids, efforts were made to conceal the handicap.

The various shapes and configurations of these ear trumpets are of interest. In general, these devices had a large opening on one end, and a small one at the other. The large end collected the sound waves and concentrated them at the small opening, which, of course, the hard-of-hearing person held to his ear canal. This general shape actually produced amplification across a restricted frequency band. However, since any hollow tube will act as a resonator, certain frequencies had higher amplification than others. That is, at the resonant frequencies, peaks of amplification would be observed at the expense of other frequencies where anti-resonant valleys in the response curve can be observed. The frequency response of an ear trumpet is shown in Figure 2-1.

Some of the shapes included the "pipe" trumpet, looking like an over-sized smoking pipe, the "banjo," so named because its sound-collecting end was shaped somewhat like a banjo; and the bell resonators or London Domes shown in Figure 2-2. They can best be described as a dome-shaped resonator with the listening tube coming out of the large end and curving up to the earpiece.

Another approach was the speaking tube, a flexible tube usually 3 to 4 feet long. The hearing-handicapped person could hand the large end to the person with whom he wished to converse and, holding the outer end to his ear, still be 3 to 4 feet away from his conversational partner who spoke into the tube.

Some of the more exotic or unusual aids were small "scoops" on a

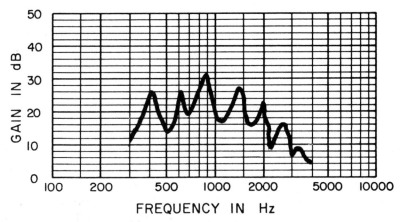

Fig. 2-1. Frequency response of an ear trumpet.

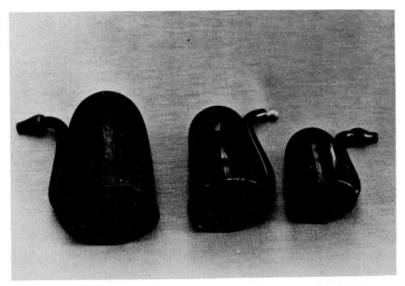

FIG. 2-2. Ear trumpets (Courtesy of Kent State University Hearing Aid Museum).

headband; an acoustic vase, which had one or more listening tubes coming out of it, the latter for group conversations; a cane with a small bell resonator or scoop at the handle; an ear trumpet of the bell resonator type in a hat. There was even an acoustic chair, as shown in Figure 2-3. The arms were sound collectors, and there was a flexible tube for listening.

Many of these devices, especially the trumpet types, were collapsible. This allowed one to have the advantage of a longer tube for listening, but a less cumbersome thing to carry, when the tube was not required.

It should also be mentioned that an artificial eardrum was developed, which appears to be somewhat dangerous. It was said to be used by those who had large tympanic membrane perforations. It was a small tube covered by a pig's bladder with a small silver rod connected to it. This silver rod was to be inserted through the perforation and located on the stapes. Its value is somewhat suspect.

For those with conductive losses, non-electric bone conduction aids were available. In general, these aids had a large sound-collecting area and a device which was either placed on the teeth or between the teeth. Figure 2-4 shows an "acoustic fan" for bone conduction.

Several texts have additional illustrations of non-electric hearing aids. These are Berger (1970), Davis (1947), and Watson and Tolan (1949).

ELECTRIC HEARING AIDS

The first hearing aids which employed electricity for amplification were introduced around the beginning of the 20th century. It is known that electric hearing aids were associated with the development of the tele-

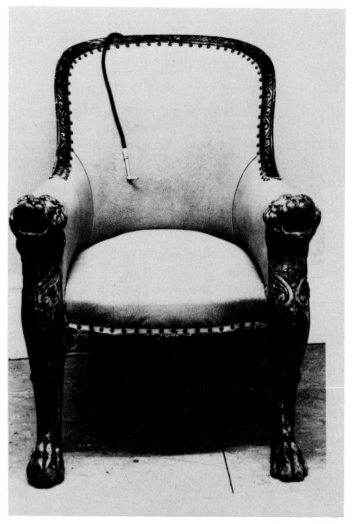

FIG. 2-3. Acoustic chair (Courtesy of Kent State University Hearing Aid Museum).

phone. Some say that Alexander Graham Bell was attempting to produce an electronic hearing aid, but ended up with the telephone (Watson and Tolan, 1949). What is interesting is that Bell invented the telephone in 1876, and the first patent on the use of the principle was granted in 1880, but the hard-of-hearing had to wait until 1903 for an electronic hearing aid to be commerically produced (Berger, 1970). The principle employed in these early electric hearing aids was a carbon granule microphone and magnetic earphone, powered by a battery. The system works like this: A current from the battery is driven through a pile of carbon granules. These carbon granules are confined in a cavity, one wall of which is a diaphragm. The diaphragm will move with the impinging sound waves, alternately compressing and releasing the carbon granules. Since these carbon granules change their electrical resistance in relation to the pressure applied, a constantly changing current will be the output. What we have described is a carbon microphone, which was called a transmitter. The changing electrical signal is led to the receiver. This is a magnetic device. The wire is coiled around metal "pole" pieces and as the electrical signal varies in the coil, it sets up a varying magnetic force which pulls on a metallic diaphragm. This diaphragm, acting on air, reproduces the signal which impinged upon the microphone diaphragm, the signal having been amplified by the carbon microphone. The frequency response of a carbon aid is compared with that of an ear trumpet in Figure 2-5.

The earlier devices were not readily portable, but time brought improvement, such that carbon aids became wearable. Several improvements were made with the carbon-type hearing aids, primarily resulting in greater amplification—for instance, the carbon amplifier: instead of leading the current from the carbon microphone directly to the receiver, the current was fed to a device similar to the receiver, except that the diaphragm was

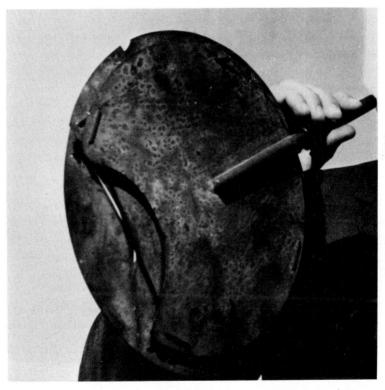

FIG. 2-4. Acoustic fan for bone conduction. The signal is transmitted from the collecting discs via the solid cylindrical handle (Courtesy of Kent State University Hearing Aid Museum).

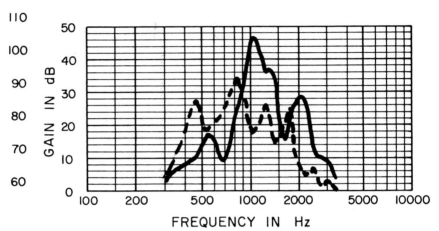

FIG. 2-5. Frequency response of an ear trumpet and a carbon hearing aid. The *broken line* represents the ear trumpet and the *solid line* the carbon aid.

made to compress additional carbon granules through which current was being driven. This effectively increased the amplification to about 35 dB gain.

Carbon aids were noisy and produced some distortion. Also, they had an annoying habit of "going off the air" when the wearer bent over. This was because the carbon granules would lose contact with the diaphragm or the wire contacts when in positions other than upright. Moisture was also a problem with the carbon granules.

Manufacturers attempted to increase output by increasing the number of microphones. Many carbon aids had two microphones, and some had even three or four. All of these aids were bulky and those persons with carbon amplification often had to carry the batteries separately, but many hearing handicapped made good use of them.

VACUUM TUBE HEARING AIDS

Vacuum tubes (radio tubes) had been around for many years before they were employed in wearable hearing aids. According to Berger (1970), the first vacuum tube hearing aid was commercially available about 1921. Produced by Western Electric for Globe Ear-Phone Company, it was a single tube amplifier in a box which was portable, but not wearable.

Western Electric then produced its own hearing aid. This hearing aid was binaural, but not the least bit portable. It required automobile-type batteries.

So, for a few years, the hearing-handicapped had some choice. They could wear a carbon-type aid, or they could use a tube-type amplifier, but they could not conceal it on their person. The advantage of the carbon aid was the wearability, but the wearer had to sacrifice gain and fidelity. The tube-type aids, some portable and some not, had greater gain and better fidelity, but, if portable, the person had to carry a large box that was comparatively heavy because of the batteries.

Tube-type hearing aids require two power supplies. Electronic tubes have filaments which must be heated to drive off the electrons. A $1^{1}/_{2}$-volt battery was used for this purpose. To "draw" the electrons through the grid to the plate, a comparatively high voltage must be applied to the plate. Hearing aids usually used either a $22^{1}/_{2}$ or a 45 volt battery for the plate voltage. The $1^{1}/_{2}$ volt battery was called the "A" battery, and the higher voltage battery, the "B" battery.

In the early 1930's, electronic tubes were reduced in size sufficiently to be placed in a case which could be worn on the body. The case usually contained only the microphone and the amplifier. The batteries had to be carried separately. Women sometimes strapped the batteries to their legs, leading the power wires to the chest where the microphone-amplifier was hung, then a wire led to the receiver at the ear or to a vibrator for bone conduction. Men would often carry the batteries in their pockets.

The microphones employed in the early vacuum tube hearing aids were of a crystal type. Rochelle salt crystals were employed. These crystals have the property of producing minute electrical currents when distorted (called the piezoelectric effect). Therefore, the diaphragm of the microphone was attached to the crystal and the tiny currents produced by sounds impinging upon the diaphragm were led to the grid of the electronic tube for amplification. The receivers, in the early wearable vacuum-type hearing aids were also crystal. Two major problems surrounded the use of crystals in hearing aids; (1) their inability to withstand high temperatures or moisture, and, (2) their fragility.

The wearable tube-type hearing aid did not immediately replace carbon aids, but their time was limited. Some hearing aid companies which produced carbon aids switched to vacuum tube models and a few are still viable. Other companies either were sold or dropped from sight.

As time passed, tubes became smaller and so did batteries. A major problem for manufacturers was battery life. The current drawn from the "A" battery to heat the filament was very high in the early aids, requiring continuing battery changes. Current drain in the "B" batteries was also high, compared to later models. During a period of 10 years, manufacturers were able to reduce current drain $4^{1}/_{2}$ times for the "A" battery and 8 times for the "B" battery (Watson and Tolan, 1949).

The first wearable aid was produced in England (where the vacuum tube was invented years before). The first wearable aid made in the United States was called the "Stanleyphone," which was introduced in 1937. One would think that a Mr. Stanley had made the aid, but it was a Mr. Arthur M. Wengel who produced it. Other manufacturers soon began to manufacture wearable vacuum tube hearing aids in the years following. The earliest were Trimm, followed by Telex, and then Maico, according to Berger (1970). Watson and Tolan (1949) mentioned only Telex as producing the vacuum tube aid in 1938 and Maico in 1939. The Aurex Company was the first to manufacture vacuum tube hearing aids on a large scale in the United States. These aids employed four vacuum tubes of the company's own design.

Those companies who were manufacturing carbon-type hearing aids such as Sonotone, Western Electric, Auraphone, Gem, Acousticon, and Radioear were slower in changing over to vacuum tube hearing aids. New names of manufacturers also began to appear; some of them are still with us today. In order of introduction date, some of these manufacturing companies were Paravox, Solo-Pak, Vacolite, all in 1938, Otarion in 1939, Beltone in 1940, Alladin in 1941, Golden Tone and Zenith in 1942, Micronic and National in 1946 and Microtone in 1947.

World War II had its effect on the hearing aid industry. Probably, as far as the hearing aid user was concerned, one of the most useful developments was the significant reduction in battery size with the introduction of the mercury battery. Beltone designed an early one piece aid (probably the first one piece wearable vacuum tube aid) which employed a mercury battery. Beltone's problem was getting these batteries released for the non-military consumer.

The "Monopac," Beltone's name for the one piece aid, was larger than the amplifier-microphone package (with separate batteries) of that date, but it found immediate acceptance because one no longer had to "wire himself up" to hear. It wasn't long before manufacturers further reduced the size of the aid, employing techniques and materials developed during World War II: for instance, the printed circuit and ceramic capacitors.

TRANSISTOR HEARING AIDS

The transistor as described in Chapter Three is a semi-conductor made of silicon or germanium crystals which have certain amounts of impurity in them. They perform many of the tasks that vacuum tubes do, sometimes better and often more efficiently. There are two major advantages that the transistor has over the radio tube: they are smaller and they do not require electric current for heating a filament. Recall that the vacuum tube in hearing aids required a $1\frac{1}{2}$ volt "A" battery to heat the filament and a higher voltage, usually $22\frac{1}{2}$ or 45 volts, to supply the plate current. The transistor is a solid, has no heater, and requires very little voltage to "drive" it. Therefore, it uses a single cell battery of 1.4 to 1.6 volts.

The first transistor, developed by Bell Telephone Laboratories in 1947, was of a point contact type which was not suitable for hearing aids. Around 1952, the junction type was introduced and was used in hearing aids. Transistors are discussed in some detail in Chapter Three.

Several manufacturers, probably looking for advertising fodder, quickly employed one transistor and two or more vacuum tubes in their hearing aids, thus being able to advertise that they were employing transistors in their hearing aids. It wasn't too long, however, before conventional aids were all transistor. The first ones were introduced in 1953 by several manufacturers.

I can recall vividly sitting in a classroom one summer morning in 1953. Dr. Raymond Carhart was lecturing and, in essence, said, "Now that the transistor has been developed, hearing aids can be built small enough to place them on the head. It's too bad," he went on, "because we could have true binaural hearing aids except that since the microphone and the receiver would be so close to each other, feed-back would be an insurmountable problem."

Late in 1954, Otarion introduced the first head-worn hearing aid. It was an eyeglass hearing aid. Perhaps, because of a concern over feedback, or maybe because of size limitations, the aid (called the "listener") had the microphone in one temple and the receiver in the other temple. The first CROS (contralateral routing of signals) aid had arrived!

In 1955, Beltone introduced the "Hear-N-See" eyeglass hearing aid with the entire hearing aid in one temple, thus true binaural hearing aids were made possible. In the same year Audiotone produced a behind-the-ear hearing aid. The early models were somewhat bulky. But, the size was quickly reduced.

At first, eyeglass-type hearing aids far outsold either behind-the-ear or conventional body aids, but as the size was reduced, behind-the-ear hearing aids became the largest seller. Everything has been getting smaller. One component, the capacitor, was significantly reduced with the introduction of the tantalum capacitor. The transducers were also being reduced in size, with the adverse effect of restricting the bandwidth of the frequency response and the creation of sharp resonant peaks and anti-resonant valleys. This continued until the introduction of the ceramic microphone. The ceramic microphone is a piezoelectric microphone without many of the problems of the rochelle salt crystal microphone. The ceramic microphone has been replaced by the electret microphone described in Chapter Three. Both the ceramic and electret microphone have wide, comparatively flat frequency responses, but the electret is much less subject to shock damage and is, therefore, the microphone of choice.

Circuit changes were equally dramatic. Developing from printed circuit boards to which transistors, resistors, and capacitors were hand-soldered, into extremely small integrated circuits or so-called hybrid circuits, the amplifier is the smallest part of today's hearing aid. Hearing aids are now so small that they can be placed entirely within the concha in an earmold fashioned for each individual ear. Manufacturers of these "all-in-the-ear" aids claim that they can satisfactorily fit severe hearing losses. Styles of current hearing aids are shown in Figure 2-6.

THE HEARING AID INDUSTRY

There has been a comparatively large number of hearing aid manufacturers, especially when the relatively small market is considered. Some companies have been quite stable, making the transition from carbon aids to vacuum tube aids to transistor aids with little difficulty. Others have dropped out with the change, while others took their place.

The list of companies which have, or which are manufacturing hearing aids is almost overwhelming. If the reader is interested in this aspect, he is referred to Berger (1970). Part II of this book (almost as thick as Part I) lists manufacturers and their products as best as Berger could gather. It is an impressive compendium.

With the exception of Sonotone, hearing aid manufacturers have sold their products to independent businesses, a large number under some kind of franchise agreement. Sonotone owned their retail outlets until 1969.

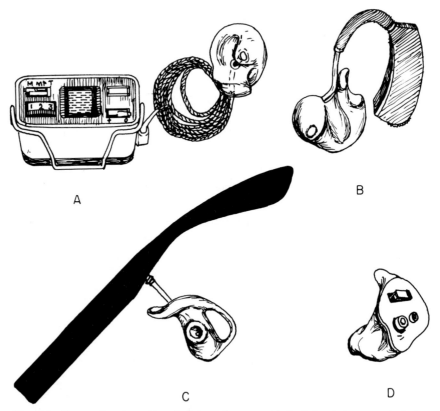

FIG. 2-6. Current hearing aid styles. A. Body-worn aid. B. Behind-the-ear aid. C. Eye-Glass aid. D. In-the-ear aid.

Periodically, throughout the years the hearing aid industry has come under attack, by Government, by consumer groups, and by professional groups. In the 1940's and the early 50's, hearing aids could be submitted to the Council on Physical Medicine of The American Medical Association. The Council tested aids submitted and "accepted" those which met certain minimum standards. Interestingly, the Council also took into account merchandising practices, financial dealings, and advertising, among other items, before accepting an aid. The Council most frequently withdrew or temporarily suspended acceptance because of advertising practices (Davis, 1947). This entire practice was discontinued in the 1950's.

The Federal Trade Commission began in the late 1940's to investigate the franchise system of the hearing aid industry. Beginning in 1949, the Federal Trade Commission (FTC) has brought action against many companies for violations of federal laws, most often the Clayton Act and the FTC Act. Early, several companies had exclusive contracts with their dealers which required each dealer to sell only those aids manufactured by the company with whom he was franchised. The FTC ordered that this be discontinued. Two companies fought the order of the Commission and lost, the others signed consent decrees which allowed all dealers to sell any hearing aid they wanted to. Also, the FTC has been putting out cease and desist orders to companies for false advertising, misrepresentation, false claims, "bait" advertising, etc.

Although companies had to give up their exclusive dealing contracts, they were still able to sell their products only to those dealers they wished. Recently the FTC brought action against this practice and most of the companies have signed consent decrees. One very large company is fighting the FTC order. At this writing a decision from the Commission is being awaited.

In 1962, Senator Kefauver, Chairman of the Sub-Committee on Anti-Trust and Monopoly of the Committee of the Judiciary held a hearing subsequent to an investigation of the "prices of hearing aids" (1962). Among the witnesses at that hearing was Mrs. Eleanor Roosevelt. No laws were a direct result of that hearing.

At the present time the FTC is holding hearings on other aspects of the delivery system and on advertising. One important proposed ruling is that a purchaser be allowed to return an aid he has purchased within 30 days for his money back less some allowances. Another ruling is that all advertisements relative to hearing aids carry the disclaimer, "Many persons with a hearing loss will not be able to consistently distinguish and understand speech sounds in noisy environments by using any hearing aid." Naturally, the industry is objecting to these proposed rulings.

The history of the hearing aid and the industry is, if we are concerned with only electric aids, three-quarters of a century old. In the 75 years, technology has made tremendous strides and the hearing aid industry has kept up technologically. New techniques were employed as they were developed and, as a matter of fact, the industry was the first to employ the transistor commercially.

Because there were no audiologists when the hearing aid industry was developing, the dispensing of hearing aids fell to the salesman. Early hearing aids were far from the sophisticated instruments of today. They were noisy, cumbersome, and the portable ones could not provide much amplification. Instrumentation for measurement of hearing loss was just being developed and was not portable. Salesmen only had to determine whether their customers were able to get some help from the products. Unfortunately, there are many itinerant salesmen who did not even make that determination. Through the efforts of the industry and its sales force, salesmen began to improve themselves. The larger companies wrote training manuals. The salesmen organized the national organization now called the National Hearing Aid Society and they have a correspondence course which must be taken and the test passed before a salesman can become a member. The larger companies have training seminars to which they invite their salesmen. The Hearing Aid Industry Conference has sponsored workshops throughout the country. In short, the industry has realized that it is, in a sense, a semi-medical field. Attempting to maintain the present delivery system, it is trying to upgrade its salespersons. Only time will tell how successful it will be.

physical characteristics of hearing aids

Wayne O. Olsen, Ph.D.

INTRODUCTION

A hearing aid may be described as "any instrument that brings sound more effectively to the listener's ear. It may simply collect more sound energy from the air, it may prevent the scattering of sound during transmission, or it may provide additional energy, usually from the battery of an electrical amplifier" (Silverman, Taylor, and Davis, 1960, p. 265). It is the last type of instrument, specifically the electronic hearing aid, that is the focus here.

An electronic hearing aid is a private, portable, public address system. As with any public address system, its purpose is to amplify, or make sounds stronger. Also like a public address system, the main components are a microphone, an electronic amplifier, a loudspeaker, and a power source. Many public address systems, however, are large devices permanently installed in buildings or stadia of various types. Nevertheless, some public address systems are portable, but they generally are not thought of as being "worn" or carried inconspicuously on the human body. Thus, the distinguishing features of electronic hearing aids are that they are carried or worn on the body and that they are "private" in amplifying sound only for the ear (or ears) of the wearer.

The writer does not presume that this chapter will provide a complete synopsis of the intricacies of hearing aid design, and makes no attempt to trace the development of hearing aids and the refinements of their components to their current state. It is hoped that those readers who are unfamiliar with hearing aid technology will become somewhat acquainted with the terminology and principles involved in the function of the various components of hearing aids. Thereby, hopefully, they will gain a better appreciation of the workings of contemporary hearing aids.

MODE OF OPERATION

As alluded to earlier, the purpose of a hearing aid is to increase the amplitude of sounds occurring in nature so that they become audible to the user. However, substantial increases in acoustical energy at the ear are not easily or inconspicuously accomplished by enlarging surface areas for collection of acoustic energy. Further, the laws of nature do not allow creation or loss of energy. Conversion of energy from one form to another form is, however, readily achieved. Hearing aids take advantage of the latter phenomenon and the fact that electrical energy is readily modified and increased by additional electrical energy provided from a different source.

The basic operation of a hearing aid is a three step process. First, the sound waves (acoustic energy) are transduced into corresponding electrical waveforms (electrical energy) by the hearing aid microphone. Second, these electrical waveforms are amplified by the electronic circuit of the hearing aid through the utilization of additional electrical energy provided by a battery. Third, the amplified electrical waveforms are transduced back to sound waves, more intense than those impinging upon the microphone, by the hearing aid earphone and delivered to the wearer's ear.

ELECTRICITY AND ELECTRONICS

Electrical energy and electronic circuitry are essential to the function of hearing aids. Therefore, a cursory review of the fundamentals of electricity and the behavior of the electronic components in hearing aids is appropriate here. This discussion cannot be complete, but it is hoped that it will suffice at least to acquaint readers with relevant terminology and give them some insight into the workings of a hearing aid.

Beginning at the molecular level, all molecules are made up of atoms, each of which consists of a nucleus and electrons which orbit the nucleus. The nucleus is made of protons and neutrons and carries a miniscule positive electrical charge, while the electrons have a minute negative electrical charge. The number of electrons possessed by an atom determines the basic element to which it belongs in the universe. Those elements which possess a greater number of electrons also have a higher number of protons in the nucleus so that each atom appears electrically neutral. The electrons are constantly in orbit around the nucleus. The orbits of these electrons are referred to as *electronic shells* or *valences* with different shells having different diameters around the nucleus. The electrons are held in their orbits by *electrostatic forces of attraction* in which unlike charges attract each other. That is, the negative charge of the electron attracts it to the positive charge of the proton. The electrons in the larger diameter orbits or shells, however, are only weakly attracted to the nucleus. Further, the outer electronic shells are not always fully occupied in metals and similar materials. In such instances neighboring atoms sometimes share one or more electrons, so called *covalent electrons*. Since these electrons in the outer shells are only weakly attracted to the nucleus, it requires only a small force or energy of some sort to detach them from the nucleus and cause them to change location. Hence the application of some external force to materials having these loosely attached or *"free"* electrons can cause them to escape the orbit of their nuclei and result in *"electron flow,"* more commonly referred to as *current flow*. Current flow is measured in units called *amperes,* one ampere being the flow of 6.3×10^{18} electrons "flowing" past a given point in one second. Materials which possess free electrons that can be readily caused to "flow" are called *conductors*. Copper is one such material that is commonly used as a conductor.

When electrons are "fed" in some way to a material, it then has an excess of electrons and takes on a *negative charge,* or potential, relative to its previous state. If electrons are extracted from a material, the shortage of electrons results in *positive charge,* or potential, in that material. If two points of any material or system have a relative excess of electrons at one point and a relative shortage of electrons at another, a *difference in potential* exists at the two points. If these two points are connected by a conductor such as described above, in electrical jargon called *"completing the circuit,"* the electrons at the negative point will flow toward the less negative or positive point through the conductor. Hence, the difference in potential at the two points has resulted in an electron flow or current flow through the conductor to equalize the charge at the two points. In view of the fact that a difference in potential can result in electron flow, *electromotive force* is another descriptive term used for this electrical entity.

The unit of measure for this electrical difference in potential or electromotive force is given the label of *"volt(s)"*; hence, the synonym *voltage* in place of the longer terms, difference in potential or electromotive force. One volt is the voltage necessary to cause one ampere of current flow through one ohm of resistance. Resistance and ohms are defined later.

One of the interesting phenomena accompanying the motion of electrons is the generation of *magnetic fields*. Apparently the magnetic fields thus developed are due primarily to the *spinning motion of the electron on its own axis* as it orbits about the atomic nucleus. Even though electrons generally orbit the atomic nucleus in pairs, in most materials the spin of each electron in the pair is usually in opposite directions. In magnetic or magnetized materials the pairs spin in the same direction setting up *magnetic domains* and *magnetic lines of force* such that magnetic *north* and *south poles* are developed. The important point for this discussion is that the electron action in current flow through a conductor is such that magnetic fields also develop around the conductor. The strength of the magnetic field is dependent upon the amount of current flow; further, the "north-south" orientation of the magnetic field is dependent on the direction of the current flow. This facet of electrical phenomena is important to hearing aids in the operation of their output transducers, that is their earphones and bone vibrators, as is seen later in this chapter.

Just as current flow in a conductor generates magnetic fields, it should be noted that *relative motion of magnetic lines of force in the vicinity of a conductor* can also *induce* a *voltage* and thereby cause a current flow in a conductor. Thus, if two conductors are placed side by side and a current is caused to flow in one of them, magnetic lines of force are developed around it. As current flow increases, more and more lines of force are developed. The action of this expanding magnetic field is to induce a small current flow in the adjacent conductor, in a direction opposite to that of the first conductor. The current flow in the second conductor is caused by the magnetic lines of force *"cutting across"* the conductor as the magnetic field is expanding. When the current flow in the first conductor has stabilized at one level, no current flow is induced in the second conductor. In other words, it is only as the magnetic lines of force are expanding, diminishing, or changing polarity and thereby cutting across the second conductor that current flow is induced in it accordingly. This principle is utilized in hearing aids in their telephone pickup coils to receive magnetic signals developed by telephone receivers and the magnetic signals developed by induction loop amplification systems used in some classrooms for the hearing-impaired.

Batteries

One electrical source of power which possesses a large number of electrons at one point and considerably fewer at another is an *electric storage cell*, commonly referred to as a *battery*. The principle of operation here is that when two different metals (*electrodes)* are placed in an acid or lye (*electrolyte)*, a chemical action takes place between the acid and metals in which electrons are liberated. These electrons collect at one of the metals, which thereby takes on a negative charge and becomes a source of free electrons. As a source of free electrons it is also called a *cathode*. The other metal now has fewer electrons, is thereby positively charged relative to the cathode and, in that state, is referred to as an *anode*. Thus, there is a difference in potential between these two metals; that is, between the negatively charged cathode with its excess of electrons and the positively charged anode with its fewer electrons. If an external conductor (described earlier as a material having free electrons which can be caused to flow) is connected between the cathode and anode, the free electrons in the cathode will displace the free electrons in the conductor toward the less negative, that is the positive metal or anode, producing current flow. Upon reaching the anode more electrons are displaced from it into the electrolyte and the chemical action again frees electrons which are collected at the opposite metal. Thus, there is a continuing current flow from the cathode through the conductor to the anode, through it and the electrolyte back to the cathode again. This process continues until the metals and/or the acid are spent or formed into new compounds no longer capable of liberating free electrons. Thus, in such an operation a storage cell or battery can be considered as a *reservoir of energy* stored in a chemical state which can be converted to electrical energy when called upon to do so.

The most popular devices of this type used in hearing aids are *mercury cells* or *silver oxide cells*. Although commonly referred to as batteries, most energy sources used in hearing aids are more accurately labelled *cells*. A *battery* is a *group of cells* interconnected to provide electrical power of proper voltage and current. Most hearing aids use a single cell capable of developing ≃1.3–1.5 volts. In the mercury cell the cathode is formed by zinc, the anode is made up primarily of mercuric oxide, and the electrolyte is a solution of potassium hydroxide and zinc oxide. The difference in potential between these two electrodes is ≃1.4 volts. The materials are encased in corrosion-proof nickel-plated containers to prevent leakage. Silver oxide cells are constructed of similar materials, but silver oxide is used for the cathode and potassium hydroxide is used for the electrolyte. The voltage developed by a silver oxide cell is ≃1.5 volts.

The above-described sources are *primary cells* in that chemical energy is converted to electrical energy without previous electrical charging. *Secondary cells* (also called *accumulators)* are used in a few hearing aids. Secondary cells require electrical charging before use. In this process electrical energy applied to the accumulator is converted to stored chemical energy. This chemical energy in turn is converted back to electrical energy when properly connected to a circuit through which current can flow. The process of applying electrical energy to the accumulator, that is, charging and recharging it, can be repeated again and again. (A car battery is a common example of a secondary cell and the charging, use, and recharging process.)

Nickel cadmium (nicad) accumulators are used in some hearing aids. The name here denotes the materials, nickel serving as the anode, cadmium as the cathode. Potassium hydroxide is the electrolyte in such accumulators.

The schematic symbol for an electric cell is ⊢⊢⌣ (A schematic is a diagram using various symbols to show electronic circuit connections. Throughout this discussion schematic symbols are introduced.) In the symbol for an electric cell, the short bar represents the cathode or negative pole and the longer bar is the anode or positive pole. When a group of cells are connected to form a battery, a series of short and long bars is used: ₊│┃│┃│ .

Resistance

The discussion so far has implied that electrons do not readily "flow" in a conductor inasmuch as some outside force is necessary to cause current flow in a conductor. All materials having free electrons offer some opposition to current flow dependent upon the material, that is, the number of free electrons, length, and cross section of the material. The opposition to current flow in a conductor is labelled *resistance,* the measurement unit of electrical resistance being *ohm(s).* According to international agreement, one ohm is the electrical resistance of a 106.3 cm column of mercury of 1 mm² cross section at 0°C.

In 1826 G. S. Ohm recognized the relationship between voltage, resistance, and current which has come to be known as Ohm's Law. Obviously, the unit of resistance is also named after him. If resistance is maintained as a constant in a material or circuit but the voltage is increased or decreased, the current flow also increases or decreases in direct proportion. Similarly, if the voltage is maintained at a constant level, but the resistance of the conductor is increased or decreased, the current flow decreases or increases in an inversely proportional manner. As mentioned earlier, one volt is the electromotive force necessary to cause one ampere of current to flow through one ohm of resistance.

At this point it seems appropriate to introduce some of the shorthand used for discussions of electricity. E represents voltage — unit of measurement: volts. I represents current — unit of measurement: amperes. R represents resistance — unit of measurement: ohms (often symbolized by Ω). Ohm's Law then can be written $I = E/R$. This equation can of course be transposed so that if the values of two of these factors are known the third can be determined. Since $I = E/R$, then $E = IR$ and $R = E/I$.

In order to limit current (I) flow to desired levels either the voltage (E) or the resistance (R) can be altered. In some electrical circuits however, it is desirable to obtain different voltages and different amounts of current flow in the various segments of the circuit. Devices simply labelled as *resistors* are one of the means by which current flow is limited to desired levels. Resistors are constructed to present an obstacle, but not an insurmountable opposition to current flow. Such devices can be constructed to offer a few ohms, hundreds, thousands, or even millions of ohms of resistance (R) to current flow.

Resistors used in hearing aids are generally of the carbon or carbon film type. Whereas carbon is a relatively good conductor, the amount of resistance offered by it is dependent upon the density of the packing of the carbon as well as the dimensions of the device. Carbon film resistors are made up of a thin film of carbon deposited on a ceramic body. The length and thickness of the carbon deposit determine the value of the resistance. Resistors of the carbon or carbon film type which are fixed in value are represented by the symbol ⊣□⊢ .

Other resistors can be varied in value simply by placing a sliding contact on the resistive element. The symbol for a *variable resistor,* also called a *rheostat,* aptly represents the principle involved: ⊣□⊦ . The position of the contact on the resistor can be moved along the length of the resistor and thereby vary the length or amount of resistance through which the current must pass. Devices such as this function as a variable control in the tone controls of some hearing aids.

A variation of this arrangement is called a *potentiometer* and follows the same principle as shown by the symbol ⊣□⊦ . It differs only in that two paths of current flow are provided so that some of the current can continue through the whole resistor to the rest of the circuit, and through the sliding contact to the circuit beyond it. Devices such as this serve as gain controls in hearing aids.

Insulators

Materials having essentially no free electrons and offering virtually total opposition to current flow are labelled *insulators.* Glass, rubber, plastics, etc. are examples of insulators. Even though such materials can be forced to conduct current if a high enough voltage is impressed across them, they are usually destroyed in the process. Insulators prevent current flow between two points.

Capacitors

One type of electrical device which incorporates both conductors and insulators in its construction is called a *capacitor* (also sometimes called a *condenser*). Capacitors are made up of two conductors, usually in the form of plates, separated by an insulator. Capacitors are aptly named for their capacity to store an electrical charge and thereby oppose changes in voltage. The larger the plates, and the better the insulator (also called *dielectric*) the greater its capacity for storing electrical charges, or *capacitance.* The symbol for a capacitor is ⊣ ⊢ .

When the negative pole (cathode) of a battery or some such source is connected to one plate of a capacitor and the positive pole (anode) is connected to the other plate, a momentary flow of electrons occurs from the cathode to the plate until it is saturated; simultaneously some electrons leave the opposite plate, being attracted to the positive pole of the battery. After this momentary flow of electrons, the capacitor is charged to the same potential as the battery and no further current flow occurs because the electrons are unable to pass through the dielectric (insulator) separating the two plates.

Circuits in which the negative and positive polarities are maintained at the same points continually have current flow in only one direction, referred to as *direct current* or *DC*. Batteries, of course, are direct current sources. Inasmuch as there is momentary but not continued current flow when a capacitor is connected to a DC source, capacitors are considered to *block* direct current flow. That is, they "*block DC*"

If, however, one were to connect an electrical source to a capacitor in the manner described above, but then suddenly reverse the polarity of the voltage applied to its plates, the excess electrons at one plate would leave it, and flow through the outside circuit connections to the opposite plate of the capacitor. That is, they would flow around the capacitor to the other plate. If this reversing process were repeated again and again, the resulting current flow would be alternating in direction, and would be called *alternating current,* or *AC*. Under such circumstances capacitors function to pass *alternating current*, in effect passing the current flow around the dielectric of the capacitor through the outside circuitry connected to the capacitor. In this manner, capacitors are said to "*pass AC*."

Both DC and AC are utilized in hearing aids. Capacitors therefore are important components in their electronic circuitry.

Transistors

Having considered conductors with free electrons, insulators which have essentially no free electrons, and capacitors which incorporate both, it is time to consider an intermediate class of materials, *semi-conductors*. Such materials are neither good conductors nor good insulators, but under certain circumstances they can conduct some current.

The atomic structure of some materials, for example, pure germanium or pure silicon, is such that electrons in the outermost shell of one atomic nucleus are simultaneously members of the outer shell of another atomic nucleus. These electrons are held in their orbits by so-called *covalent bonds*. With these shared electrons, there is seemingly full occupancy of the outer electronic shells of the nuclei. However, if a different material or *impurity*, with a different number of electrons, is added, the stability of the previously pure germanium or silicon is upset.

If atoms of the material added, for example, *arsenic*, have more electrons than the atoms of the semi-conductor material, the extra electrons are unable to enter covalent bonds, and are free electrons. These electrons can be caused to flow, that is, to contribute to current flow upon application of voltage from some external source. Semi-conductors having had impurities added to produce an excess of free electrons are referred to as *N-Type* materials.

On the other hand, if *indium*, a material which has fewer electrons than germanium or silicon, is added as the impurity, there is a shortage of electrons. That is, spaces or holes occur in the structure where electrons are "absent." Once again, an electrical instability is created and the electrons can be caused to move by the application of an external force. Semiconductor materials having had impurities added to produce holes or spaces allowing electron movement are called *P-Type* materials.*

In the construction of transistors both N- and P-types of materials are used in sandwich fashion. They are arranged to form either an *NPN*- or *PNP*-type transistor, this nomenclature describing the manner in which the materials are sandwiched. These materials are labelled further in transistor terminology with the middle component always being the *base*, the outer components being called *emitter* and *collector*. When drawn in schematics the base is drawn as a bar, the emitter as an arrow, and the collector as a line. NPN-types are drawn —⨂   and PNP —⨂   .

Connections are made such that current flow is toward or into the arrowhead of the emitter. In the NPN-type the current flow is from the emitter to the base and to the collector. In the PNP-type the direction of the current flow is from the collector and from the base into the emitter. This fact is mentioned only to alert the reader to the different types of transistors and their arrangement in circuits since both types are used in hearing aids.

The important point to be kept in mind is that the application of a voltage between the base and one of the other elements strongly influences the current flow in the other element. Actually then, the transistor should be considered as a current-controlling device, or as a conversion device; it converts the current supplied by a power source — for example, a battery — into a desired output current under the control of an input current. In hearing aids, the microphone develops an input current by transducing acoustic energy into electrical energy, which is applied to the transistor. This input current strongly influences the current flow from the battery through the transistor. In essence a small signal from the microphone effects a much larger change in the current flow from the battery, through the transistor and the remainder of the circuitry, and hence a small input signal is amplified to a larger output signal.

Refinements in transistor production and so-called solid state electronic

---

* Although germanium was mentioned as a semi-conductor material used in transistors, it has been found to be quite sensitive to temperature changes. That is, its performance fluctuated as a function of the temperature of the environment in which it was operating. Silicon was found to be less sensitive to temperature variations. Therefore, silicon became more popular as the semi-conductor material to which impurities were added.

circuitry have led to the development of *integrated circuits*, variously referred to as *chips, micromodules, microcircuits* or *microlithic circuits*. Regardless of what they are called, thin films of the desired materials are deposited on a substrate, tiny canals and holes are etched into the film deposit, and other materials in minute quantity are added, all under precise automated control. This process can be repeated layer by layer with necessary patterns of etchings until transistors, connections, and other components as well are created, all in place and appropriately connected as a single unit. Provision for making appropriate connections to other components which cannot be built into the integrated circuit are, of course, included in the production process. For hearing aids provisions for such connections are made for capacitors, etc. which are too large physically to be incorporated into the integrated circuit, for the microphone, for the battery, for the controls, and for the earphone.

Integrated circuits have the advantages of small power requirements, low electronic noise characteristics, small size, fewer connections which might break, hermetic sealing against external influences, and manufacture under uniform conditions and mass production techniques. All of these advantages are important to the electronics industry in general, including the manufacture of hearing aids.

Microphones

A *microphone* is probably best defined as an *acoustic mechanoelectric transducer* in that it converts acoustic energy to mechanical energy which in turn is converted to electrical energy. The acoustic to mechanical conversion is accomplished by a diaphragm responding to the compressions and rarefactions of the sound waves with corresponding to-and-fro motions. This action of the diaphragm in turn activates some type of mechanism capable of converting these mechanical vibratory motions into a corresponding flow of electrical energy. In current *electret*-type hearing aid microphones, the mechanical to electrical conversion takes the form of capacitor-like action similar to that in the high quality condenser microphones used for calibrating audiometers and accurate sound level measurements.

A word about the construction of electret type microphones is in order. Electrets are actually *dielectric materials* in the form of *teflon* or *polycarbonate* strips which are heated and placed in a strong electrical field. Upon cooling the electrical charge is maintained to some extent. A thin metal coating is then deposited on these strips. This metal coating serves as a diaphragm and one plate of a capacitor. A metal backplate serves as the other plate of the capacitor. In order to insure low inherent noise characteristics, the diaphragm must be very close to the backplate. For this reason, the backplates have been designed so that the diaphragm makes contact with its supports at several points, dividing a single diaphragm into several diaphragms (Figure 3-1).

When a sound wave impinges upon the diaphragm, the effect is that the distance between the plates (diaphragm and backplate) is reduced during the compression phase of the sound wave and increased during the rarefaction phase. These changes in distance between the plates alter the capacitance, or ability of the capacitor to store electrical charges, accordingly. Thus, the voltage at the plates changes as a function of the motion of the diaphragm, thereby creating a small electrical voltage corresponding to the impinging sound wave.

This tiny voltage is delivered to a special type of transistor, called a *field effect transistor* or *FET*. In these devices there is virtually no current flow at the input portion of the transistor. This is an important feature since essentially no current flow is available from the electret microphone. Recall from the previous discussion of conventional transistors that the output current flow—for example, collector current—is controlled by an-

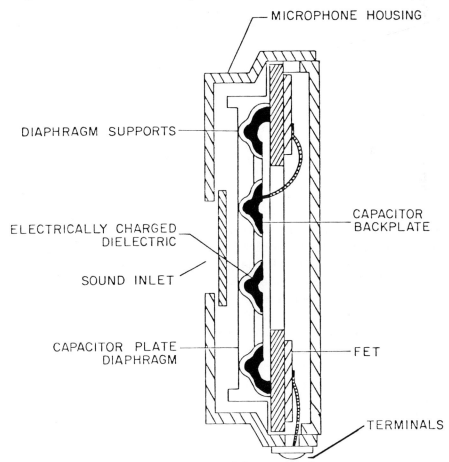

FIG. 3-1. Cross-section of electret microphone.

other current flow, between the base and emitter. In FET devices, the control of output current is by a voltage or an *electric field* input rather than by current flow. Thus, the output of the FET is controlled by the variations in the electric field of the electret microphone. In turn, the output of the FET is delivered to a conventional transistor for control of the transistor's output current. The FET is built into the housing containing the electret microphone itself. In this way the coupling of the electret microphone, a device which has essentially no current flow capabilities, to a conventional transistor whose output is controlled by an input current, is accomplished by an intermediate device, the field effect transistor.

The advantages of the electret microphones to hearing aid applications are many. First of all, their response to frequencies across the audio range can be essentially constant, that is, a flat *frequency response*. The response can, of course, also be altered or tailored somewhat for special purposes. Second, construction such as shown in Figure 3-1 results in very small diaphragm mass. Small mass permits excellent sensitivity since only a small amount of acoustic energy is needed to set it into motion. The small mass also has the advantage of being less sensitive to damage from high gravity forces which occur if the instrument is dropped onto a hard surface. Similarly, because of its reduced mass it is not necessary to mount an electret microphone in as much shock absorptive material, thereby reducing space requirements for the microphone. Furthermore, in spite of using less cushioning in their mounting, electret microphones are less sensitive to body-borne vibratory motions in the hearing aid case set up by the earphone. Third, with construction such as shown in Figure 3-1 it is not necessary that the diaphragm be stretched or held taut. Therefore, its performance is less sensitive to temperature changes. Fourth, magnetic fields are not involved in the transduction process of electret microphones (magnetic fields are involved in previously used magnetic microphones and are also necessary for the earphones used in hearing aids). Therefore magnetic coupling and feedback between the microphone and earphone is no longer a problem. The microphone and earphone can now be mounted in closer proximity to one another, allowing forward facing microphones in ear level instruments and further development of all-in-the-ear hearing aids. Ceramic microphones developed just previously to the electret microphones offered many, but not all, of the above advantages. Electret microphones are used most commonly in the current manufacture of hearing aids.

From the above, it is obvious that the development of the electret microphone was important to recent developments and changes in hearing aid design. Of course, the above-indicated advantages of electret microphones have applications not only in hearing aids but in virtually all other audio amplification, recording, and communication applications as well.

Another innovation is the development of *directional microphones* for hearing aids. Directional microphones are those which are more responsive to sound from certain angles of incidence than from other angles, for example, more responsive to sounds originating from the front of the microphone than from behind it. Such devices have been used for public address systems, etc. for some time, but they were, of course, considerably larger physically than those employed in hearing aids. Recent developments have allowed the application of the principles of directional microphones to miniature hearing aid microphones as well.

Microphones which do not have directional preference in their response to sound waves are generally referred to as *pressure-type microphones*, that is, they respond to sound pressure fluctuations (compressions and rarefactions) and have the same sensitivity for all angles of sound incidence. Directional microphones on the other hand are also called *gradient microphones* because their output is dependent on a pressure *gradient* or *difference* between two points in a sound field. For this purpose two *acoustic inlets* or "microphone openings" are utilized, one on either side of the diaphragm. The motion of the diaphragm is dependent on the pressure difference on the two sides of the diaphragm.

In the construction of directional electret microphones for hearing aids, the rearward facing sound inlet is extended with tubing so that the separation of the front and back sound inlet is approximately 13 mm ($^1/_2$ inch). Alternatively, an acoustic delay element is placed at the back sound inlet. The intent is to create a 40 μsec delay in the sound entering the back opening, about the same length of time it takes sound to travel 13 mm. (Sound velocity is about 340 m/sec or 1100 ft/sec.) The effect is that the sounds from the back are delayed in reaching one side of the diaphragm through the rearward facing inlet by about the same amount as the sound traveling from the rear inlet to the front sound inlet and the other side of the diaphragm. Under this circumstance, the sound waves on the two sides of the diaphragm essentially cancel one another. Such cancellation does not occur for sounds originating from the front since the sounds must travel 40 μsec more to reach the back sound inlet than to reach the front sound inlet and then after reaching the back inlet, it must pass through a tube or an acoustic delay element for an additional 40 μsec delay. The directional effect thus accomplished irregularly covers a range of about 200–2000 hertz and the microphone is about 15–20 decibels more sensitive to sounds originating from its front than to sound originating from the back.

Telecoil

A different mode of input is accommodated in some hearing aids by a "telephone coil," more commonly called a *telecoil*. The initial purpose of the telecoil was to allow hearing-impaired individuals to utilize their hearing aids to amplify signals transmitted via the telephone. Since the telecoil is not sensitive to acoustic signals, its use results in amplification of the telephone message, but not competing room noise. This telecoil feature also has been used for hearing-impaired youngsters in classrooms with induction loop group amplification systems.

The principle of operation is the induction of current flow by magnetic lines of force cutting across a conductor. Recall that earlier in this chapter it was stated that a magnetic field was created around a conductor carrying current. Further, it was indicated that current flow would be induced in a nearby conductor as the magnetic field expanded, diminished, and reversed polarity, that is, as the magnetic lines of force cut across the conductor. A telecoil is simply a conductor wound into a tight spiral or coil to allow a high concentration of conductor material into which current flow is induced when a magnetic field and its attendant lines of force are introduced in its vicinity. The schematic symbol for a coil is —mm— .

Telecoil and Telephone Variations

Until 1965, the *G-type handset* with its *U-type magnetic receiver* or *earphone* was used almost exclusively in the Bell Telephone System. One unexpected benefit from this particular device is that in addition to its acoustic output it also produces a strong *stray magnetic field*. It is this strong stray magnetic field that induces corresponding current flow in the telecoil of the hearing aid, which is then magnified by the hearing aid amplifier, delivered to the hearing aid earphone, and transduced to corresponding acoustic signals at the user's ear. It should be pointed out that other telephone companies in the United States and abroad do not use this particular type of handset. Considerably less stray magnetic field emanates from the handset utilized by the other telephone companies. Consequently, hearing aid telecoils do not function adequately with telephone handsets other than the Bell Telephone G-type unit.

However, in 1965, the Bell Telephone System announced that it had begun to employ a different handset, with an L-type magnetic receiver or earphone which, unfortunately, did not develop a strong magnetic field. This new receiver had been designed for their Slimline series, but it was also found that it was more rugged and less expensive to manufacture than the U-type receiver. Therefore, in 1972, Bell Telephone began installing handsets with the L-type receivers in coin operated telephones also.

In order to allow hearing aid users to utilize the telecoil feature in their hearing aids, the Western Electric Company, the manufacturing and supply subsidiary for the Bell Telephone Company, developed an adapter called a *100 A Coupler*. It is a small battery-operated device which the user places between the earphone of the telephone handset and his hearing aid.

The adapter is held in place by an elastic band around the handset. The adapter is actually an acoustic-to-magnetic field converter, which develops the strong magnetic field needed to induce adequate current flow in the telecoil. The device is distributed by the Bell Telephone System on a non-profit basis for about $7.50/unit. It can be used effectively with the L-type receivers of the Bell Telephone System and will, of course, work equally well with the handsets of other telephone companies also.

Another modification recently introduced by the Bell Telephone System consists of a magnetic field-generating device installed in the handset with the L-type receivers. It generates a magnetic field approximately equivalent to that developed by the older U-type receiver.

Different handset cords are used to identify the type of receiver in coin-operated telephones. Handsets with the old U-type receiver have the usual metal-covered or armored cable which enters directly into the microphone end of the handset. Handsets with only the L-type receiver have the armored cable entering the handset through a black or charcoal gray rubber grommet. In handsets with the L-type receiver and added magnetic field generating unit the armored cable enters the handset via a blue rubber grommet (Smith, 1974).

Independently, a new telephone coil and amplifier arrangement which can be built into present day hearing aids has been devised. The device has approximately twice the volume of other telephone coils, but also incorporates a 28 dB amplifier in it to overcome the difference in magnetic signal between the L-type and U-type receivers (Goldberg, 1975). The success of this device and the acceptance of it by hearing aid manufacturers for incorporation into their hearing aid design remains to be seen.

Earphones

Just as microphones were defined as acoustic mechanoelectric transducers, the same definition can be applied to earphones, but in reverse, *electromechanical acoustic* transducers. Hearing aid earphones are frequently called *receivers* in the literature. However, with the advent of radio frequency auditory training units, in which the unit worn by the student is correctly called a radio receiver, but more commonly a "receiver," this writer prefers to refer to the electromechanical acoustic transducers of hearing aids as *earphones* in order to avoid some confusion and ambiguity in terminology.

As mentioned earlier, current flow through a conductor sets up a magnetic field, the north pole-south pole orientation of the magnetic field being dependent upon the direction of the current flow. At this point it is well to keep in mind that the current flow at the earphone of a hearing aid is an amplification of the electrical events begun at the microphone. Hence, the magnetic field at the earphone is also changing its polarity in sequence with the input sound wave at the hearing aid microphone. This magnetic field, in effect, attracts and repels a metal sheet or diaphragm, setting it into mechanical motion. This movement of the diaphragm creates, of course, motion in the air medium around it, and ergo, sound waves akin to those at the microphone, only larger in amplitude and concentrated at the ear of the wearer.

At this point, it is worthwhile to describe the different types of earphones utilized in hearing aids. The most common type of earphone used in body-type hearing aids or some of the more powerful ear level-type hearing aids is the *moving iron magnetic* earphone. In Figure 3-2 it can be seen that a conductor is wound into a coil around a magnetic material. Many more turns than shown here are wrapped around the *pole piece*. Winding the conductor into a coil in this fashion increases the amount of conductor in a small area and thereby increases the strength of the magnetic field in its immediate vicinity. With no current flow in the coil the permanent magnet at the back exerts a constant magnetic attraction to the diaphragm. Current flow in the coil also develops a magnetic field. Current flow in one direction produces a magnetic field which enhances that of the permanent magnet and thereby attracts the diaphragm toward the back of the earphone. The greater the current flow the stronger the magnetic field and the greater the attraction of the diaphragm. Current flow in the opposite direction sets up a magnetic field which is in opposition to that of the permanent magnet and hence diminishes its attraction of the diaphragm. Under these conditions the diaphragm moves forward or away from the back of the earphone. In this way, the direction and magnitude of the current flow in the coil enhances or diminishes the influence of the permanent magnet on the diaphragm and its to-and-fro movement corresponds to the current flow in the coil.

Figure 3-3 shows a cross section of the earphone arrangement used in most ear level hearing aids, so-called internal receivers or earphones since

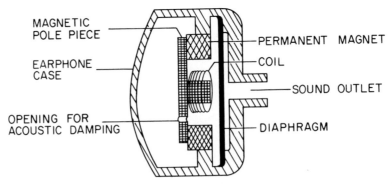

Fɪɢ. 3-2. Cross-section of external type hearing aid earphone (connections to coil not shown).

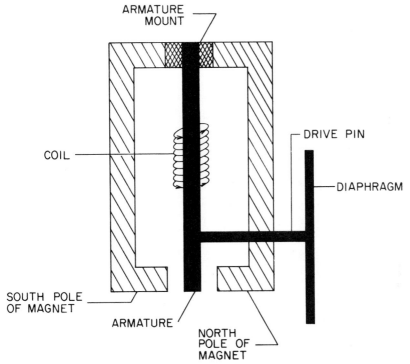

FIG. 3-3. Cross-section of internal type hearing aid earphone (earphone housing and connections to coil not shown).

they are mounted inside the hearing aid case. In this configuration a coil is wrapped around a *metal reed* or *armature* fixed at one end. The free end of the armature is positioned between the two poles of a permanent magnet. Current flow through the coil in the direction of the *arrows* results in the establishment of a magnetic field with a south pole at the lower end of the coil. This south pole is attracted to the north pole of the permanent magnet (unlike magnetic fields attract one another, like fields repel each other) and hence the armature moves toward it. Current flow in the opposite direction produces a north pole at the lower portion of the coil and a consequent opposite direction in motion on the part of the armature. A *drive pin* connects the armature to a diaphragm so that motion by the armature results in like motion of the diaphragm. Again, this motion creates a disturbance in the air molecules around the diaphragm and thus the propagation of sound waves from the earphone through the tubing coupling it to the wearer's ear.

All earphones have, of course, a *natural* or *resonant frequency*, that is a frequency at which they are most efficient, determined primarily by a combination of the mass and elasticity of their mechanical system. Acoustic damping in the form of tubes, holes, so-called Helmholtz resonators, parallel channels, and various acoustic damping materials are used in the earphone assembly to smooth and extend its response. These tubes, cavities, channels, and damping material are built into the casing of the earphone and the hearing aid case and are not shown in Figure 3-3.

Earphones such as described above are used as the output transducers for the vast majority of hearing aids. *Bone vibrators* are used in those instances when the hearing-impaired individual cannot benefit from amplified air-conducted sound for some reason, such as atresia of the ear canals. The same electrical and magnetic principles operate in the bone vibrator, but in this instance the diaphragm is rigidly attached to a plastic case (Figure 3-4). The magnetic system is supported by the edge of the diaphragm. Here too the pull of the magnet varies with changes in the electric current flow through the coil. The end result is that the magnet and case move in relation to one another, and since the mass and inertia of the magnet is appreciably large, the case vibrates considerably. It is this vibration of the case held tightly against the skull that sets the skull into like vibration and stimulates the inner ear.

Controls

As mentioned earlier, the frequency response of the hearing aid can be manipulated somewhat by the use of tubes, cavities, acoustic damping materials, etc. in the construction of the microphones and earphones. However, some hearing aids also employ electronic controls to change the hearing aid frequency response characteristic from that inherently developed by the combined response of the microphone and earphone.

Electronic tone controls used in hearing aids are generally made up of combinations of resistors and capacitors which are switched into or out of the circuitry as desired, or a potentiometer may be used in combination with other resistor and capacitor combinations. Capacitors are used in such circuitry because in addition to blocking DC, another electronic property of capacitors is the ability to allow high frequencies to pass

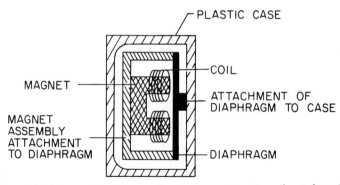

Fig. 3-4. Cross-section of bone vibrator (connections to coil not shown).

"through" them more easily than low frequencies. The effect is that low frequencies are somewhat attenuated by the action of the capacitor; thus, "high frequency emphasis" is, in actuality, low frequency suppression.

The volume or gain control of the hearing aid is also a resistor, but a variable resistor—that is, a potentiometer—as was pointed out earlier. Its function is to control the amount of current flow from the output of one transistor delivered to the input of the next transistor. Recall that it is the current flow at the input of a transistor that controls the amount of current flow at its output. The smaller the resistance, the greater the input current to a given transistor and hence the greater its output.

There are, of course, limitations to the amount of current that a transistor (and its power supply) can develop at its output. When this limit is reached, the output of the transistor does not increase in spite of greater inputs to it. Under this circumstance, the transistor is "forced" into *non-linearity* in that an increased input does not result in an increase of its output. This nonlinearity is also called *peak clipping*, because the transistor continues to follow the input signal or current as long as it can, but beyond a certain point it is unable to do so. It is the *tops* or *peaks* of the signal that are eliminated or "clipped off," hence the term peak clipping. In hearing aids it is the peaks of the current fluctuations corresponding to the input sound waves that are eliminated when the sound input is too strong resulting in too much current flow for the transistors to handle. This limitation usually takes place at the last transistor or so-called *output stage* leading to the earphone. It is one effective means of limiting the output of the hearing aid so that sounds are not amplified to levels that are uncomfortably or painfully loud for the hearing aid user. Of course peak clipping can also occur if the earphone diaphragm is driven to the limits of its mechanical motion or excursion ability, or if the armature shown in Figure 3-3 is driven sufficiently hard that it "bumps against" the magnet poles on either side at the extremes of its excursions.

Another means of limiting the hearing aid output to acceptable levels and one which seems to be incorporated into more and more hearing aid models is labelled *automatic gain control* (*AGC*) or sometimes *automatic volume control* (*AVC*). AGC is used here since it seems to be the more popular acronym at this time. In AGC circuitry part of the electrical signal at the earphone is delivered to a *diode* or *rectifier*, an electronic device which changes or *rectifies* the alternating current (AC) signal at the earphone to direct current (DC). This rectified signal is then delivered or *fed back* to one or more of the transistors (that is, *amplifying stages*) preceding the output stage in such a way that it will oppose the regular current flow at one or more of the transistors in the hearing aid. When the sound input to the hearing aid is weak and the consequent electrical signal at the earphone is not excessively large, the rectified signal fed back to the appropriate stages of amplification is also very small and has no influence on their operation. On the other hand, when the sound input to the hearing aid is very strong, the electrical signal at the earphone is also considerably larger; if transduced to an acoustic signal in the wearer's ear, the sound could be uncomfortably loud. Thus, when the electrical signal at the earphone exceeds a predetermined level, the rectified signal fed back to the preceding amplifying stages is also larger. Its action then is to diminish the current flow of these particular transistors and thereby reduce the magnitude of the amplification they develop for the signals delivered to their inputs by the preceding transistor or by the microphone. The advantage of output limiting of this type is that it more accurately reproduces the intended signal than does peak clipping.

In discussing the performance of such circuits, the terms *attack* and *release times* frequently are encountered. *Attack time* refers to the length of time required for this controlling action to take effect after a strong signal is present at the earphone. *Release time* refers to the length of time required for the amplification stages to return to full amplification after the strong signal is no longer present at the earphone. Attack and release times are usually only a few msec and are reported in specific values.

Regardless of whether the output limiting in a given hearing aid model is by peak clipping or AGC, the upper limits of output level are predetermined and are part of the overall design of the hearing aid. Components are chosen with known efficiencies and current carrying capabilities for peak clipping instruments, and by design, appropriate amounts of electrical signal are fed back to early amplification stages from the signal at the earphone in AGC hearing aids.

Hearing Aid Operation

Figure 3-5 is a schematic diagram of a hearing aid circuit. It is, by no means, the only possible design. It is not totally complete, nor necessarily one that will work perfectly; it is intended only to illustrate the function of the different components in a hearing aid and to serve as a summary for this chapter. The sine wave $\sim$ shown throughout is the signal passing through the hearing aid.

Closure of switch S_1 completes the circuit for the battery (B_1) to provide the current flow necessary for the operation of the transistors. The electret microphone (EM) and its resistors (R) and field effect transistor (FET) within the *dashed lines* are unnumbered since all are constructed as a single unit in the microphone housing. The compressions and rarefactions of the sound wave (SW)—that is, acoustic energy—impinge upon the diaphragm of the electret microphone which transduces it to a corresponding electrical wave (EW)—that is, electrical energy. Since the electret microphone is incapable of developing the necessary current flow for

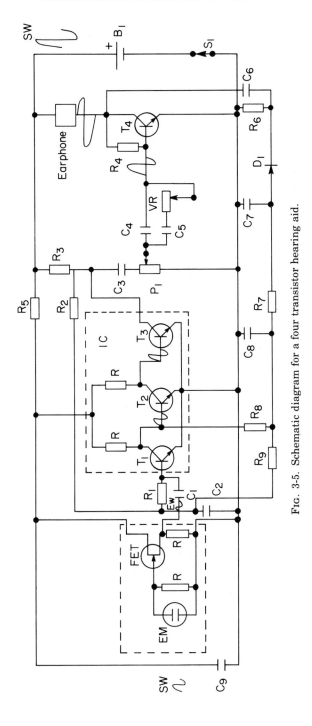

FIG. 3-5. Schematic diagram for a four transistor hearing aid.

control of current flow in conventional transistors, the output of the electret microphone is delivered to a field effect transistor (*FET*) in which the voltage or electric field developed by the microphone controls the current flow in the FET. The FET in turn develops the necessary current flow to deliver to the next transistor in the amplifying sequence. It is coupled to the next stage via a capacitor (C_1). Recall that capacitors block DC but pass AC.

The next three transistors and two resistors are shown enclosed by another set of *dashed lines*. These components are incorporated in a "chip" or an integrated circuit *IC*). A three transistor/two resistor chip such as this has an area of about 1 mm² and has a thickness of about 0.1 mm. The signal from the FET is delivered between the base and emitter of the first transistor (T_1). It is this small current flow that controls the larger current flow at the collector of T_1 resulting in an amplification of the input signal through utilization of the energy provided by the battery. This process is repeated at the next two transistors (T_2 and T_3) in the *IC* as well. The symbols used for all the conventional transistors in the schematic indicate that they are of the NPN type. The resistors in the chip and R_3 serve to set the operating levels and acceptable levels of current flow in these transistors. R_1, R_2, and C_2 serve to stabilize the operating level of the transistors in the chip. Note that there are no capacitors in the *IC*. As mentioned earlier, capacitors appropriate for hearing aids are physically too large to be incorporated into the small dimensions of the chip.

C_3 serves as a coupling capacitor between the last transistor in the chip and the potentiometer (P_1) or gain control. If the contact is near the top of the potentiometer more current will be delivered to the fourth transistor (T_4) and hence more amplification will be delivered from it. With the contact further "down" on the potentiometer, the current must flow through a greater amount of resistance, less current will be delivered to the transistor, and thus its amplification will be less. From the potentiometer the signal is delivered to C_4 and C_5 and a variable resistor (*VR*). If the contact of *VR* is at the far right most of the signal will be passed through C_4 because of the high resistance to current flow presented by *VR*. Recall that in addition to blocking DC and passing AC, proper selection of capacitor values can result in passing higher frequencies more efficiently than low frequencies, and low frequency signals in effect are suppressed. However, as the contact of *VR* is moved to the left, less resistance is offered to signals through that branch of the circuit. The action of the two capacitors in combination is to be less suppressive to low frequency signals. Hence, low frequency and high frequency signals may be passed on to T_4 almost equally well when the contact of *VR* is at the far left. Thus manipulation of *VR* and its function in combination with C_4 and C_5 serves as a tone control to either suppress low frequencies or to pass low and high frequencies almost equally.

The *Earphone* and R_4 serve to set the operating level and acceptable level of current flow for the output stage T_4. Of course, it is at the earphone that the electrical signal is converted back to an acoustic signal that is stronger than the one impinging upon the microphone.

If the input to the microphone is very strong, the corresponding electrical signal at the earphone will also be very large. Under this circumstance, the electronic network consisting of C_6, C_7, C_8, diode 1 (D_1) and R_6, R_7, R_8, and R_9 serves as the automatic gain control (AGC) and will act to decrease the amount of amplification developed by the hearing aid. A portion of the AC signal is passed by C_6 to the diode (D_1) where it is rectified to DC, then fed to T_1 and T_2 and is in opposition to the ongoing events there. That is, it changes the operating levels of these two transistors such that the magnitude of the amplification they develop is reduced. The other components mentioned above as being part of this network serve to smooth the control signal being fed back to T_1 and T_2 and develop the attack and release times of this control.

R_5 and C_9 have not been mentioned in the previous discussion because they do not participate directly in the signal amplification or AGC circuit. Instead these two components serve to stabilize the performance of the hearing aid as the energy of the battery is used.

Although not shown in this schematic, telecoils, when incorporated in a hearing aid for pickup of magnetic signals from telephones or from induction loop group amplification systems, are coupled to the input of T_1. A switch at the input of T_1 allows selection of the signal from either the microphone or telecoil. When the telecoil is switched into the circuit, the magnetic signal from the telephone (or induction loop amplification system) induces a current flow in the telecoil which is then amplified by T_1 through T_4 and transduced to an acoustic signal by the earphone in the same manner as a signal from the microphone. In some instruments a three position switch is used to allow the hearing aid user to pick up the desired acoustic signal from the microphone, or the magnetic signal from the telephone, or pick up from both simultaneously. The latter is particularly advantageous for use with induction loop group amplification systems used in some classrooms for hearing impaired students. It allows them to receive the signal from the classroom group amplification system and still monitor their acoustic environment as well.

Another variation in hearing aid design not shown in Figure 3-5, but which should be mentioned, is the *push-pull output stage*. Such output stages are often used and cited in the literature provided by hearing aid manufacturers. Basically a push-pull output stage consists of two transistors operating side by side to develop more current flow at the earphone. Consequently, a push-pull stage is capable of providing more amplification than is a so-called *single-ended* output stage such as shown in Figure 3-5. Push-pull output stages are commonly used in the more powerful ear level and body type hearing aids.

SUMMARY

In the above this writer has attempted to describe that: (1) Electrical energy is the movement of electrons along a path (current flow) resulting from a difference in potential (voltage), due to an excess of electrons at one point relative to another point; (2) electrical and electronic circuits are designed to create such differences in potential and to control the current flow to achieve desired effects; (3) a microphone transduces acoustic energy to electrical energy (or a telecoil converts magnetic energy to electrical energy) at the input of a hearing aid; (4) the small amount of electrical energy thus produced controls current flow in transistors in such a manner that the transistor utilizes electrical energy provided by a battery to enlarge the small electrical signals developed by the microphone or telecoil; (5) it is these enlarged electrical signals which are transduced to stronger acoustic signals by the hearing aid earphone and delivered directly to the ear of the hearing aid user; (6) the acoustic energy from the earphone is greater than that present at the microphone (or telecoil) because, in effect, energy from the battery has been added to it.

RECOMMENDED READINGS†

PHYSICAL CHARACTERISTICS OF HEARING AIDS

BAUER, B., Electroacoustic transducers. Chapter 3, pp. 50–72, in *Introductory Hearing Science*. Gerber, S. (ed.), Philadelphia: W. B. Saunders Co. (1974).

BERGER, K., *The Hearing Aid: Its Operation and Development* (2nd. ed.). Livonia, Mich.: National Hearing Aid Society (1974).

BRITE, R., et al., *Transistor Fundamentals,* vol. 1, *Basic Semiconductor and Circuit Principles and Basic Transistor Circuits*. Kansas City: Bobbs-Merril (1972).

CARLSON, E., Smoothing the hearing aid frequency response. Paper presented at 48th Audio Engineering Society Convention (1974).

CARLSON, E., AND KILLION, M., Subminiature directional microphones. *J. Audio Eng. Soc.,* 22, 92–96 (1974).

DE BOER, B., Tolerance of components for hearing aids. *J. Audiol. Tech.,* 9, 142–150 (1970).

HEYNE, K., Construction and function of sound transducers. Chapter 5.6 in *Hearing Instrument Technology*. Compiled by Hans-Jürgen von Killisch-Horn, Median Verlag, Heidelberg, West Germany (1975).

KILLION, M., AND CARLSON, E., A wide-band miniature microphone. Paper presented at 37th Audio Engineering Society Convention (1969).

KILLION, M., AND CARLSON, E., A subminiature electret-condenser microphone of new design. *J. Audio Eng. Soc.,* 22, 237–243 (1974).

NIELSEN, T., Information about: The directional microphone. Oticongress 2 (1972).

NIEMOLLER, A., SILVERMAN, S., AND DAVIS, H., Hearing aids. Chapter 10, pp. 280–317, in

---

† References cited in this chapter are included in the bibliography at the end of the Book.

Hearing and Deafness (3rd ed.). Davis, H., and Silverman, S. (eds.). Chicago: Holt, Rhinehart, and Winston (1970).

OBNESORGE, H., Introduction to functional principles of a hearing aid. Chapter 5.1 in *Hearing Instrument Technology*. Compiled by Hans-Jürgan von Killisch-Horn, Median Verlag, Heidelberg, West Germany (1975).

PIKE, C., *Transistor Fundamentals*, vol. 2, *Basic Transistor Circuits*. Kansas City: Bobbs-Merrill (1974).

SESSLER, G., AND WEST, J., Electret transducers: A review. *J., Acoust. Soc. Am.,* 53, 1589–1600 (1973).

TRUAX, R., Amplifier to prosthesis. Chapter 1, pp. 3–39, in *Interpreting Hearing Aid Technology*. Donnelly, K. (ed.). Springfield, Ill.: Charles C Thomas (1974).

VIET, I., A short introduction to the circuitry and function of hearing aid amplifiers. Chapter 5.7, in *Hearing Instrument Technology*. Compiled by Hans-Jürgen von Killisch-Horn, Median Verlag, Heidelberg, West Germany (1975).

VIET, I., Short introduction to electrical science. Chapter 4.1, *Hearing Instrument Technology*. Compiled by Hans-Jürgen von Killisch-Horn, Median Verlag, Heidelberg, West Germany (1975).

earmolds and hearing aid accessories

Kenneth E. Smith, Ph.D.

INTRODUCTION

Over the past several decades, manufacturers and scientists have expended considerable effort toward improvement of the electronic components and characteristics of hearing aids. With the development of new materials and renewed interest in the amplified signal as it reaches the human ear, clinicians and researchers are directing attention to hearing aid accessories, such as earmolds and power supplies.

Both the earmold and the power supply for the hearing aid can have a profound effect on the acoustic signal reaching the human eardrum. The purpose of this chapter is to describe the current technology relative to earmolds and to describe other types of hearing aid accessories which may affect the efficiency with which sound reaches the impaired ear.

EARMOLDS

The earmold, sometimes called the earpiece, is generally a plastic insert device designed to conduct amplified sound from the hearing aid receiver into the ear canal with as much efficiency as possible. Considering current technology, the functions of earmolds may be described as:

1. Sealing the ear, in many cases, so that amplified sound is not fed back to the microphone of the hearing aid.

2. Modification of the electroacoustic characteristics of the hearing aid allowing for greater control over the amplified signal reaching the ear.

3. Providing a manner of coupling the hearing aid receiver to the ear which is comfortable for the hearing aid user.

An additional purpose often described by the hearing aid dispensers and manufacturers is for the earmold to be aesthetically pleasing. Particularly with adult hearing aid users, the aesthetic consideration may become very important.

EARMOLD MATERIALS AND IMPRESSION TECHNIQUES

According to Berger (1970), the most common earmold material is lucite (metyl metacylate), a hard, clear or slightly tinted plastic. Many other materials including vinyl polyethylene and silicone are also used for the construction of hard, semi-hard, or soft earmolds. Lybarger (1958) reported that the type of material used in custom-fitted earmolds has no significant effect on the frequency response delivered to the ear.

A custom-fitting process usually precedes earmold manufacture. In this process, an ear impression is obtained and sent to a laboratory which returns a finished earmold. The procedure for obtaining an adequate impression is critical. The following is an abbreviated, but acceptable procedure for taking an impression for the preparation of a custom-made earmold:

1. The pinna and canal should be examined for infection, wax, collapsed canals, or abnormal growths. The purpose of this observation is to identify any abnormality which should be referred for medical management before the impression is taken. A few persons will exhibit canals of abnormal dimensions because of old surgical procedures, such as a fenestration operation. If the operated ear must be aided, caution is necessary to obtain an impression which can easily be removed from the abnormal canal. The resulting limitation may be an earmold canal shorter than would otherwise be desired.

2. A small piece of cotton is tied to a string, and inserted into the canal, just beyond the first bend. This cotton and string, called a "canal stop," serves to plug the canal so that the tip of the impression is blunted. Otherwise the finished earmold tip may be rounded, possibly causing acoustic feedback problems.

3. Materials for obtaining an impression should be prepared according to the manufacturer's specifications.

4. The impression material is inserted into the canal, using either a syringe or hand-pressing method. The canal, concha, and helix are filled with impression material (Figure 4-1).

5. The impression is removed after the material has hardened slightly, following the manufacturer's instructions.

6. The canal should be re-examined for any residual impression material or irritation.

7. The earmold impression is sent to the laboratory with instructions regarding type, color, bore, and venting desired for the final product.

8. If the impression was not adequate a defective earmold will result and

the entire process must be repeated until an acceptable fit is obtained. The characteristics of a good earmold impression are shown in Figure 4-2.

A recent improvement in earmold fitting has been the development of the instant earmold. Instant earmolds are generally made of silicones,

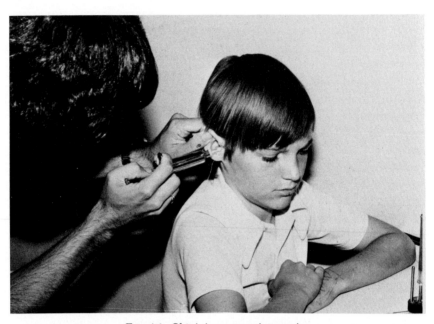

Fig. 4-1. Obtaining an ear impression.

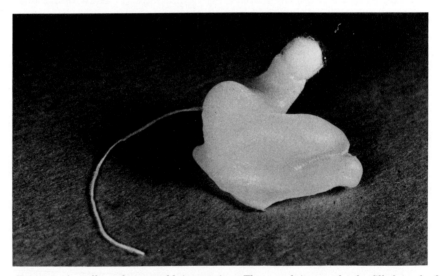

Fig. 4-2. A well made earmold impression. The canal is completely filled, and of appropriate length, resulting from proper placement of the cotton block. The helix and concha are clearly outlined, resulting from proper filling of those areas.

acrylics, or rubber polymers. According to Raas (1972), soft earmolds of this type provide a better acoustic seal than hard earmolds since they tend to expand slightly upon exposure to body heat.

The first instant earmold appeared on the market in 1957 and was made from acrylic. The most widely used material is silicone which is vulcanized by the addition of two catalytic agents. Curing time is approximately 10 minutes, resulting in an unbuffed, soft, and non-allergenic earmold.

The addition of antioxidant material, aplastizer or hydrocarbon oils (mineral oil or petroleum jelly) to the silicone mixture weakens the mold and may lead to a variety of skin reactions. These additives may cause the temperature of the ear canal to rise more quickly than normal, resulting in excessive sweating in the ear. These impurities may also migrate to the surface of the earmold causing shrinkage and an increased probability of feedback.

The new synthetic polymer earmolds require only one catalyst hardener, require only 10 minutes of curing time, and have excellent performance under a variety of temperature conditions. These rubber earmolds do not absorb body odor, and are easily cleaned with soap and water. While these types of instant earmolds allow the patient to leave the dispenser's office with a hearing aid in place, there is still a lack of technical data on techniques for venting and attaching various types of receivers to these earmolds.

The stock earmolds used in hearing clinics as well as the earmolds worn by hearing aid users should be routinely cleaned. Lankford and Behnke (1973) investigated the bacterial population of stock clinic earmolds. While they did not isolate many harmful bacteria, they recommended a routine cleaning procedure for clinics as follows:

1. Place the dirty mold in bacteriostatic or bacteriocidal solution (Cetyl-cide, Effer-Kleen, soapy water).

2. At the end of the day wash the earmolds, using a small brush and a pipestem cleaner for the sound bore. Rinse thoroughly.

3. Dry the earmold carefully, making sure that the tubing and bore are free of water.

4. Place the earmold in a container to await reuse.

Individuals are probably best advised to clean their earmolds routinely with soapy water. They should, of course, be careful not to get the hearing aid wet, and to dry the earmold thoroughly.

Audiologists who deal with children are frequently concerned about allergic reactions to earmold material. The incidence of allergic reactions to earmold material is approximately one in 10,000; reactions may include rash, swelling, heat buildup, and possible fluid dishcarge from the ear. Allergic reaction to earmold material can be identified through a patch test (Sullivan, 1973a) in which filings of earmold material are taped to the skin just above the elbow. If an allergic reaction is suspected, the audiologist can specify allergy-free or chemically inert materials. Daily cleaning of the earmold, removal of the earmold for short periods of time during the day, and allergy-free materials can reduce the incidence of abnormal reaction to the earmold.

Adult patients sometimes complain of discomfort due to the insertion of the earmold. In such cases, the audiologist may find it useful to use an earmold tip of soft plastic material. Tipping the earmold with a plastic material can reduce the possibility of abrasion of the external canal through improper insertion of the earmold.

TYPES OF EARMOLDS

A variety of earmold types is available to the hearing aid user. The type of earmold used is generally determined by the nature of the hearing loss and the needs of the hearing aid user. In the past, conflicting terminology has resulted in confusion about the various types of earmolds. To reduce such confusion, standard terminology was agreed upon at the 1970 Annual Meeting of the National Association of Earmold Laboratories. Figure 4-3 shows the parts of the earmold according to standard terminology published in 1972.

Figure 4-4 shows various earmold styles. Many of these styles have evolved for cosmetic, rather than acoustic purposes. Some are not practical for hearing aid use.

EARMOLD CONNECTORS

Earmold connectors, couplers, or receiver connectors are all terms which are applied to that part of the hearing aid which connects the earmold and/ or receiver to the hearing aid tubing. A variety of plastic materials is used in the manufacture of these connectors, including lucite (a hard clear material which is very durable), polyethylene (a white, hard milk-colored plastic), and vinyl. According to earmold laboratories, both hard and soft vinyl will withstand considerable abuse and will not crack, break, or lose resiliency with age.

Earmold connectors can be attached to the earmold and receiver by a variety of methods. They can be snapped into the earmold through the use of plastic bushing, glued into the earmold, or screwed into the receiver.

To assure a tight fit between the tubing and earmold connector, commercial liquid products designed to soften the tubing are applied. As these fluids dry, the tubing contracts slightly, and a tight fit is possible. The clinician should be familiar with such products before disassembling the patient's hearing aid. Without chemicals to soften the tube, tubing connectors and receivers can be very difficult to rejoin.

By themselves, the length of earmold connectors have a minimal influence on varying the frequency response of the hearing aid. In some cases,

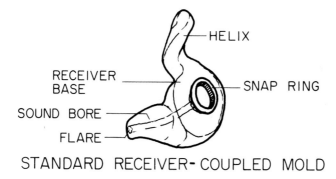

STANDARD RECEIVER-COUPLED MOLD

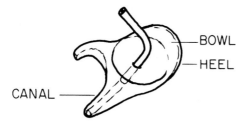

SHELL TUBING-COUPLED MOLD

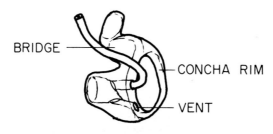

SKELETON VENTED MOLD

FIG. 4-3. Standard earmold terminology. *Bowl:* The portion of a shell mold which inserts into the concha. *Bridge:* The part between the canal and the junction of the concha rim and the helix. *Canal:* The part which inserts into the ear canal. *Concha rim:* The portion of a skeleton mold which fits into the concha. *Flare:* The enlargement of the sound bore at the end of the canal. *Heel:* The part between the tragus and the anti-tragus. *Helix:* The segment which fits into the helix of the ear. *Receiver base:* The area of a receiver-coupled mold in contact with the receiver. *Sound bore:* The channel in the canal through which sound energy passes. *Vent:* An opening permitting passage of air via the sound bore to the ear canal.

however, variation in the frequency response may be affected through the use of sintered metal pellets, plastic inserts, or lamb's wool inserted into the earmold connector. The effects of inserts will be discussed later in this chapter.

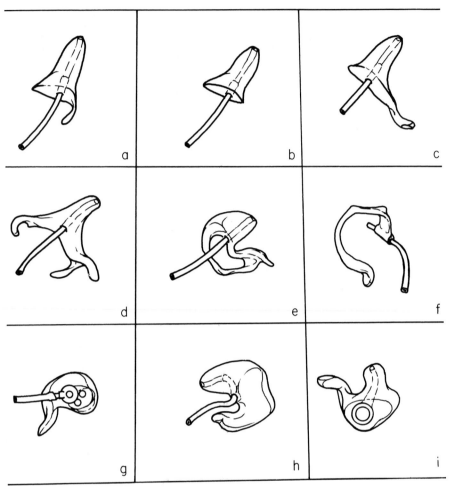

Fig. 4-4. Various styles of earmolds. (a) Canal-lock style. Consists of canal and lower half of concha rim. Unless very well fitting, retention and feedback may be problems. (b) Canal style. Retention problems render practicality of this style questionable. (c) Semi-skeleton style. Consists of canal, bridge, and helix. (d) Three-quarters skeleton style. Skeleton mold without center part of concha rim. (e) Skeleton style. A comfortable and effective earmold. (f) Open, non-occluding type. Designed without a canal for purposes of acoustic modification discussed later in this chapter and in Chapter Ten. (g) Vented type. Canal is short, sound bore diameter is wide, and one or more vents permit passage of air between canal and outside air. This mold is also designed for acoustic modification of the hearing aid's response, as discussed later. Venting can also be used in skeleton-style earmolds. (h) Shell style. There is a full canal, and a concave shell fills the concha. This style is effective to reduce feedback with higher gain instruments. (i) Standard receiver-coupled type. Full solid mold with snap ring to take receiver. Most effective for reducing feedback with highest gain aids. Used with body-worn or other aids with external receivers. May also be coupled to internal receiver aids via a nubbin attached to the hearing aid's sound tubing.

Not all receivers and earmolds require an external connector. A connector makes the earmold more conspicuous and in many cases the tubing is inserted directly into the earmold. The type of earmold connector used with a particular hearing aid is usually specified by the company manufacturing the aid. Often, however, the audiologist is presented with a choice.

EARMOLD MODIFICATION: CANAL LENGTH, TUBING, BORE, AND FILTERS

A discussion of earmold modification must include a basic understanding of the cavities which are created by and associated with earmolds placed in the ear. These cavities are indicated by V (volume of air), as shown in Figure 4-5. The cavities are discussed in detail by Lybarger (1972). $V1$ is an essentially invariant volume between the receiver diaphragm and case. The basic cavities of concern are labelled $V2$ (where the nubbin inserts into the earmold), and $V3$ (a theoretical 2 cc cavity between the tip of the earmold and the tympanic membrane). The size of these critical cavities varies from one individual to another, but the effects of earmold modification through alteration of these cavities is similar. For example, when a small filter is placed in the nubbin cavity, the earphone exhibits a response which shows a smoothing of the peaks or a damping effect. If the area between the nubbin and the hole of the earmold is too large, an adverse effect will result on the high frequency response of the receiver. If the characteristics of $V3$ are altered by either the earmold tip or some type of abnormality in the external auditory canal, there will also be a noticeable effect on the frequency response. Normal cavity range in the unoccluded ear is between 0.4 and 1.0 cc. The standard volume $V3$ used in measurement procedures is 0.6 cc.

Finally, because of the friction of the vibrating air within the walls of the

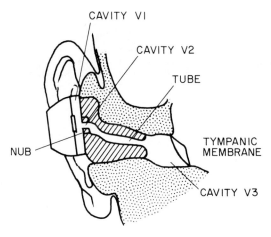

Fig. 4-5. Critical volumes in the aided ear.

tube of the earmold, the tube is said to have an acoustic resistance. Therefore, the diameter and the length of the hole affect the overall response of the system. To demonstrate modification of electroacoustic characteristics, one must first consider a typical frequency response curve from the earmold receiver measured in a 2 cc coupler with a standard earmold hole 18 mm in length and 3 mm in diameter (Figure 4-6). Three areas of major importance are: (*A*) a low frequency response, (*B*) the primary peak (between 800 and 2000 Hz), and (*C*) the secondary peak (2000 Hz and above). The following is a summary of the major effects of the modification of canal length, tubing, bore, and filters on the three primary frequency areas of the response curve.

A. *Low Frequency Response*

    1. Cavity size alterations (area between earmold tip and tympanic membrane).

        a. Shorten earmold tip—increase *V3*. The entire low frequency response drops about 2 dB; other factors remaining constant (Figure 4-7).

        b. Lengthen earmold tip—decrease *V3*. The entire low frequency response increases about 4 dB.

B. *Primary Peak*

    1. Bore diameter (hole through earmold—change diameter, length remains constant), (Figure 4-8).

        a. Smaller diameter (less than 3 mm)—lower primary peak frequency.

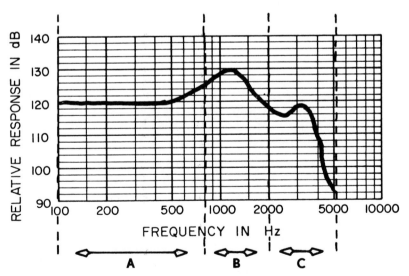

FIG. 4-6. Areas of importance for modification by earmold changes. (*A*) constitutes the aid's low frequency response, (*B*) the aid's primary peak, and (*C*) the secondary peak.

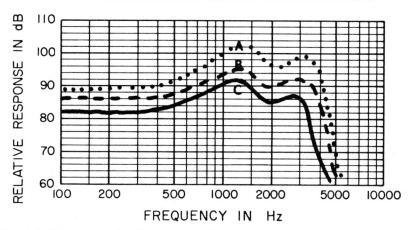

FIG. 4-7. Effects on the low frequency response of modifying cavity *V3*. *(A)* small cavity achieved by long earmold canal. *(B)* standard cavity. *(C)* large cavity associated with short earmold canal.

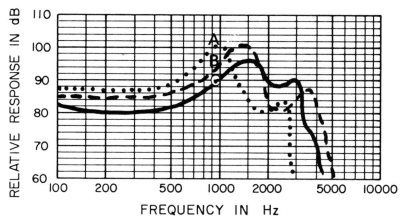

FIG. 4-8. Effects of bore diameter on primary peak response. *(A)* narrow bore *(B)* standard bore *(C)* wide bore.

    b. Larger diameter (more than 3 mm)—higher primary peak frequency.

  2. Bore length (tube through earmold)—change length, diameter remains constant (Figure 4-9).

    a. Longer length (more than 18 mm)—lower primary peak frequency.

    b. Shorter length (less than 18 mm)—higher primary peak frequency.

Lybarger (1972) states that, "the inertance of the bore contributes only about a fourth of the total mass that determines the primary peak. Thus the peak is not critically sensitive to moderate departures from the standard earmold size."

  3. Acoustic damping devices (chokes or filters).

The effect of acoustic damping devices like chokes or filters placed in the earphone nub, or loose cotton or felt in the earmold tube, will be to reduce or flatten the primary peak (Figure 4-10). Discs with very small holes placed in the nub of the earphone are very effective acoustical damping devices. The damping effect generally becomes larger when the damping element is placed nearer the ear canal (Figure 4-11).

C. *Secondary Peak*

    1. Bore diameter.
        a. Smaller diameter (from 0.118 inch) — the high frequency cutoff is extended by 500 cycles, when the length of hole remains constant (Figure 4-12).

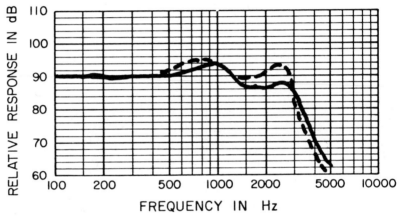

FIG. 4-9. Effects of bore length on primary peak response. The *broken line* represents reduced length; the *solid line* is standard.

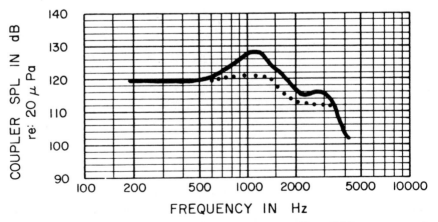

FIG. 4-10. Effect of filter inserts on primary peak response. The *solid line* represents the standard (unfiltered) response. The *broken line* shows effect of the filter.

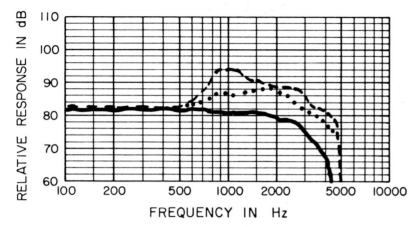

FIG. 4-11. Effect of position of the filter on frequency response. *Dashed line,* unfiltered; *dotted line,* filter in receiver nub of aid with external receiver: *solid line,* filter in flare of earmold canal.

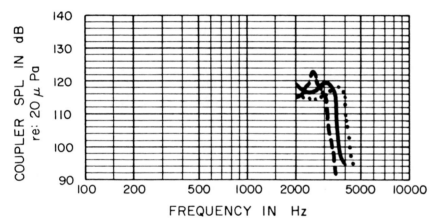

FIG. 4-12. Effect of bore diameter on secondary peak. The *solid line* represents the standard bore response, the *dotted line* the narrowed bore response, and the *dashes* represent the widened bore response.

     b. Larger diameter (bore diameter increased 1.4 times its original diameter)—the high frequency response is lowered by 500 cycles (Figure 4-12).

  2. Bore length

     a. Shorter length—The high frequency cutoff is extended.

     b. Longer length—The high frequency cutoff is lowered.

  3. Cavity size alterations

     a. *V2*: The importance of maintaining a constant *V2* cavity was demonstrated by Lybarger (1972) by hollowing out the entire interior of an earmold. The secondary peak disappeared, along with much of the output above 2000 Hz. Low frequency performance also suffered because of the greatly increased air volume. The primary peak increased markedly in frequency because the acoustic mass of the earmold hole almost disappeared, and the peak increased in height because the acoustic damping provided by the earmold hole was no longer present.

4. Acoustic damping devices

Damping devices placed in the nub of the earphone have a substantial smoothing effect on the secondary peak. The damping effect of a filter is generally somewhat less for the secondary peak than for the primary peak.

5. Tubing

The effects of tubing used to connect the earphone to the earmold are directly related to both the length and width of the tubing. In many earmolds the tubing is continuous through the mold to the earmold tip.

   a. Length—As tubing length increases, high frequency response decreases and as length decreases the high frequency response increases (Figure 4-13).
   b. Diameter—As tubing diameter increases, the high frequency response increases; as diameter decreases, the high frequency response decreases (Figure 4-14).

From a review of the preceding data, it should be apparent to the clinician that the electroacoustic characteristics of the hearing aid can be modified significantly through alteration of the characteristics of the ear-mold.

VENTING

The clinician can effect significant changes in the frequency response of the hearing aid through manipulation of canal length, bore tubing, and filters. Additional flexibility is provided through the use of venting.

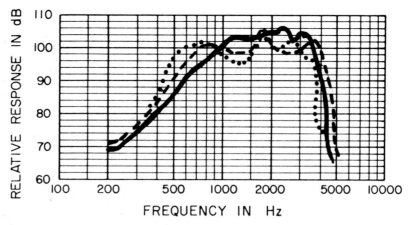

FIG. 4-13. Effect of tubing length on hearing aid frequency response. The *solid line* reflects the effect of 1¹/₄ inch length tubing; the *dashes*, 2 ³/₄ inch length; and the *dots*, 3¹/₂ inch length.

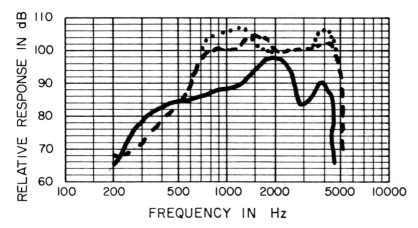

FIG. 4-14. Effect of tubing diameter on hearing aid frequency response. The *solid line* reflects the effect of 0.032 inch diameter tubing; the *dashes*, 0.077 inch diameter, and the *dots*, 0.095 inch diameter.

The earmold vent is a channel drilled between the cavity adjacent to the eardrum (*V2*) and the outside atmosphere. The earmold vent serves three basic purposes:

1. It serves to equalize pressure in *V2* and to relieve feelings of pressure reported by patients. Pressure equalization requires a very small vent and does not materially affect the frequency response of the aid (Lybarger, 1972).

2. Moderate size vents are commonly used with the intent of reducing the low frequency response delivered to the ear.

3. Wide, short vents are used to provide even more reduction of the low frequency response. This type of venting is seen in the "acoustic modifier" type of earmold. These vents are covered with damping material which allow low frequencies to be shunted out of the ear with a minimal effect on the high frequencies.

In general, the use of either moderate or large vents in the earmold leads to an increased probability of acoustic feedback. Therefore, the amount of gain which can be supplied with a vented earmold is limited, particularly in ear level hearing aids.

With custom earmolds, the diameter of the vent may be specified and is fixed by the earmold manufacturer. However, two procedures are available which allow adjustment of vent size: (1) Variable Venting Valves (VVV), and (2) Select-A-Vents (SAV).

Griffing (1971, 1972) describes the VVV as a valve which is turned in a 540° rotation allowing full closure to a full open position of about 1.5 mm. The advantage of the VVV is that the listener has control over the output of his hearing aid for the low frequencies by self-adjustment.

The SAV also allows for modified venting size. This procedure requires a selection of one of six plastic inserts of the following diameters: 3.96 mm, 3.18 mm, 2.38 mm, 1.59 mm, 0.79 mm, and an occluding plug. The desired vent size is then inserted into a 4.62 mm diameter vent which is drilled into the earmold (Sullivan, 1973b). A study by Sung, Sung, and Hodgson (1975) reported increased low frequency attenuation as SAV vent size was increased. However, unexpected resonance peaks and reduction of midfrequency output also occurred. This study emphasized the importance of considering the entire amplifying system as an operating unit – the aid, the ear-hook, connecting tubing, and so forth – as well as the earmold. Cooper, et al. (1975) reported that the loudness reduction, in phons, afforded by VVV was small, and concluded their utility was questionable.

Two common positions for the placement of the vent in the earmold are the side branch (conventional) vent and the lateral vent (Figure 4-15). The side branch vent intersects with the sound bore of the earmold before terminating at the earmold tip, whereas, the lateral bore vent parallels the sound bore of the earmold. According to Cooper et al. (1975), the side branch vent resulted in increased effectiveness in influencing the low frequency response as compared to the lateral branch vent. Additionally, there tends to be more precision in drilling side branch vents.

Sullivan (1973b) states that varying the angle of the vent or multiventing makes little difference in the response. According to Berger (1970), two vent holes seem to have the same effect as one vent of the combined diameter.

The direction of the vent should be determined by the placement of the microphone. Feedback tends to be a problem because of escaped acoustic energy through the vent which is picked up by the microphone (Weatherton and Goetzinger, 1971). A vent directed at the microphone will increase the chances of feedback, and therefore, should be avoided (Sullivan, 1973b). The size of the vent will also affect the amount of feedback (Lybarger, 1972). A high gain hearing aid with a moderate to large vent can lead to excessive acoustic feedback and thus, dissatisfaction to the wearer.

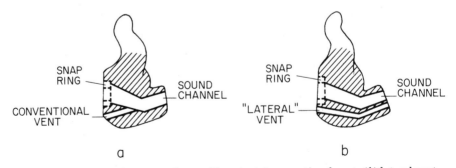

FIG. 4-15. Common placement of earmold vents. (a) conventional vent, (b) lateral vent.

Smaller vents (0.32 mm to 0.125 mm) fitted for mild to moderate hearing losses tend to eliminate acoustic feedback (Sullivan, 1973b).

According to Lybarger (1972), only a very small vent is required for pressure equalization. Sullivan (1973b) states that a vent of 0.090 mm diameter is effective in relieving pressure and, thus, eliminating discomfort to the wearer. A vent of this size has little effect on the frequency response except for frequencies below 300 Hz. Smaller vent diameters can also relieve pressure, but keeping the vent open becomes a problem because of cerumen, moisture, etc. Larger vents introduce noticeable changes in the frequency response of the aid.

According to Sullivan (1973b), the accumulation of pressure within the auditory canal results in a resonance or standing wave between the eardrum and hearing aid receiver. The result is an influence upon the frequency response which, according to Van Winkle (1975), can be identified by the hearing aid wearer as overamplification of background noise. The vent serves to allow this energy to escape. Thus, the transmission of low frequency sounds is not as effective as with a tight acoustic seal.

A review of the literature indicates many discrepancies concerning vent size and the resultant frequency responses. Past studies have measured sound pressure levels by artificial ear couplers or with probe tube microphones. Van Winkle (1975) attributes the discrepancies of the data to the variability between measurement methods.

Despite conflicting data, it is generally agreed that increased vent size is correlated with increased attenuation of the low frequencies (250 and 500 Hz) (Studebaker and Zachman, 1970). In order to appreciate this attenuation, consideration must first be given to the effects of the standard earmold. According to Van Winkle's study (1975) with five hearing-impaired and five normal subjects, the standard earmold enhanced sensitivity for low frequencies (250 to 500 Hz) by as much as 15 dB relative to earphone thresholds. Increasing vent size to 4.62 mm in the high frequency earmold led to progressive attenuation of the low frequencies up to 20–25 dB at 250 Hz and 10–15 dB at 500 Hz relative to the standard earmold. Little change was noticed for frequencies beyond 500 Hz with the exception of 3000 Hz. At this frequency, thresholds were approximately 5 to 10 dB more sensitive as compared with standard earmold thresholds. This increase in sensitivity was explained as the result of natural, closed tube resonance at 3000 Hz.

Several studies have reported improved speech intelligibility with the vented molds compared to the standard mold for high frequency losses. McClellen (1967) found that the vented earmold improved discrimination of W-22 words in noise by as much as 15%. Hodgson and Murdock (1970) found consistently better PB-50 scores with an open, non-occluding mold as compared to the standard earmold in quiet and in noise. Jetty and Rintel-mann (1970) found a 10% improvement in discrimination with all modified earmolds compared to standard earmolds. Davis and Green (1974) reported an average improved discrimination performance of 16% for subjects.

In summary, it appears that venting is an effective procedure for the relief of pressure in the external canal and attenuating low frequencies for the sloping sensorineural loss. According to Van Winkle (1975):

> The combined effect of low frequency attenuation, high frequency resonance, and the ability to control attenuation and feedback with graduated vent size would tend to recommend the high frequency controlled venting earmold as an effective hearing aid coupler for sloping sensorineural losses.

LIMITATIONS ASSOCIATED WITH THE USE OF EARMOLDS

Much of our data on hearing aid response is based on the 2 cc couplers described in Chapter Five. These couplers have become a standard and simulate the closed earmold. They simulate the volume of the enclosed space between a standard receiver and the eardrum, assuming a standard closed earmold (McDonald and Studebaker, 1970; Studebaker and Zach-man, 1970; Briskey, Greenbaum, and Sinclair, 1966; Van Eysbergen and Groen, 1959).

The 2 cc coupler consists of a single cylindrical cavity with an acoustic tube located on the axis of the cylinder connecting it to the earphone. The dimensions of the acoustic tube depend on the type of earphone and the manner in which it is coupled to the ear. Studebaker and Zachman (1970) suggested that a metal 2 cc coupler is not a satisfactory device for use in the evaluation of the extent and influence of earmold modifications on the acoustic signals delivered to the real ear. Their assumption is based on the fact that the acoustic damping provided by the simple metal cavity is much less than that provided in the ear canal.

Alternatives to the 2 cc coupler as a standard measuring device are the Zwislocki coupler described in Chapter Fifteen and the use of probe tube measurements in the external auditory canal. In this procedure, a thin tube is introduced into the cavity, through the earmold, and is positioned near the eardrum. The subject's head is held in a fixed position. Briskey et al. (1966) indicated that the frequency of the secondary peak is lower in the human ear cavity than in the 2 cc coupler. They suggested that the 2 cc coupler records a distribution of sound pressure at higher frequencies than indicated by the probe tube measurements made in a human ear.

In summary, the actual effects of earmold modification in the human ear are difficult for the clinician to measure using standard electroacoustic measurement equipment. This lack of precision in measurement may account for variability in patients' responses to a given hearing aid-earmold combination even though the audiologist has made what he considers to be accurate recommendations.

Acoustic feedback is a common problem in hearing aids where both venting and/or high gain are required. Acoustic feedback is an annoying, high pitched squeal resulting from reamplified sound leaking from the receiver back to the microphone of the same aid.

With standard earmolds, acoustic feedback is an indication that the earmold is not tight, and the canal length is too short, or that the canal tip is rounded instead of blunt. Acoustic feedback can occur from leakage at any point of connection outside of the body of the hearing aid. While both acoustic and mechanical feedback may occur, only the acoustic type of feedback is appropriate in a discussion of earmolds.

One method of determining the source of feedback is to occlude the tip of the earmold with the hearing aid in an "on" position. In theory, if the feedback continues under these conditions, then the leakage is occurring at some point beyond the tip of the earmold. However, Sullivan (1973a) states that this method of defining the source of feedback is invalid. According to Sullivan, sound can be amplified within the ear canal and reflected back and forth between the eardrum and the hearing aid receiver.

As intensity increases, vibration is intensified in the air and in the material surrounding the ear canal such as the earmold material, bone, and hearing aid. This type of feedback is not an "acoustic leak" but a reported acoustic phenomenon which can be corrected with a better selection of frequency response. This phenomenon may occur when the earmold is too tight.

The problem of feedback in vented earmolds was discussed earlier. One solution for this problem is the use of CROS amplification, in which the microphone and receiver are separated by the head.

Acoustic feedback can be a frequent problem in hearing-impaired children because of rapid growth of the ear. It may be necessary to change the earmold every 3 months in children under the age of 4. Beyond that age, it may be necessary to change the earmolds on an annual basis until the child reaches 8 or 9 years.

A buildup of cerumen (wax) in the ear canal which clogs the earmold can also lead to acoustic feedback. Obviously, regular and thorough cleaning of the earmold provides a simple solution to this problem.

As tubing ages in ear level hearing aids, it not only discolors, but it may crack. The result of this cracking is a leakage of sound and an increase in acoustic feedback. According to Sullivan (1973a), feedback may also occur in ear level hearing aids because of the resonance characteristic of the pinna. Alteration in microphone placement or in the position of the hearing aid may alleviate this problem.

CLINICAL ASSESSMENT OF EARMOLD PERFORMANCE

The following is a series of suggestions for the clinician who evaluates a patient wearing a hearing aid-earmold combination:

1. Check for irritation of external ear or external auditory canal. Irritation may indicate the presence of allergies, sharp edges on the earmold, or improper insertion technique.

2. Check the earmold to make sure that the canal is an appropriate length (the canal should be longer in a standard earmold where high gain is required).

3. Check for feedback with the aid in an "on" position. If feedback is encountered, check earmold fit, check whether or not the end of the earmold is blunted, and check the receiver-earmold or tubing-earmold connections for leaks.

4. Evaluate the ability of the ear to hold or retain the earmold. This lack of retention can be a problem in children where the external ear is hypoplastic and incapable of holding a heavy earmold-receiver combination. In these cases, ear hooks (plastic coated wires inserted in the earmold and looped over the top of the ear) may hold the earmold and receiver in place.

5. Be sure that the patient knows how to place the earmold properly in the ear. If the patient is a child, encourage parents or teachers to train the child in insertion and removal of his own earmold.

HEARING AID ACCESSORIES

In general, hearing aid accessories are designed to fulfill one of three basic functions: (1) extend the life of the aid, (2) increase the probability that the aid is working properly, and (3) provide added convenience to the hearing aid user.

Hearing-impaired patients who are capable of telephone conversation may use aids which contain a telephone coil. Telecoil operation is described in Chapters Three and Seven. While there are advantages to a properly working telephone coil in an ear level hearing aid, there are also several disadvantages:

1. The telecoil may not be compatible with the induction system used by the telephone company.

2. A telecoil is an additional circuit inserted into the body of the hearing aid, increasing the probability of breakdown.

3. The use of the telecoil can be inconvenient for the hearing-impaired patient who lacks sufficient fine motor skills.

A simple solution to the problems associated with the telecoils is the installation of a telephone amplifier. The telephone amplifier is a small loudspeaker with a separate gain control which is attached directly to the telephone. It provides amplification of the telephone signal without manipulation of the hearing aid.

In some cases, the hearing-impaired individual may wish to listen to a record player, radio, or television without causing discomfort to other normal-hearing listeners in the same room who would be exposed to a high level of output. In these cases, a variety of manufacturers provide earphone jacks and receivers which can be coupled directly to the ear, or routed through an FM connection directly to the hearing aid. For children whose hearing aids are equipped with telephone coils, it may be desirable for parents to "loop" defined areas in which the child can listen to an audio signal through his own hearing aid. Detailed and practical instructions for installation of a loop are presented by Ling (1967). The use of telecoils in classroom amplifying systems is considered in Chapter Thirteen.

A third type of accessory which is essential to the hearing aid user who lives in a warm, humid climate is the Dry Aid Pac. Moisture is one of the biggest enemies to the hearing aid, since it causes corrosion and shorting of electrical connections. The Dry Aid Pac consists of silica gel crystals and a plastic bag. The hearing aid and earmold are placed in the bag with the crystals when the aid is not in use. Silica gel crystals absorb moisture, and dry the aid and earmold completely in a time period ranging between 4 and 7 hours. When the silica gel crystal is saturated with moisture, it changes color, and can then be baked in an oven, dried out, and used again. Drying packs are particularly critical when a hearing aid user is fitted with an ear level hearing aid. Ear level hearing aids are much more susceptable to perspiration, and the use of a Dry Aid Pac can extend hearing aid life appreciably.

Finally, hearing aid users, and particularly parents of hearing-impaired children should be encouraged to purchase battery testers. The battery tester is an inexpensive, portable, no-load voltage meter which can help the parent determine whether or not the battery is capable of delivering adequate voltage for the use of the hearing aid. Since the measurement is a no-load measurement, it does not draw power from the battery. It is a well known fact that batteries may recover part or all of their voltage potential after a period of rest. Therefore, while the battery may test within normal range in the morning, in a few hours the battery may have discharged to the point where it no longer allows the transduction of speech by the hearing aid. Therefore, a battery tester must be used in conjunction with listening to the battery in the hearing aid, and training the child to notify his parents or teacher when the battery is no longer serviceable.

BATTERIES

The battery is designed to supply current or voltage to the hearing aid and may be activated by an on/off switch on the hearing aid or by proper insertion of the battery in ear level hearing aids. Miniaturization of hearing aids and hearing aid components has been accompanied by a reduction in size and increased efficiency in batteries. Currently, the hearing aid user has access to a relatively stable power supply, capable of operation in all types of temperatures, with a relatively long life and low impedence characteristics. Battery composition is discussed in Chapter Three.

The voltage at which the battery operates in the hearing aid is called the nominal voltage. That voltage potential is measured with a battery tester. The nominal voltage of the silver oxide cell is 1.5, that of the mercury cell, 1.4 volts. Typical voltage discharge curves for silver oxide and mercury cells are presented in Figure 4-16. Note that the mercury oxide cell shows a gradually sloping discharge curve, whereas the silver oxide cells show a relatively flat curve with an abrupt cutoff. It is notable that fresh batteries may show an initial no-load voltage higher than the nominal voltage under which they are supposed to operate. This higher voltage is related to a substance called manganese dioxide which the manufacturer placed in the battery for stability purposes. Once the battery is activated, the manganese dioxide burns off and the power cell operates at its nominal voltage.

Note also that corresponding to a gradual decrease in nominal voltage is a gradual increase in internal impedance of the battery. At the point where the internal impedance of the battery reaches 0.7 ohms, the hearing aid will no longer transduce speech clearly. It is possible to obtain a normal voltage reading with mercury oxide cells even though internal impedance is high enough to preclude efficient battery operation. Therefore, it is important to complete both no-load voltage measurements and to listen to the hearing aid. This problem is not critical with silver oxide cells, since its voltage discharge curve is relatively flat and loss of power from the battery is very abrupt.

Despite the wide variety of power cells available to the hearing aid user, relatively little is known about the effects of battery life on the electroacoustic characteristics of the hearing aid. It is well known (Lotterman and Kasten, 1967b) that as the power supply fades, the hearing aid user tends to rotate the gain control upward to compensate for the drop in hearing. As he does, harmonic distortion in the hearing aid increases.

Two studies (Smith, Baldwin, and Hetsel, 1971; and Rosenthal, 1975) examined the effects of the power cell on the electroacoustic characteristics of the hearing aid. Using a continuous monitoring method (Figure 4-17), variability in sound pressure level output in new hearing aids using mercury oxide, silver oxide, and nickel cadmium power supplies were studied. In both studies, new hearing aids which met manufacturers' specifications were measured continuously with complete electroacoustic analysis of hearing aid performance taken every 24 hours until the sound

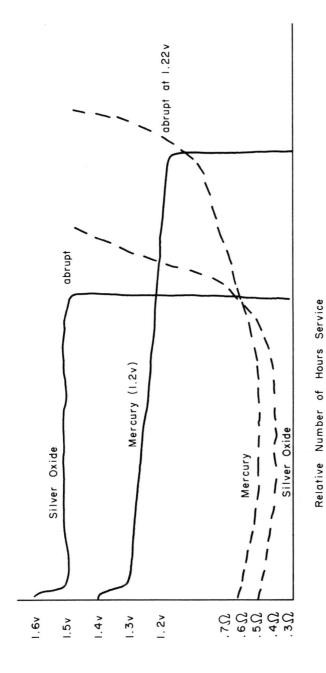

FIG. 4-16. Voltage discharge and internal impedance curves for silver oxide and mercury oxide batteries.

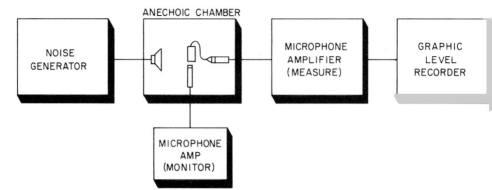

Fɪɢ. 4-17. Instrumentation for continuous monitoring method used to examine the effects of power cells on the electroacoustic characteristics of hearing aids.

pressure level output from the aid dropped 10 dB below the initial output level of the hearing aid. Measures of frequency response, gain, and harmonic distortion were plotted along with the actual sound pressure level discharge curve of each hearing aid.

Major conclusions from both of these studies were:

1. Sound pressure level (SPL) output in hearing aids using mercury cells tends to be gradual, unpredictable, and highly variable (Figure 4-18).

2. SPL discharge curves from hearing aids using silver oxide or nickel cadmium cells tends to be highly consistent, and show an abrupt termination of service.

3. The number of hours of service life and variability between aids and discharge characteristics was related only to the type of aid used in the experiment.

4. Consistency of battery life is not related to the source of battery purchase. In other words, batteries purchased from a discount department store with an undefined stock rotation policy performed just as well as batteries from a hearing aid dealer who rotates his stock every 3 months.

5. Whereas decrease in gain and maximum power output are evident as the efficiency of the power supply decreases, the frequency response of the hearing aid is not affected. In other words, the frequency response of the hearing aid remains constant despite the quantity of power delivered by the power supply.

6. Harmonic distortion does not increase as a function of battery life when the gain control of the hearing aid remains constant.

7. Except for the actual number of service hours delivered by the hearing aid, nickel cadmium and silver oxide cells perform in a very similar manner. Their SPL discharge characteristic is flat, with an abrupt cutoff. SPL discharge curves typical of silver oxide and nickel cadmium cells are presented in Figure 4-19. The curves shown are for the silver oxide cell, but the discharge characteristic is identical to the nickel cadmium cells.

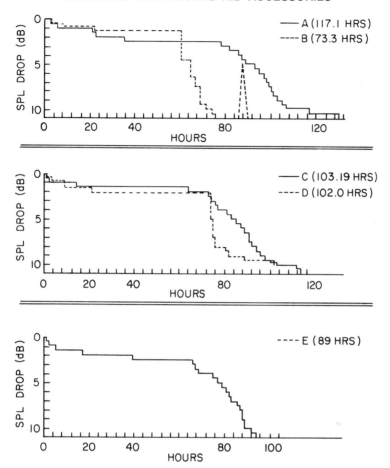

FIG. 4-18. Sound pressure level discharge curves for five mercury oxide batteries.

Results of these studies indicate that the silver oxide cell and nickel cadmium cells are preferable power supplies in modern hearing aids. This conclusion is based on their service life across numerous batteries. Nickel cadmium has the additional advantage of being rechargeable, thus reducing the overall cost to the hearing-impaired patient.

One common fallacy among hearing aid users is that batteries should be stored in the refrigerator. Except for the nickel cadmium cells (which are inaccessible to the hearing aid user), batteries operate through the interaction of their chemical components and oxygen. This means that the can, or shell of the battery is vented. Refrigeration cools the battery so that when it is brought out into normal temperature conditions, condensation forms on the outside of the battery leading to corrosion and premature shorting of the battery. If batteries are refrigerated, they should be stored in an airtight plastic bag. When the bag is taken from the refrigerator and allowed to warm to room temperature, condensation forms on the bag

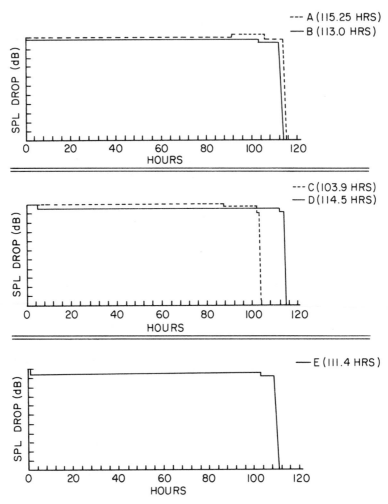

FIG. 4-19. Sound pressure level discharge curves for five silver oxide batteries.

instead of the battery can. For additional information which hearing aid users should have regarding battery usage, refer to Chapter Eleven.

SUMMARY

This chapter has presented a brief overview of earmolds, hearing aid accessories, and power supplies for modern hearing aids. With a thorough understanding of the variables presented in this chapter, the audiologist can specify an amplifier for the hearing-impaired patient which is tailored to the hearing loss, the patient's comfort, and his need for amplification.

chapter 5

electroacoustic characteristics

Roger N. Kasten, Ph.D.

INTRODUCTION

The measurement of the electroacoustic characteristics of hearing aids is a complicated and frustrating task. Many pitfalls face the routine measurer of electroacoustics (Briskey, Greenbaum, and Sinclair, 1966). Artifact appears to abound within the measurement equipment and the hearing aids themselves. Indeed, in a carefully controlled round-robin testing sequence conducted by members of the American National Standards Institute (ANSI) Writing Group for hearing aid characteristics under laboratory conditions, the variability seen among hearing aids and between laboratories was considered high. It is important to realize that this variability in measureable characteristics existed even though the laboratories conducting the measurements are considered to be some of the most sophisticated in the country.

Not wishing to paint an overly dismal picture in terms of the precision of measurement, we must also take into consideration the use that will be made of these measured characteristics. Unfortunately, it seems that altogether too many people are measuring hearing aid characteristics in a hard-walled 2 cc coupler and applying the results directly for the fitting of a hearing aid on a human being. This direct application of hearing aid performance characteristics is a gross misapplication of results. The previous American Standard, the International Standards, and the new American Standard, are all designed to facilitate comparison of measurement from one laboratory to another or from one facility to another. No attempt was made in the preparation of any of the standards to apply the measured data to conditions of real use. This type of activity must be accomplished carefully and cautiously and should be done only with a full understanding of the difference between real ear and coupler measurements of hearing aid characteristics.

INSTRUMENTATION FOR MEASURING ELECTROACOUSTIC CHARACTERISTICS OF HEARING AIDS

Coupling

Initially a standard device is needed to couple the aid to the microphone of the measuring system. Traditional couplers are shown in Figure 5-1 (ANSI, 1973). These devices incorporate about the same volume of air, 2 cc, as is contained in an ear canal occluded by a hearing aid earmold. Thus they are called "artificial ears." However, differences exist in the acoustic properties of these hard-walled cavities and the human ear canal. Some substantial differences which may occur between coupler-obtained and real ear measures were explained by Briskey et al. (1966). One example is shown in Figure 5-2. Real ear measurements of hearing aid function are obtained by inserting a probe tube through the earmold into the ear canal. This tube carries the signal to a measuring microphone. Obviously this procedure is not feasible in all cases and coupler measurements remain popular. A new coupler-artificial head arrangement, which permits more representative measure of hearing aid function, is described in Chapter Fifteen.

Establishing and Calibrating a Free Field

Many hearing aid measurements involve the use of pure-tones and require an essentially echo-free test space. Therefore, an anechoic chamber or a commercially available hearing aid pressure test box is used. Provision must be made for a standard test point for placement of the hearing aid microphone and for measurement of the sound pressure level (SPL) in the field during testing of the hearing aid.

Measurement of Input-Output Characteristics

Electroacoustic measures are basically measurements of input-output functions. That is, they are concerned with how the output signal differs from the input signal. Therefore, a means is required of generating and specifying an input signal and of measuring the output from the hearing aid. The instrumentation shown in Figure 5-3 is often used, and is described below.

Signal Generator

A continuously variable beat frequency oscillator is desirable for generation of pure-tones. Provision should also be made for generation of complex signals.

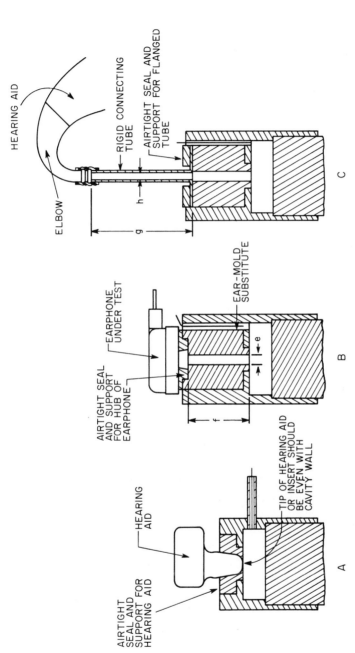

FIG. 5-1. Two couplers. (*A*) HA-1-type coupler. (*B*) HA-2-type coupler. The bore diameter is represented by *e* and the bore length by *f*. (*C*) HA-2-type coupler with entrance through tubing. Tubing diameter is represented by *h* and tubing length by *g*.

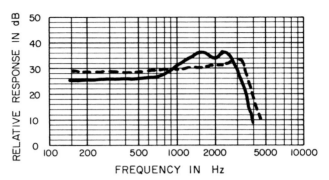

FIG. 5-2. Real ear versus coupler measurement. The *solid line* represents a real ear (probe tube) measurment. The *broken line* designates the 2 cc coupler response for the same condition. Data from Briskey, Greebaum, and Sinclair (1966).

Hearing Aid Test Box

The hearing aid may be placed in an anechoic chamber – an expensive "dead" room free from reverberation and vibration. More commonly measurements are made in a small insulated box containing a substantially anechoic space. The box also contains a loudspeaker, or "artificial voice," which transduces the test signal.

Regulating System

The test space contains a microphone attached to its complement, with which the input sound pressure level at the hearing aid microphone is monitored. There is another common use for this system. The frequency response of the loudspeaker is usually not entirely flat. Therefore, for automated measures – in which frequency changes rapidly – a compensatory method is needed to keep intensity of the input signal constant. The regulating system is commonly attached to a compressor amplifier in the signal generator. This device can then modify voltage to the loudspeaker to compensate for its frequency response irregularities.

Measuring System

Another microphone in the test space receives the output signal from the hearing aid, via the 2 cc coupler described above. Thus, the output can be read visually from the associated microphone amplifier, or recorded graphically if a permanent record is needed. For automated measures, the motor of the level recorder commonly drives the sweep-frequency oscillator so that, in synchrony, the input frequency is changed and the output results are recorded.

Harmonic Analysis

If distortion measures are needed, provision is called for to reject unwanted signals and accomplish frequency analysis of distortion products.

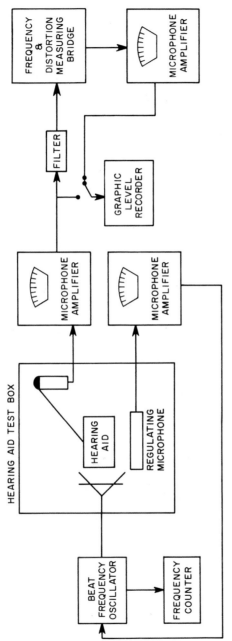

FIG. 5-3. Instrumentation for electroacoustic analysis.

This provision may be achieved with a variable band rejection filter which eliminates from the test signal the fundamental (input) frequency and thereby permits measuring the remaining energy in the output signal — distortion products generated in the hearing aid. More detailed measurement of harmonic distortion is possible with a series of band-pass filters which reject all other energy and permit measurement of each individual harmonic generated within the hearing aid. With compatible systems, the filters may be driven electronically, in synchrony, with the signal generator and graphic level recorder, to permit automated recording of distortion across frequency.

Here is a summary performance of the instruments shown in Figure 5-3: The electric signal from the oscillator generates an acoustic signal within the test box. The regulating microphone system measures the SPL in the test space and, if the oscillator's compressor is activated, attempts to achieve essentially unvarying intensity in the test space as frequency changes. The measuring system receives the output of the hearing aid, which may be read visually or recorded graphically. Filters additionally permit measurement of distortion products generated within the aid.

COMMON ELECTROACOUSTIC CHARACTERISTICS

The performance characteristics of a hearing aid — that is, the changes effected in a signal as it is transduced from acoustic to electric to acoustic energy — are known as electroacoustic characteristics. Hearing aid manufacturers release specification sheets describing the electroacoustic characteristics of given hearing aid models. The characteristics commonly reported are described below.

Gain

The amount, in decibels, by which the sound pressure level developed by the hearing aid earphone in the coupler exceeds the sound pressure level in the free field into which the hearing aid, or its microphone, if separated, is introduced is termed the gain. That is, gain equals output minus input. Maximum gain is the gain of the hearing aid with the volume control turned full on.

Frequency Response

Because of the nature of the components of a hearing aid, some frequencies are amplified more efficiently than others. Thus, the relation between frequency and amplification constitutes one area of interest in specifying the electroacoustic behavior of hearing aids. This relationship may be shown by graphing the acoustic output delivered by a hearing aid against the frequency of the input sound. The procedure for determining the frequency response characteristics of a hearing aid consists of measuring the sound pressure developed by the hearing aid receiver in an artificial ear when a known sound pressure for a given frequency is applied to the hearing aid microphone. That is, a frequency response graph shows how the output of an aid changes across frequency when the intensity of the input is held constant and frequency is changed. The *frequency range* of an aid refers to the useful range of the frequency response. It is expressed by two numbers, one representing the low frequency limit of amplification and the other the high frequency limit with both numbers expressed in Hz.

Saturation Sound Pressure Level (Maximum Power Output)

This value represents the maximim root mean square sound pressure level obtainable in the coupler from an earphone of a hearing aid. That is, each hearing aid has an output ceiling that cannot be exceeded regardless of how far the gain control is turned or how intense the input is made. This maximum output limitation is a safety factor against sounds that might be harmful or uncomfortable.

Harmonic Distortion

Harmonic distortion (amplitude distortion) is a result primarily of over-loading the hearing aid amplifier. It occurs when the instantaneous output sound pressure of the hearing aid earphone is not directly proportional to the instantaneous sound pressure at the microphone (Nichols et al., 1945). This distortion results from peak clipping. When output limiting, as discussed above, occurs in its commonest form, the strongest peaks of the signal are clipped, changing the waveform of the signal. Weak components of the signal are amplified and otherwise unaltered. The clipped energy reappears in the output signal, as frequencies which are multiples, or harmonics, of the input signal. This harmonic distortion further changes the waveform of the input signal. Psychologically, it results in change in the perceived quality and, if sufficiently severe, in loss of identifiability of the signal.

In one form or another the above characteristics, totally or in part, are usually expressed on hearing aid specification sheets. Measurement of these characteristics, and some others, are discussed in detail in this chapter.

STANDARDS

At the present time, individuals who are seriously interested in making accurate measurements of hearing aid characteristics must be willing to cope with at least four separate major standards or recommendations. Other standards also exist that deal with specific aspects of hearing aid construction or measurement. Two of the four standards that must be taken into consideration are Publication 118 of the International Electrotechnical Commission (1959) and the *American Standard Methods for Measurement of Electroacoustical Characteristics of Hearing Aids* (1971). These two documents deal with specific measurement techniques and procedures that should be followed when making electroacoustic measurements. The two standards that deal with procedures for committing the measured data to paper are the USA *Standard Method of Expressing Hearing Aid Performance* (1971) and the Hearing Aid Industry Conference *Standard Method of Expressing Hearing Aid Performance* (1974).

The contents of these standards have been discussed in detail elsewhere (Kasten, 1968; Kasten, 1972; Lybarger, 1974) and the readers are referred to these other coverages for detailed descriptions. These narrative coverages of the contents of the standards or recommendations present clear and easily followed descriptions of methods for both measurement and expression of hearing aid characteristics.

FROM YESTERDAY TO TODAY

Several years ago, a committee was formed to evaluate the accuracy and appropriateness of the American standard for hearing aid characteristics and recommend improvements. This committee was called S-3-48, American National Standards Institute Working Group For The Measurement And Specification of Hearing Aid Characteristics. It has been made up of approximately 10 hearing aid industry representatives and five or six audiology and government representatives (government representatives are from the Veterans Administration and the National Bureau of Standards). This writer joined the Working Group during 1967.* Since that time the group has actively investigated modifications or total alterations to many of the provisions of the then existing American standard. The group was comprised of dedicated and knowledgeable individuals who were all interested in effecting the most meaningful change in the standard. It soon became apparent, however, that each of these dedicated and knowledgeable individuals had his own interpretation of what the most meaningful change ought to be.

Valuable research was evaluated and the results were frequently interpreted in such a way as to permit more than one set of conclusions. Honest differences existed among Working Group members regarding actual procedures for measurement and regarding the interpretation of results.

---

* Members of the ANSI Writing Group included: Mr. Richard Brander – Beltone, Mr. Mahlon Burkhard – Industrial Research Products, Mr. Edwin Burnett – National Bureau of Standards, Dr. G. Donald Causey – Veterans Administration, Mr. William Ely – Qualitone, Mr. Michael Gluck – Food and Drug Administration, Mr. W. F. S. Hopmeier – Dealers Association, Dr. James Jerger – Texas Medical Center, Dr. Roger Kasten – Wichita State University, Mr. Hugh Knowles – Knowles Electronics, Dr. Arthur Niemoeller – Central Institute for the Deaf, Mr. James Nunley – Vicon, Dr. Wayne Olsen – Mayo Clinic, Mr. David Preves – Starkey Labs, Dr. John Sinclair – HC Electronics, Dr. Gerald Studebaker – City University of New York, Mr. Harry Teder – Telex.

Discussions were long and laborious, and progress was measured in milli-meters rather than meters.

In the spring of 1974, the Working Group was visited by a representative of the Food and Drug Administration (FDA). This individual indicated that the FDA was interested in preparing a standard for the measurement and specification of hearing aid characteristics, and he had come to the Working Group to benefit from their experience and expertise.

The Working Group responded. Information was shared, ideas were explained, and procedures were discussed. The Working Group met again during early fall of 1974. At that time, the Food and Drug Administration representative passed out the third draft of a proposed standard for hearing aids (FDA-MDS-071-0002, 1974). This third draft included techniques for measuring electroacoustic characteristics, tolerances for every measured characteristic, and rigorous environmental tests that had actually never been used before with hearing aids. This included environmental stresses such as altitude, heat and cold, humidity, shock, and vibration. It was the consensus view of the Working Group that, if this FDA draft were put into effect, there probably would not be any hearing aids that could qualify under it and be sold in this country.

The sentiment was expressed by the FDA representative that it would be necessary for the FDA to continue in its efforts to prepare a standard if the ANSI Writing Group would not be able to move with haste. Needless to say, what appeared to be a proposed intolerable government standard was a great incentive for action.

The Working Group then began a series of meetings that were character-ized by cooperation and concession. Research biases and vested interests on the part of individual group members were dropped. Concerted efforts were made to establish measurement techniques that would provide informa-tion useful to both the engineer and the dispenser or user. At the same time, tolerances for all measured electroacoustic characteristics were de-termined that would be both rigorous and livable. In short, the Working Group worked as a group in an effort to prepare a document that would be meaningful and realistic.

By the Spring of 1975, the Working Group had actually prepared a finalized draft for a new standard. This proposed standard, like its prede-cessors, contained measurement and specification procedures, but also contained tolerances for measured characteristics. The document was sub-mitted to the American National Standards Institute and, upon receipt of their comments, was further revised during the fall of 1975. At the same time, a seventh draft of the proposed FDA standard was prepared which was essentially identical to the ANSI draft in terms of techniques, specifi-cations, and tolerances (FDA-MDS-071-0002, 1975).

The new standard was approved by the American National Standards

Institute on July 23, 1976. It previously had received approval from the Acoustical Society of America (ASA). The standard is designated as ASA Standard 7 - 1976/ANSI Standard S3.22 - 1976, Specification for Hearing Aid Characteristics. Copies are available from ASA Standards Secretariat, 335 E. 45th Street, New York, NY 10017. The price at the time of this printing is seven dollars.

TOMORROW AND BEYOND

The new standard has called for many changes in measurement technique. In addition, care was taken to define carefully the characteristics of the test space, sound source, and measurement system.

The definition of the test space is relatively similar to that described in ANSI S3.3-1960 (R-1971). The test space is to have high sound absorption, while unwanted stimuli, such as ambient noise or electrical or magnetic fields, shall remain at a low enough level that they do not affect the test results by more than 0.5 dB.

The sound source, including the control microphone, will need to be able to maintain a stable sound pressure level at the hearing aid sound entrance opening within ±1.5 dB between 200 and 2000 Hz and within ±2.5 dB between 2000 and 5000 Hz. The sound source will also be able to deliver calibrated SPLs between 50 and 90 dB re 20 micro Pascals (μPa) at the position of the hearing aid sound entrance opening. Total allowable harmonic distortion in the sound source shall not exceed 2% for frequency response measurements or 0.5% total harmonic distortion when harmonic distortion measurements are to be made. The control microphone system is also required to have a frequency response that is flat within ±1 dB over the frequency range from 200 to 5000 Hz. The frequency actually being delivered must be within 2% of the sound source indicator, and the indicated frequencies on a recorder chart need to be accurate within ±5%.

A real need was felt to establish some type of control over paper speed of the apparatus recording the test results in order to eliminate differences that can appear as a result of control manipulation. It was ultimately decided that, rather than deal with specific speeds, it would be more appropriate to specify that the indication at any given paper and writing speed does not differ by more than 1 dB from the steady state value over the standard frequency range. This particular specification will still leave those who measure aids freedom in the selection of equipment speeds, but will place an ultimate restriction in terms of the accuracy of the results.

Within the measurement system, the earphone coupler is critical in the containment and specification of the hearing aid output. Following extensive discussion, it was decided that the new standard would call for the continued use of the standard 2 cc hard-walled coupler. Figure 5-1, taken from ANSI S3.7, presents both the Type HA-1 and the Type HA-2 couplers that are discussed in the new standard. Also recommended is the Type HA-2 with entrance through a rigid tube. A flexible tube may be used with the Type HA-2, but it will be necessary for both the coupler and the tubing type to be specified. The pressure microphone, used in conjunction with the earphone coupler, along with the microphone amplifier and readout device, will need to be uniform within ± 1 dB over the standard frequency range.

It should be pointed out that the conventional hard-walled coupler was selected over newer innovations, such as the Zwislocki coupler, for a variety of reasons. To begin with, conventional couplers are well understood and are inexpensive. Of primary importance, however, was the consideration that the purpose of a standard is to provide methods to exchange information reliably. No attempt was made on the part of the Writing Group to relate the results measured in the hard-walled coupler to actual performance in the human ear canal. Rather, it was clearly pointed out that the primary purpose of a standard is to allow measurements to be made from laboratory to laboratory in a very standardized and stylized fashion.

Standard ambient environmental conditions were also specified. Temperature in the test room shall be between 64 and 81° Farenheit, relative humidity shall be between 0 and 80% and atmospheric pressure shall be between 610 and 795 millimeters (mm) of mercury. The actual conditions at the time the tests are conducted will need to be measured and recorded. In addition, the type of power source used, the supply voltage and, in the case of a power supply, the internal impedance, will need to be stated.

Finally, the various controls of the hearing aid being measured should be set to give the widest possible frequency range, the greatest saturation sound pressure level, and the highest full-on gain. If all three are not possible, then the controls should be set to give the highest saturation sound pressure level. When measuring an aid with varying degrees of compression available, the instrument should be adjusted to the greatest amount of automatic gain control (AGC), even if this setting results in a somewhat reduced saturation.

ELECTROACOUSTICS

This portion of this chapter will deal with the new specifications and tolerances for electroacoustic characteristics. Some comparisons will be made to the previous standard, but primary consideration will be given to the changes that have been adopted and to the new concepts that have been described. Also, it should be borne in mind, for gain, frequency response, or saturation sound pressure level, the results shall be plotted on a grid having a linear decibel ordinate scale and a logarithmic frequency abscissa scale. The determination of grid size and proportion will be made by having the length of one decade on the abscissa equal to the length of 50 ± 2 dB on the ordinate. Table 5-1 presents a summary of the various recommendations and the tolerances applied thereto. The reader should refer to Table 5-1 for a quick summary and for an examination of the interrelationships among the various characteristics.

SSPL 90

The traditional procedure for measuring saturation sound pressure level (SSPL), or maximum power output, has involved a three step procedure: (1) The gain control is turned full on and the aid is placed in the test position. (2) At a given frequency the free field SPL is increased until additional increase results in no increase in the coupler SPL (the hearing aid output). (3) The procedure in step 2 may be repeated at enough frequencies across the range 200-5000 Hz to define the shape of the saturation curve. The ANSI and Hearing Aid Industry Conference (HAIC) procedures for specifying saturation sound pressure level have been to average the maximum output, as measured above, for the frequencies 500, 1000, and 2000 Hz.

Saturation sound pressure level will no longer be measured using the point-by-point manual method. Instead, the hearing aid gain will be set to full on and a saturation curve will be obtained in the range from 200 to 5000 Hz using a constant input SPL of 90 dB. Average saturation sound pressure level will be calculated from the values at the frequencies of 1000, 1600, and 2500 Hz. The resultant figure shall be referred to as high frequency (HF)-average SSPL 90. This particular term was chosen in order to differentiate clearly between the new value and the value calculated according to the previous standard. The tolerance applied to HF-average SSPL 90 is such that the value shall be within ±4 dB of the manufacturer's specified value for the model. Figure 5-4 gives an SSPL 90 curve for a randomly selected hearing aid from clinic stock along with the conventional saturation value measured according to the previous standard.

Gain

Maximum gain was previously measured by the following procedure: (1) The hearing aid gain control is turned full on. (2) The free field input SPL is adjusted to 50 dB. (3) Sound pressure levels are measured in the coupler, covering the range 200-5000 Hz. The ANSI and HAIC method of expressing maximum gain has been to average the values for 500, 1000, and 2000 Hz.

It is now stipulated that gain shall be measured with the volume control of the hearing aid turned to full on. A sinusoidal input signal shall be used at an SPL of 60 dB, or, if necessary to maintain linear input-output conditions, at an SPL of 50 dB. The 50 dB level should always be used when measuring gain in AGC aids. In any case, the magnitude of the input SPL

TABLE 5-1. Condensed outline of tests in ANSI standard for hearing aid specification

CHARACTERISTIC	INPUT SPL dB re 20 μPa	FREQUENCY Hz	GAIN CONTROL SETTING	PRESENTATION	TOLERANCE REQUIREMENTS
SSPL90 (Saturation)	90	200-5000	Full on	Curve	Basic test equipment tolerance
Maximum SSPL90	90	Any frequency between 200 & 5000	Full on	Number (dB)	Mfr. to state max. value for model
Average SSPL90	90	1000, 1600, 2500	Full on	Number (dB) (3-freq. average)	+ 4 dB
Average full-on gain	60 or 50 (State which) 50 for AGC	1000, 1600, 2500	Full on	Number (dB) (3-freq. average)	+ 5 dB
Reference Test Gain Control Position*	60	100, 1600, 2500	Set gain control back to give output SPL 17 dB less than average SSPL 90, or full on for low gain aids.		17 + 1 dB
Frequency Response	60	200-5000 or to -20 dB below 3-freq. avg.	Reference test position	Curve	Low band + 4 dB High band + 6 dB
Total Harmonic Distortion	70	500, 800, 1600	Reference test position	Number (%)	Mfr. to state max. value for model
Equivalent Input Noise Level, L_n	60	1000, 1600, 2500 (Avg. to get L_{av})	Reference test position	Number (dB) $L_n=L_2-(L_{av}-60)$ **	Mfr. to state max. value for model
Telephone Pickup (Induction coil)	10 mA/m rms magnetic field	1000	Full on	Number (dB)	Within + 6 dB of mfrs. specified value
Battery Current	70	1000	Reference test	Number (mA)	Not to exceed mfrs. specified maximum for the model
Input-Output Curves (AGC only)	50 to 90	2000	Full on	Curve Input=abscissa Output=ordinate	Match at 70 dB input then to be within + 4 dB of specified
Attack and Release times (AGC only)	Abrupt 55 to 80; 80 to 55	2000	Full on	Numbers (ms)	To be within values specified by mfr.

* Reference test gain control position for AGC aids is full on.

** L_2 is the noise reading in the coupler with the input signal turned off.

will need to be stated. Full-on gain is then calculated as the difference between the input SPL and the output coupler SPL. Full-on gain is calculated as the average of the values at 1000, 1600, 2500 Hz. This figure will be referred to as HF-average full-on gain. This HF-average full-on gain shall have a tolerance of within ±5 dB of the manufacturer's specified value for the model.

These three frequencies, rather than the previously required 500, 1000, and 2000 Hz, were chosen for the computation of gain and saturation in an attempt to obtain a value that might be more meaningful in terms of fitter or user application. There is an increasing tendency for manufacturers to construct instruments that have no measurable gain at 500 Hz. Also, as technology improves, there is an increasing tendency to shape frequency responses so that the real emphasis lies in the range above 1000 Hz.

Figure 5-5 contains a full-on gain curve from a randomly selected aid of our clinic stock. The difference between the previous calculation and the new calculation for full-on gain is clearly apparent. Obviously, most hearing aids will end up with a slightly larger full-on gain value using the HF-

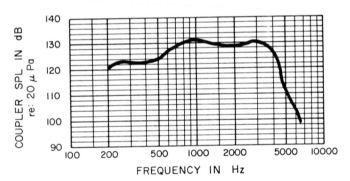

FIG. 5-4. SSPL (saturation sound pressure level) 90 curve. The SSPL 90 average (1, 1.6, and 2.5 kHz) is 130 dB. The conventional SSPL average (0.5, 1, and 2 kHz) is 128 dB.

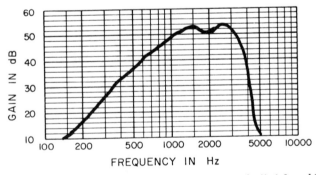

FIG. 5-5. Full-on gain curve. The high frequency average gain (1, 1.6, and 2.5 kHz) is 51 dB. The conventional average gain (0.5, 1, and 2 kHz) is 48 dB.

average method since most hearing aids tend to have greater amplification in the higher frequencies.

Reference Test Gain

A totally new concept in the new standard is that of the reference test gain at which the hearing aid gain control will be set for frequency response measurement. This gain setting is established, using an input SPL of 60 dB, by adjusting the gain control so that the average of the 1000, 1600, and 2500 Hz gain values are equal to the HF-average SSPL 90 minus 17 ± 1 dB. If some aids do not have sufficient gain to achieve this level, then the gain control is set to full on. The full-on gain control is also used for all AGC aids. It is further stipulated that the reference test gain, regardless of how established, be stated on the specification sheet.

The rationale for the establishment of a reference test gain is that the long-term average SPL for speech at a distance of about 1 meter approximates 65 dB re 20 μPa. Additionally, speech peaks are typically considered to be approximately 12 dB above the long-term average level. Using a 65 dB input level with the gain control adjusted to give a coupler output 12 dB less than saturation, it can be assumed that the speech peaks should not exceed the saturation sound pressure level in any particular aid. The use of a 60 dB input and a 17 dB gain control setback would result in essentially the same value but it will be easier to accomplish with the generally used test equipment. Also, the reference test gain position gives a more realistic approximation of a probable use setting than any other setting in previously written standards.

Frequency Response Curve

The traditional measure of frequency response involved these steps: (1) The free field input SPL is adjusted to 60 ± 1 dB at 1000 Hz. (2) The hearing aid gain control is adjusted to give an output SPL in the coupler of 100 ± 2 dB. If the aid does not have enough gain to permit this adjustment, the gain control is set at maximum. If the aid has more minimum gain than will permit the adjustment, the SPL in the coupler is set at 110 dB. (3) The gain control is not changed thereafter. (4) The frequency of the test signal is varied from 200 to 5000 Hz. Keeping the free field SPL constant at 60 dB, measurements of coupler SPL are made at each frequency. (5) With the gain control held constant, input intensity is changed to 50, 70, 80, and 90 dB, and response curves are obtained at each intensity level. These are then plotted, along with the basic curve, to provide a family of curves to describe the frequency response characteristics of the aid. Needless to say, the frequency response measure is usually accomplished by an automated procedure with automatic recording of the resulting coupler SPL versus frequency.

The HAIC method of expressing the useful range of frequency response, or frequency range, is as follows: (1) The average of the 500, 1000, and 2000 Hz on the frequency response curve is determined and plotted on the 1000 Hz ordinate. (2) A point is plotted on the 1000 Hz ordinate 15 dB below the average point. (3) Through this "15 dB down" point a line is drawn, parallel to the frequency axis (the abscissa). (4) The low frequency limit of the hearing aid is defined as the frequency where the line first intersects the response curve, moving in the direction of decreasing frequency from 1000 Hz. If the curve dips below the "15 dB down" line and returns above it, the second downward crossing of the line may be considered the low frequency limit, provided (a) that the band width of the following rise above the "15 dB down" line is 15% or more of the frequency of the first upward crossing, and (b) that the band width of the dip does not exceed 15% of the frequency of the first downward crossing. The purpose of this exception is to avoid penalty where a single notch of inconsequential effect on the hearing aid's performance may exist. (5) The high frequency limit of the aid is defined as the frequency where the "15 dB down" line first intersects the response curve, moving in the direction of increasing frequency from 1000 Hz. The same exception that applies to "notching" in specifying the low frequency limit also applies to notching considerations in specifying the high frequency limit.

The new standard requires that a single frequency response curve shall be recorded using a 60 dB input with the hearing aid set to the reference test gain. The curve shall be measured through the range from 200 to 5000 Hz but may extend above or below these limits if the instrument has such capability (see Figure 5-6). For hearing aids operating with AGC circuitry, the input level for frequency response shall be 50 dB.

The frequency response curve also has tolerances placed upon it. These are calculated by determining the average of the 1000, 1600, and 2500 Hz response levels. From this average, 20 dB are subtracted and a line is drawn parallel to the abscissa at this reduced level. The lowest frequency at which this straight line intersects the response curve is labeled "f_1." The highest frequency at which this straight line intersects the response curve (but not greater than 5000 Hz) is labeled "f_2." The response curve is then broken into a low band and a high band. The frequency limits for the low band are 1.25 f_1 to 2000 Hz. In this frequency region, the response curve must be within ±4 dB of the manufacturer's curve for that model. The high band extends from 2000 to 4000 Hz or 0.8 f_2, whichever is lower. In the high band, the response curve must be within ±6 dB of the manufacturer's curve for that model. It is important to realize that 4000 Hz (0.8 f_2 when f_2 = 5000 Hz) is the absolute top of the high band. Since the higher frequency region of the response curve is by far more difficult to control than the lower frequency region, it was felt that a tolerance which extended to 0.8 f_2

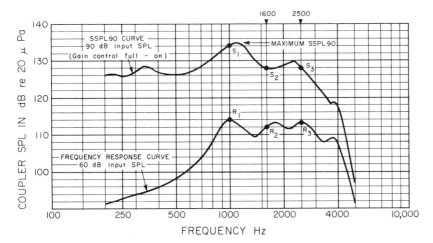

FIG. 5-6. SSPL 90 and frequency response curves. The high frequency (HF)-average SSPL 90 = $(S_1 + S_2 + S_3)/3$. The reference test gain control setting is determined by $S_1 + S_2 + S_3)/3 - (R_1 + R_2 + R_3)/3 - 17$ dB.

without any restriction would be punitive to those manufacturers who attempted to extend the high frequency response of their instruments. By placing a tolerance limit at 4000 Hz, the most central part of the response curve will be controlled and manufacturers can still experiment with extended high frequency instruments.

It was felt that compliance with these tolerances could be determined using a template derived from the manufacturer's response curve for the model. Figure 5-7 pictures such a template and provides instructions for the use of the template. Note that vertical adjustment of the template would be permitted as would horizontal adjustment up to 10% in frequency. After making these two adjustments, it would then be necessary for the response curve of the instrument to lie between the upper and lower limit curves.

Harmonic Distortion

The following procedure is the traditional measure of harmonic distortion, representing the percentage of the total output sound pressure which resides in harmonics generated by the hearing aid: (1) The free field SPL is adjusted to 75 dB at 500 Hz. (2) The gain control of the aid is adjusted so that the total SPL in the coupler is approximately 80 dB, or some higher level if 80 dB is not possible. (3) The sound pressure is measured in the harmonics of the signal from the coupler, using an harmonic wave analyzer. The gain control of the aid is advanced and the sound pressure is measured in the harmonics at a sufficient number of coupler sound pressure levels, including the maximum available, to define the curve of harmonic distortion versus coupler SPL. (5) The above procedures are

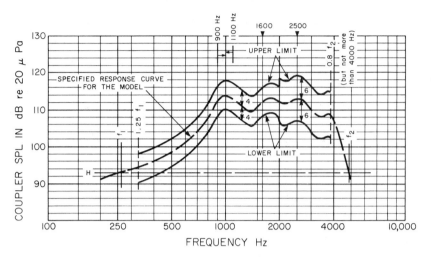

FIG. 5-7. Tolerance template for frequency response curve. The *horizontal line H* is 20 dB below the average of the 1, 1.6, and 2.5 kHz levels on the specified response curve. In use, the template must be kept square wiᴛh the graph of the curve being measured, but may be adjusted vertically any amount and horizontally up to +10% in frequency. Lines on the template at 0.9 and 1.1 kHz show the maximum allowable horizontal movement referred to the 1 kHz ordinate on the measured curve. After adjustment of the template, the measured curve must lie between the upper and lower limits of the template.

repeated at 700 and 900 Hz. (6) The percent total harmonic distortion is determined according to:

$$100\sqrt{\frac{p_2{}^2 + p_3{}^2 + p_4{}^2 + p_n{}^2}{p_1{}^2 + p_2{}^2 + p_3{}^2 + p_n{}^2}}$$

where: p_1 = the amplitude of the SPL at the fundamental frequency in the coupler and p_2, p_3, p_4, etc. = the amplitudes of the sound pressure levels at the harmonic frequencies. The data are plotted with per cent distortion as ordinate, sound pressure as abscissa, and frequency as the parameter.

Alternative measures are to specify different harmonics as × dB below the fundamental at a given gain setting, or to record the basic frequency response curve and harmonic curves on a frequency response chart. A quick measure of harmonic distortion can be obtained with a "distortion bridge," a band rejection filter which eliminates the fundamental frequency and permits measure of total harmonic distortion without gaining information about the energy present in specific harmonics.

Rather than construct a curve of harmonic distortion as is called for in the previous standard, the new standard specifies a single point distortion measurement. Harmonic distortion will be measured with the hearing aid set in the reference test position and with an input SPL of 70 dB. Total harmonic distortion will be measured in the coupler output for input frequencies of 500, 800, and 1600 Hz. Any one of these frequencies may be omitted from the measurement scheme if the frequency response curve rises 12 dB or more between the distortion test frequency and its second harmonic. This stipulation was placed in the standard so as not to penalize instruments that have a steeply rising frequency response which may cause an artifact in the distortion measurement resulting solely from the shape of the frequency response curve. With each model of hearing aid the manufacturer shall specify maximum total harmonic distortion using the above test conditions, and no instrument shall exceed the maximum stated by the manufacturer.

Equivalent Input Noise Level

This particular characteristic relates to the magnitude of internal noise generated by the hearing aid. The gain control shall be set in the reference test position and, with an input SPL of 60 dB, the coupler SPLs at 1000, 1600, and 2500 Hz shall be recorded. The acoustic input signal shall then be removed from the test chamber and the coupler SPL shall be recorded in the absence of the acoustic input. If we now define L_{ave} as the average SPL in the coupler resulting from the 1000, 1600, and 2500 Hz signals, and L_2 as the SPL in the coupler due to internal noise, we may then compute the equivalent input noise level as: $L_n = L_2 - (L_{ave} - 60)$ dB. This measure equivalent input noise level shall not be greater than the maximum level specified by the manufacturer for that model.

Induction Coil

For those instruments constructed with a telephone or induction coil system the controls shall be set for that operating mode. The gain control shall be turned full on, and the hearing aid should be placed in a 1000 Hz alternating magnetic field with a magnetic field strength of 10 milliamps per meter and the instrument shall then be oriented to produce the greatest coupler output level. This SPL is then recorded and it will need to be within ±6 dB of the manufacturer's specified value for these test conditions for that model.

Automatic Gain Control Characteristics

The input-output characteristics of AGC aids shall be measured using a 2000 Hz pure-tone. Input SPL is varied from 50 to 90 dB in 10 dB steps and the coupler output SPL is recorded at each step. Output SPL is plotted on the ordinate with corresponding input SPL on the abscissa. Values will be plotted on a grid using linear decibel scale with equal-sized intervals for both ordinate and abscissa. The five curves are then matched at the point corresponding to the 70 dB input SPL and the measured curves at the two input extremes shall not differ from the manufacturer's specified curve by more than ±4 dB.

The dynamic AGC characteristics are measured with the gain control of the hearing aid turned to full on and with a 2000 Hz square wave modulated pure-tone input signal that can alternate abruptly between 55 and 80 dB SPL. Both attack and release times can be determined from an oscilloscopic pattern. Attack time is defined as the time between the onset of the abrupt increase from 50 to 80 dB and the point where the output has stabilized to within 2 dB of steady state for the 80 dB input signal. Release time is defined in the same fashion using the abrupt decrease from 80 to 55 dB. The tolerance for the attack and release time shall be within ±5 milliseconds (msec) or ±5%, whichever is larger, of the values supplied by the manufacturer for that model.

ENVIRONMENTAL TESTS

Although some manufacturers have conducted some environmental testing on their own hearing aids, the concept of consistent environmental testing for hearing aids is not a common one in this country. This statement is not made in criticism of the manufacturers of hearing aids. Environmental tests can be extremely costly. In addition, environmental tests can be very time consuming. Each of the above items can potentially add markedly to the cost of a hearing aid unit. Finally, however, until recently, there has really been no advocate for environmental tests for hearing aids.

If one thinks of the well-traveled hearing aid user, it is easy to imagine someone moving from the heat of Tucson, Arizona, to the cold of Anaktuvak, Alaska, from the humidity of the Amazon jungle to the dryness of the Sahara desert and from the depths of Death Valley to the heights of Mount Everest. Until now, we have assumed that our hearing-impaired traveler would receive equivalent performance from his amplification system at all of the above-mentioned locations. The validity of the previous statement has only recently been seriously questioned.

Throughout most of the earlier drafts of the FDA proposals, sections appeared with detailed requirements for environmental tests. Since the specifics of the tests tended to change somewhat from one draft to another, this writer will attempt to present a somewhat composite view of the tests that were proposed by FDA. The tests did not become a part of ANSI S3.22. These tests are not being discussed because they, specifically, will become a part of some formal proposal. Rather, it is the feeling that environmental tests, of some sort, are definitely a thing of the future. With this in mind, it behooves all of us to become somewhat more aware of environmental testing procedures.

Temperature Testing

Figure 5-8 shows the variations in the time and temperature parameters for this environmental test. Note the temperature is varied between −20 and +140° Farenheit. This would be somewhat equivalent to the difference between our winter extreme and the glove compartment of an automobile in the middle of a desert. While the actual time of a temperature test can vary markedly, the particular one displayed in Figure 5-8 was scheduled to last somewhat over 30 hours. Commercially available equipment can be obtained that can traverse these extremes and automatically cycle through the sequences. It is particularly important in the construction of a temperature test to have test apparatus that will provide a rapid transition between the temperature extremes.

Shock Tests

It was proposed that the hearing aids be exposed to a shock loading of 1500 gravities peak amplitude of a 2 msec duration with a half-sine pulse wave form. This is an extremely high shock level for a very sort duration and, presumably, is designed to simulate the fall of a hearing aid into a hard surface. This shock should be applied to each aid in each direction (from both the botto and the top) along three axes of the hearing aid. For hearing aids having two parallel transducers, one of the axes will be parallel to the transducer axis and the other two axes will be orthogonal to this axis. For non-parallel transducer systems, each transducer axis shall form a shock axis with the third shock axis orthogonal to the two transducer axes. Thus, since each aid will be shocked in each direction, a total of six shocks will be applied. This writer knows of no facility anywhere that has attempted shock testing of this magnitude with hearing aids.

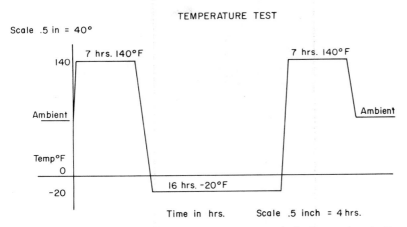

Fig. 5-8. Variations in the time plus temperature parameters for temperature testing.

Humidity Testing

Figure 5–9 shows the variation in the time, temperature, and humidity parameters for this environmental test. It is important to realize that humidity cannot be varied independently but must be varied in conjunction with temperature. Therefore, appropriate instrumentation must be obtained that will provide a continuous indication of the accuracy of the relative humidity within the test chamber along with the accuracy of the temperature.

Humidity tests are, by necessity, generally rather lengthy. The test outlined in Figure 5–9 is a 24 hour test that would be recycled four different times. Some proposals for humidity tests for hearing aids have gone as high as 240 hours in length. A primary concern during humidity testing is that the hearing aid be positioned in such a way that condensate will not drip upon the actual instrument and provide damage through the physical contact of quantities of water.

Vibration Tests

It is presumed that these tests are devised to simulate the many movements of a hearing aid as it would be worn on a human body. Specifically, the hearing aid would be mounted to a shaker apparatus in the same set of axes that were established for the shock tests. During the vibration tests, each hearing aid will be subjected to a 1.6 mm peak-to-peak amplitude vibration at 50 Hz for a period of 2 hours along each of the axes. Again, this writer is not familiar with any facility that has been doing this type of vibration testing with hearing aids.

Several statements should be made in summarizing this section relating

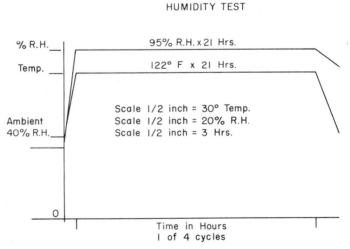

HUMIDITY TEST

FIG.5-9. Variations in the time, temperature, and humidity parameters for humidity testing.

to environmental testing. First of all, the reader should remember that the environmental tests described above are simply examples from a broad universe of tests that could conceivably be used. The examples were presented because they represented something of a composite of the FDA proposals. In particular, the reader should be aware that no one is sure, at this point in time, whether existing hearing aids could survive this type of testing. Extensive research will need to be done to verify the type of environmental stresses that hearing aids should be able to withstand and the types of tests that should be devised to simulate these stresses.

Finally, in the particular sequence of testing described above, the over-all time for tests would be approximately 12 days. This would move everyone connected with hearing aids out of the era of the 15 second frequency response test. The equipment and personnel needed for the conduct of this type of environmental test, could markedly increase the production cost of hearing aids. It would be hoped, before environmental tests become a required reality, that a determination of cost per unit test could be carefully evaluated.

OTHER CONSIDERATIONS

From this brief summary of the new ANSI standard, it can be seen that many significant changes have been made from the previous standard. It is anticipated that the new standard will promote greater accuracy and ease in measurement and generally more meaningful information. There will naturally need to be a transition period as we move from our comfortable and well understood conventional measurements to a new set of measurements that will give us a new set of data.

Importantly, this new standard—for the first time—provides tolerances for measured characteristics. It has been known for some time that there can be some rather sizable variability in the electroacoustic characteristics of instruments within given models (Kasten, Lotterman, and Revoile, 1967; Lotterman and Kasten, 1967a). The preparation of the new ANSI standard represents a real milestone in hearing aid development since it will call for a level of product uniformity not previously observed.

This writer is also aware that many other items could be discussed in a chapter that deals with electroacoustic characteristics. Indeed, the list could be exhaustive and the discussion could be unending. Instead, it seems appropriate to mention the other characteristics and provide the reader with references to existing written material. The list should include such items as intermodulation distortion (Pollack, 1975; Harris et al., 1961; Kasten, Lotterman, and Burnett, 1967), transient distortion (Pollack, 1975; Witter, 1971), use of noise signals for hearing aid measurements (Veterans Administration, 1975; Brander, 1974) or KEMAR (Preves, 1976; Burkhard and Sachs, 1973). This listing is certainly not exhaustive, but will give the reader a place to begin.

Chapter 6

Speech acoustics and intelligibility

William R. Hodgson, Ph.D.

INTRODUCTION

Acoustic events transfer meaning from speaker to listener. Information about these events contributes to understanding of the intelligibility of speech and intelligibility problems experienced by hearing-impaired individuals. Speech intelligibility is a complex function of intensity, frequency, and time factors. In the following pages, the overall intensity of speech is discussed. The frequency characteristics of speech are presented, both in terms of overall spectrum and the spectra of individual speech sounds. The interaction between hearing loss and these variables is considered. Of the factors which contribute to speech intelligibility, the role of intensity is simplest, and will be considered first.

INTENSITY

The overall intensity of speech at a representative distance of one meter from the talker's lips is likely to be 65–70 dB sound pressure level (SPL). Fletcher (1953) reported that a person talking as loudly as possible may produce a sound pressure level of about 86 dB while the softest level may approximate 46 dB. Excepting the influence of reverberation, sound pressure drops 6 dB with each doubling of distance between source and receiver.

The sensation level required by normal ears for maximum intelligibility varies according to the type of message and production characteristics of the speaker. The more homogeneous and easy to understand the message, the lower the required sensation level. Davis and Silverman (1970) reported maximum intelligibility for the recorded W-22 version of phonetically balanced (PB) lists at about 25 dB above the threshold of intelligibility for spondees. This figure agrees fairly well with what would be expected from Fletcher's analysis of the power of individual speech sounds (1953). He reported a range of 680-1, or 28 dB, between the strongest and weakest sound. The relative power of speech sounds, as determined by Fletcher, is shown in Table 6-1.

Certain precautions should be observed when interpreting these data. First, depending on the position in word or sentence, the emphasis on a given sound varies from time to time. Second, these values represent the ratio between sounds spoken at conversational level. As overall intensity of the voice increases, the range in dB between the strongest and weakest sound also increases. Therein lies, in part, the futility of "shouting at" a hearing-impaired listener. The speaker runs the risk of intensifying the strong sounds the listener is probably already hearing without making the weak sounds audible. This situation may cause perceptual masking or an increase in harmonic distortion by the listener's hearing aid, further deteriorating the listening conditions. For these reasons, and also to improve overall signal-to-noise ratio (SNR), lower intensity speech near the listener, or near the microphone of the amplifying system, is better than higher intensity speech originating at a distance.

Strictly speaking, according to Fletcher's data, a presentation level would be required 28 dB above threshold of the strongest sound in order for the weakest sound to be audible and intelligibility to reach maximum. The relationship between intensity and intelligibility may be described in two ways. First, Figure 6-1 shows a typical performance-intensity (PI) function

TABLE 6-1. **Relative phonetic power of speech sounds as produced by an average speaker***

Sound	Power	dB	Sound	Power	dB	Sound	Power	dB
ɔ	680	28.3	r	210	23.2	t	15	11.8
ɑ	600	27.9	l	100	21.0	g	15	11.8
ʌ	510	27.0	ʃ	80	19.0	k	13	11.1
æ	490	26.9	ŋ	73	18.6	v	12	10.8
ou	470	26.7	m	52	17.2	ð	11	10.4
ʊ	460	26.6	tʃ	42	16.2	b	7	8.5
EI	370	25.6	n	36	15.6	d	7	8.5
ɛ	350	25.4	j	23	13.6	p	6	7.8
u	310	24.9	ʒ	20	13.0	f	5	7.0
I	260	24.1	z	16	12.0	θ	1	0
i	220	23.4	s	16	12.0			

*After Fletcher (1953).

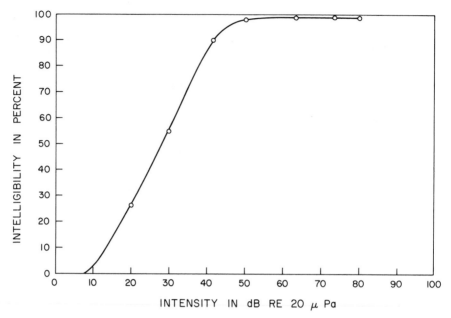

Fig. 6-1. Performance-intensity function.

for PB-lists. This function describes the relationship between overall intensity and intelligibility. Second, the contribution to intelligibility of intensity as a function of frequency can be evaluated. Table 6-2 shows this power-intelligibility relationship. The frequencies below 500 Hz contain 60% of speech power but contribute only 5% intelligibility. The frequencies above 1000 Hz contribute 5% of the power and 60% of the intelligibility. In practical terms, these data mean that vowels, the intense low frequencies, are less important for intelligibilty than consonants.*

As Carhart (1965) pointed out, the relationship described above between speech reception threshold (SRT) and PB max may not obtain for pathologic ears. The most obvious contributor to the difference is the configuration of the audiogram. Most sensorineural losses show a configuration sloping toward a more severe loss in the higher frequencies. There is less deficit for lower frequencies, important for audibility, than for higher frequencies critical for intelligibility. Therefore the relationships between SRT and discimination score may be changed, and a higher sensation level may be required for PB max. Because of this consideration it is conventional to test discrimination at a sensation level of 40 dB, or as close to that level as comfort permits.

A similar relationship exists when subjects listen to speech in noise.

---

*This statement should not be mistaken to mean that only energy below 500 Hz is important to vowel intelligibility or that consonants carry 95% of the intelligibility of speech.

Harris et al. (1961) concluded for subjects listening to speech in noise through hearing aids, that no further improvement in SNR over 25 dB will increase intelligibility. At less favorable signal-to-noise ratios, however, there is evidence that individuals with sensorineural loss fare poorer than normals. Watson (1964) reported a condition in which, for normal listeners, intelligibility was reduced 46% by a masking noise. Discrimination of subjects with sensorineural loss dropped 64%. Olsen and Tillman (1968) reported a difference in intelligibility between normal and sensorineural impaired subjects of 12% when listening in quiet. At a SNR of +18 dB, the difference was 15% and at a SNR of +6 dB the disparity widened to 28%.

There are also differences at the other end of the intensity continuum between normals and some patients with sensorineural loss. That is, beyond the intensity required for maximum intelligibility a reduction in discrimination scores may occur. Jerger and Jerger (1971) and Gang (1976) observed this rollover effect in patients with retrocochlear disorder. It may be expected in patients with eighth nerve tumor and in some presbycusics with retrocochlear degeneration. Figure 6-2 compares the PI function of 2 patients; (A) a 47 year old individual and (B) an 84 year old person who exhibits marked rollover. Both have sensorineural loss. In addition to possible diagnostic importance, the presence of rollover in an individual complicates evaluation of discrimination ability and use of amplification.

In summary, study of the relationship between intensity and intelligibility reveals these important factors: Normals achieve maximum intelligibility of discrete monosyllabic words at a sensation level of 25 dB. Hearing-impaired individuals may require a higher sensation levels for best discrimination but for some, discrimination scores may decline beyond a given presentation level. Finally, a disproportionate drop in intelligibility, compared to normals, commonly results when subjects with sensorineural loss listen to speech in noise.

The contribution of intensity to speech intelligibility was considered separately above. The role of the other contributors—frequency and durational factors—is more tightly interwoven. Therefore these factors are considered together in the following paragraphs.

TABLE 6-2. **Percent speech power and intelligibility***

Frequency Range in Hz	Per Cent Speech Power	Per Cent Intelligibility
62–125	5 ⎫	1 ⎫
125–250	13 ⎬ 60 ⎫	1 ⎬ 5
250–500	42 ⎭ ⎬ 95	3 ⎭
500–1000	35 ⎭	35 ⎫
1000–2000	3 ⎫	35 ⎬
2000–4000	1 ⎬ 5	13 ⎬ 60 ⎫ 95
4000–8000	1 ⎭	12 ⎭

*From Gerber (1974), with permission.

LONG-TERM SPECTRUM

The relationship between intelligibility and frequency is straightforward when the overall speech spectrum is considered. The sounds of speech contain energy between about 100 and 8000 Hz. This frequency range is determined by measuring the long-term speech spectrum. That is, if all the speech sounds are thrown together and spectral analysis made, results similar to those shown in Figure 6-3 will occur. Most of the energy is below 1000 Hz and the peak of energy in this instance is between 500 and 600 Hz.

Audibility of this entire range is not required for good intelligibility of

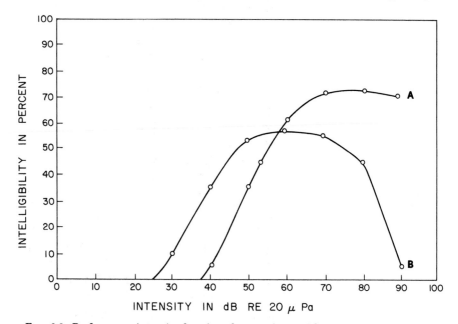

FIG. 6-2. Performance-intensity function of two patients with sensorineural loss; (A) 47 year old with sensorineural loss and (B) 84 year old with sensorineural loss and indication of retrocochlear disorder.

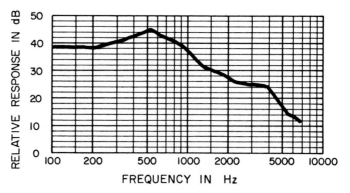

FIG. 6-3. Long-term speech spectrum (after Rudmose, 1948).

speech. Hirsh, Reynolds, and Joseph (1954) measured intelligibility of the monosyllabic words constituting the Central Institute for the Deaf Auditory Test W-22. The signal was sent through high- or low-pass filters with a fairly sharp rejection rate of 60 dB/octave to 5 normal hearing listeners. Presentation was at an overall 95 dB SPL and it should be kept in mind that some energy below the nominal cut-off frequency was available to the listeners. Results are shown in Figure 6-4. For low-pass filtered speech, intelligibility dropped only a little when frequencies above 1600 Hz were removed. There was a further drop of about 25% when the filter setting was moved downward to 800 Hz. For high-pass filtering, intelligibility remained normal when frequencies below 1600 Hz were eliminated, but dropped about 25% when all frequencies below 3200 Hz were filtered out. Stated differently, the subjects enjoyed nearly normal and nearly equal intelligibility when they could hear the frequencies below 1600 Hz or those above 1600 Hz.

In an earlier study, French and Steinberg (1947) found a similar rela-

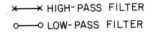

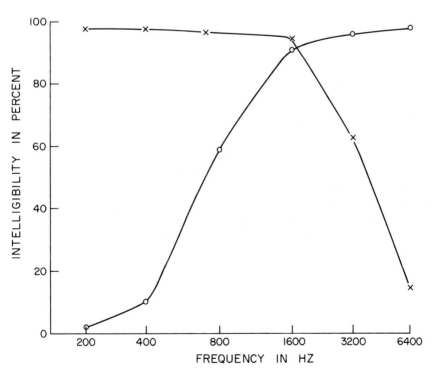

FIG. 6-4. Relationship between high- and low-pass filtering and intelligibility of speech (After Hirsh, Reynolds, and Joseph, 1954).

tionship between intelligibility and frequency. Their scores were generally lower than those of Hirsh, Reynolds, and Joseph, probably because French and Steinberg used a filter with a sharper rejection rate. They found intelligibility to be near 70% when subjects listened to speech with only frequencies above or below about 1900 Hz present.

The clinical correlate of such studies as these causes us to expect near normal discimination scores in patients with normal hearing sensitivity to 2000 Hz and a substantial reduction if sensitivity falls sharply above 1000 Hz. Minimal intelligibility of monosyllabic words is expected if there is no useful hearing above 500 Hz.

INDIVIDUAL SPEECH SOUNDS

The contribution of individual speech sounds to intelligibility is a very complex consideration. Frequency, intensity, and temporal characteristics interact and contribute to the intelligibility of speech. The spectral pattern of each sound can be established. Vowel sounds are described in terms of formant patterns; the center frequencies of conspicuous peaks of intensity and their bandwidths in the acoustic spectrum. Consonants are described in terms of the frequency characteristics associated with the quasi-random signal produced by constriction of airflow and the additional quasi-periodic contribution of the vocal folds in voiced consonants. As mentioned earlier, English consonants are more important to speech intelligibility than are vowels.

The average frequency pattern of the individual speech sounds is well established and available in several published articles, for example that of Jeffers (1966). Utility of such information to predict the effect of hearing loss affecting different frequencies is limited by several factors. First, the effect of coarticulation renders speech sound spectra significantly different in context from those of sounds in isolation. Coarticulation is defined as the effect on one sound of the sounds which precede and follow it. The same influence causes substantial spectral changes of a given sound in different phonetic contexts. That is, the effects of coarticulation vary with context. Second, there is marked variability in patterns of speech sound spectra from individual to individual. An example of this variability is shown in Figure 6-5. Variation also occurs as an individual repeats a speech sound in the same context, but this variability is much less than that observed among different speakers (Peterson and Barney, 1952).

Because of the variability mentioned above and other factors affecting individual subjects, the discrimination ability of each hearing-impaired person must be established individually. Investigators have tried to predict discrimination scores from other auditory tests. Elliott (1963) could not obtain useful correlations between speech discrimination scores and various audiometric data. She concluded that "speech discrimination among

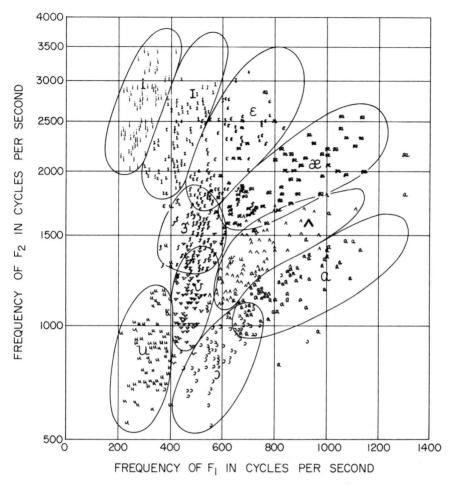

FIG. 6-5. Frequency of second formant versus frequency of first formant for 10 vowels spoken by 76 speakers (from Peterson and Barney, 1952, with permission).

ears with perceptive loss is qualitatively different from that among normal ears" (Elliott, 1963, p. 44).

Prediction of intelligibility on the basis of residual hearing and speech sound spectra must be limited to the following rather crude generalizations:

1. Persons with flat loss will probably have better discrimination than those with sloping high frequency loss.

2. Individuals with good low frequency hearing and a high frequency loss, will hear vowels well and consonants poorly. Vowels are relatively intense low frequency sounds and consonants high frequency in nature. The effect on discrimination of varying high frequency losses is shown in Figure 6-6. The individual in audiogram A with good hearing to 1000 Hz,

AUDIOLOGICAL   RECORD

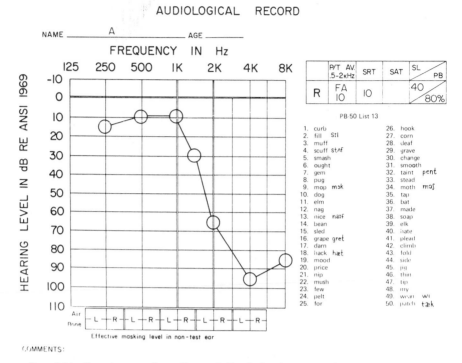

NAME _____ A _____ AGE _____

FIG. 6-6A. Pure-tone configuration and discrimination scores for patient with hearing loss above 1000 Hz.

makes only consonant errors. The patient in audiogram *B* has essentially normal hearing only to 500 Hz. He makes vowel as well as consonant errors.

3. There is no impressive evidence that individuals with profound loss, fragmented audiograms, and no measurable sensitivity over the "speech range" (500–2000 Hz) can learn to discriminate speech independent of visual clues (Hudgins, 1954).

With these limitations in mind the following analysis of speech sounds is presented.

Speech sounds result from acoustic filtering by the vocal tract of sounds generated within the vocal tract. The filtering process is called resonance. The acoustic result is the link between speech production and speech perception. Miller and Nicely (1955) suggested five features that serve to characterize and distinguish the different phonemes. These distinctive features are voicing, nasality, affrication, duration, and place of articulation.

Minifie (1973) reports that in speech of adult males vowel energy is present between 100 Hz and 4500 Hz. This spectrum is filtered by the vocal tract resulting in the resonant patterns typical of the individual vowel sounds. As a generalization, these patterns are determined by the place

AUDIOLOGICAL RECORD

NAME B AGE

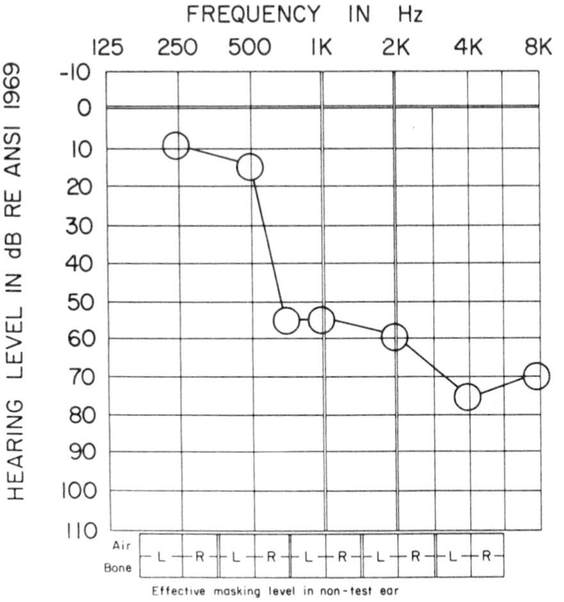

	P/T AV. .5-2kHz	SRT	SAT	SL / PB
R	FA 32	30		40 / 24%

PB-50 List 16

1. closed NR	26. ink
2. dub bɛg	27. cliff NR
3. map ma	28. crews triz
4. soar	29. had hɔg
5. suit sup	30. hook
6. rock hwat	31. thou laɪ
7. gab gæd	32. tire NR
8. sheik	33. thresh NR
9. leash liʃ	34. louse læf
10. dame dʌm	35. ton tʌŋ
11. drape brek	36. aid ɛg
12. part pat	37. knee mi
13. pitch pʌt	38. three fri
14. barge dɔg	39. din
15. stress stʌf	40. hose haɪt
16. gas	41. sang sɔŋ
17. rogue rʌg	42. cheese
18. hash haʊs	43. fifth fɪks
19. lay	44. stab
20. sheep ʃit	45. kind NR
21. pump	46. tuck pʌt
22. nap mat	47. turn tʌŋ
23. droop grup	48. next
24. rye hwaɪ	49. wield jild
25. fright faɪt	50. rug

COMMENTS:

FIG. 6-6*B*. Pure-tone configuration and discrimination scores for patient with hearing loss above 500 Hz.

where restriction occurs in the vocal tract, the amount of constriction, and the shape of the lips. The result is creation of formant patterns which, on the average, are like those shown in Table 6-3 (Peterson and Barney, 1952). Ling (1975) points out that the second formant as well as second formant transitions are important for vowel intelligibility and also lend useful intelligibility clues about adjacent consonants. Minifie (1973) mentions that only the first three formants appear to be used by listeners in differentiating vowel sounds. The data in Table 6-3 (Peterson and Barney, 1952) show the first three formants to contain energy between 270 and 3010 Hz for male voices. Experimental evidence and clinical experience certainly indicate that individuals with normal hearing sensitivity across this range will enjoy unimpaired vowel intelligibility. The range for the first two formants is from 270 to 2290 Hz. Normal sensitivity across this range would also be expected to produce unimpaired vowel discrimination ability.

Vowels appear to be differentiated, not on the basis of absolute formant frequency information, but from the ratio relationships among the formant frequencies. These patterns are similar when the same vowel is spoken by different speakers of the same sex, or when spoken by men, women, and children.

Vowels with similar F_1/F_2 ratios tend to be mistaken for each other. For

TABLE 6-3. **Averages of fundamental and formant frequencies from 6 speakers***

		i	ɪ	ɛ	æ	ɑ	ɔ	ʊ	u	ʌ	ɝ
Fundamental	M	136	135	130	127	124	129	137	141	130	133
frequencies (cps)	W	235	232	223	210	212	216	232	231	221	218
	Ch	272	269	260	251	256	263	276	274	261	261
Formant											
Frequencies (cps)											
	M	270	390	530	660	730	570	440	300	640	490
F_1	W	310	430	610	860	850	590	470	370	760	500
	Ch	370	530	690	1010	1030	680	560	430	850	560
	M	2290	1990	1840	1720	1090	840	1020	870	1190	1350
F_{21}	W	2790	2480	2330	2050	1220	920	1160	950	1400	1640
	Ch	3200	2730	2610	2320	1370	1060	1410	1170	1590	1820
	M	3010	2550	2480	2410	2440	2410	2240	2240	2390	1690
F_3	W	3310	3070	2990	2850	2810	2710	2680	2670	2780	1960
	Ch	3730	3600	3570	3320	3170	3180	3310	3260	3360	2160

*From Peterson and Barney (1952), with permission.

example there is only 22 Hz difference between these ratios for the sounds [ɑ] and [ɔ], and Peterson and Barney (1952) found the highest confusion between these two vowels. The F_1/F_2 difference for [ɝ] (363 Hz) is similar to that of [u] and [æ] but, according to Peterson and Barney (1952) the [ɝ] is not confused with these sounds because its F_2/F_3 ratio is quite different from those vowels.

Martin, Pickett, and Colten (1972), and Danaher (née Martin), Osberger, and Pickett (1973) conducted experiments using synthetic vowels to determine discrimination of formant frequency transitions in normals and subjects with sensorineural loss. These transitions, it should be remembered, give clues for consonant intelligibility. The experimenters found that, when the second formant (F_2) was presented alone, there was not much difference in performance of normal and sensorineural subjects except that for transitions of short duration, the normals performed better. A much greater difference was found when subjects listened to F_2 transitions in the presence of F_1 energy. Performance of the sensorineural subjects was much poorer, although there was marked variability, than that of normals. Presentation was at the most comfortable listening level (MCL). When the normals listened at high presentation levels, comparable to the SPL required by the hearing-impaired subjects for MCL, their performance also deteriorated. Therefore the authors concluded the effect of strong F_1 energy on F_2 discrimination was associated with spread of masking occurring at high presentation levels. Regarding practical amplification for the hearing impaired, F_1 cannot be eliminated for it also contributes to intelligibility. However the experimenters recommended, in individual aid selection, reduction of amplification in the region where F_1

energy occurs. This range encompasses approximately 250–750 Hz for male voices, 300–600 Hz for females, and 350–1050 Hz for children's voices. Unfortunately, F_1 overlaps the F_2 range in adults for some sounds. However, attention to F_1 attenuation might be useful to hearing aid users. As suggested later in this chapter, it may be that the current trend toward increased low frequency performance in many hearing aids creates a problem in this respect, and also increases the masking of speech by other low frequency non-speech environmental sounds.

Consonant sounds are products of a relatively restricted vocal tract. Depending on the degree of constriction, consonants are classified as fricatives or stops. Fricatives result when constriction permits continued passage of the air stream. Minifie (1973) mentions that the natural resonance frequency of the vocal tract increases in fricative production the closer the sound source is to the lip opening. Therefore [θ] and [ð] have their largest amplitude in the range from 7000 to 8000 Hz, and are the highest frequency fricatives (Strevens, 1960). Fant (1960) describes the [f] and [v] as broad band sounds (800–10000 Hz) with minor resonance peaks at 6000–7000 Hz. The [s] and [z] have little energy below 4000 Hz, and have a resonance peak between 7000 and 8000 (Hughes and Halle, 1956). The [ʃ] and [ʒ] are reported to have peak intensity near 2500 Hz, considerably lower than that of [s] and [z] (Hughes and Halle, 1956). Harris (1958) and La Riviere, Winitz, and Herriman (1975) reported that the [s] and [ʃ] and the [z] and [ʒ] sounds are sufficiently different in spectral composition for consistent correct identification on the basis of spectral clues only. The other fricative pairs, [f] and [θ], and [v] and [ð] can be consistently differentiated only when transitions involving adjacent vowels give additional information. Fricatives that differ in both voicing and spectrum are the easiest to differentiate.

Stops occur when the breath stream is completely stopped by the occluded vocal tract. The momentarily impeded air stream is then released either orally as in [tu] or nasally as the [t] in [bʌtn]. In English, stops are strongly exploded when they occur initially in words, and ordinarily not exploded when they occur in the final position. Thus the acoustic clues for identification of unvoiced final stops must belong entirely to the transition period of the preceding vowel.

Halle, Hughes, and Radley (1957) reported on the acoustic properties of stops. They found the greatest energy in [k] and [g] between 1500 and 4000 Hz. The sounds [t] and [d] had energy in a region around 500 Hz and above 4000 Hz. The [p] and [b] had energy mostly between 500 and 1500 Hz.

Another clue to differentiating voiced versus voiceless stops relates to the time of onset of voicing. According to Lisker and Abramson (1967), the onset of voicing in voiced stops occurring initially in words may be about 100 msec in isolated words and 50 msec in words in sentences before explosion of the sound. In voiceless stops occurring initially, voicing of the following vowel starts about 35 to 150 msec after explosion. For voiceless stops which occur in the medial position, and are therefore unaspirated, the onset of voicing is 0 to 50 msec after explosion. In voiced medial stops, voicing across the stop and the following vowel is usually continuous. Clues that differentiate these sounds are related to voice onset time and thus may be more important than the traditional classification of voiced and voiceless. The delay in voice onset following unvoiced stops is considered to help differentiate them from their voiced counterparts. However, Winitz, La Riviere, and Herriman (1975) concluded that aspiration is the primary clue to detect voicing, and that voice onset time is a relatively unimportant secondary clue. They systematically altered voice onset time for English stops and found that perception of voicing was not much affected. However, unvoicing could be detected with only very short (10 msec) aspiration following release.

Several sounds are recognized as the result of transitions from one sound to another. The diphthongs ([eɪ], [aɪ], [aʊ], [ɔɪ], [oʊ]) are examples. The perceptual characteristics of the intervowel glides [l], [r], [w], and [j], sometimes called semi-vowels, also result from the glide action. The diphthongs are "receding" intervowel glides. That is, the origin position is stressed and the movement is away from that position to a briefer unstressed vowel. The semi-vowels are approaching intervowel glides. To produce [j], for example, the articulators move from the high front vowel position to some other vowel and the terminating position receives the greater stress.

Vocalic transitions between vowel sounds in the production of diphthongs are relatively slow. The transition between vowels to produce semi-vowels is a little faster, and the transition between vowel and stop consonant is very rapid. According to Liberman et al. (1956) the speed of transition assists the listener in differentiating between diphthongs, semi-vowels, and stops.

When stops and fricative sounds made in about the same articulatory position occur together a special sound occurs. The results is called an affricate. We generally recognize the affricates [t] and [d] and have separate International Phonetic Alphabet symbols for them, probably because they have conventional spelling or letters assigned to them in the regular alphabet ('ch' and "J"). The combinations [ts] and [dz] are affricates also. Minifie (1973) reports that the temporal or durational pattern of stops, and therefore also of affricates, is more important to intelligibility than that of fricatives.

The nasal sounds, [m], [n], and [ŋ] have resonance characteristics and formant patterns similar in some ways to vowels, although their amplitude is usually less. According to Minifie (1973) the formant pattern of these sounds is sufficient to identify them as nasals, and the formant transitions associated with coarticulation are adequate to differentiate the three sounds.

The [h] sound is the result of glottal friction. The friction is caused by vocal fold approximation prior to the adduction required for phonation in the production of a vowel. Since the [h] is produced with the oral cavity set for production of the following vowel, that vowel's characteristics become imposed on production of the [h]. The same circumstances no doubt sometimes *follow* vowel production, but the result is not phonemic, and tends not to be noticed. Minifie (1973) reports that the output spectrum of [h] ranges between 400 and 6500 Hz, with peaks near 1000 and 6500 Hz.

Regarding overall duration in speech, Gerber (1974) reports the average speaking rate of American English to be 440 syllables per minute, or 165 words per minute. Average phoneme duration in connected speech is 70–80 msec. with vowels usually lasting for 200 to 300 msec and consonants being briefer than the average given above (Liberman et al., 1967).

COARTICULATION AND SUPRASEGMENTAL FACTORS

The actual spectrum of given sounds in speech varies with the influence of coarticulation. As defined earlier, coarticulation is the effect on one speech sound of the sounds which precede and follow it. Minifie (1973, p. 280) cautions " . . . context-dependent variations in articulatory behavior, constrained by the rules of our phonology and the mechanics of our articulatory mechanism, allow substantial variations in acoustical output – and yet, these variant signals evoke similar perceptual responses." One resulting implication is that an absolute prediction of intelligibility cannot be made on the basis of spectral characteristics of speech sounds and the configuration of an individual hearing loss. Minifie (1973) also points out that, in addition to the effects of coarticulation, the spectra of speech sounds are further changed by the resonance characteristics of the conductive mechanisms of the receiver's ear.

Suprasegmental aspects of speech involve changes and conditions which occur across a number of phonemes. These phenomena are (1) changes in the intonational pattern, or melody, of the voice, (2) changes in stress or relative emphasis on syllables, and (3) changes in duration, including patterns of pausing, tempo, and rate of syllable utterance. Limited meaning is associated with suprasegmental factors. For example, interrogative, declarative, and exclamative sentences can be differentiated. Also, differentiation is proved in sentences which have the same words but not the same meaning. The distinction between "Good-bye, God, we're going to Arizona;" and "Good, by god, we're going to Arizona," depends on suprasegmental events.

Ling (1964) has shown that extended low frequency amplication for profoundly impaired children with only low frequency residual hearing can improve reception of suprasegmental information, much of which is generated by the low frequency part of the speech spectrum. However, Martin and Pickett (1970) illustrated that upward spread of masking can impair intelligibility and concluded that, while there is great variability, use of an extended low-frequency response hearing aid might even reduce intelligibility in some individuals with sensorineural loss. In a reply to Martin and Pickett, Ling (1971) pointed out that extended low-frequency aids were intended for use with subjects who had little or no residual hearing above 1000 Hz, and were meant to be used in controlled acoustic conditions with high input and low gain in a relatively quiet environment. Sung, Sung, and Angelelli (1971) confirmed that extended low-frequency emphasis aids did, in fact, render poorer intelligibility in noise than aids with conventional response, for normals and subjects with mild-to-moderate cochlear losses.

In addition to auditory clues, linguistic rules are involved in the learning and the production of speech sounds. To improve articulation of the hearing-impaired individual, the teacher should choose units depending on the learner's problem — large units if possible, progressing to larger units as rapidly as possible. Winitz (1975) contends that training in articulatory production should begin at least at the syllable level. He points out that, in fact, only continuants can truly be produced "in isolation," and that there is no advantage in teaching even these sounds as isolated elements. He presents evidence that acquisition of sounds and transfer of their use to diverse phonetic contexts is facilitated by teaching the sound in an environment of one or two syllables. Problems peculiar to the speech of the deaf may be related to three associated elements: (1) Concentration of study on isolated phonemes, (2) not enough emphasis on the effects of coarticulation in connected speech, and (3) too little attention to suprasegmental variables which contribute both to intelligibility and natural-sounding speech.

Perhaps, also, matters of semantics should be considered in assisting a hearing-impaired person to speak intelligibly. That is, given a choice of words, some may be produced intelligibly with greater ease than others. If a hearing-impaired individual knows the rules that govern production and intelligibility, he may use them to improve his speech. Additionally, the use of relatively simple syntax may improve intelligibility of the hearing-impaired speaker.

CONCLUSION

Knowledge of the acoustics of speech is the basis for predicting intelligibility of speech for either the normal or hearing-impaired listener. This knowledge does not permit one to predict an intelligibility score associated with a given hearing impairment. It does provide information about the type and magnitude of error to be expected. It permits generalization about the kind of remediation that is feasible and implements prognostic statements. It is part of the knowledge needed for effective hearing aid recommendation and audiologic habilitation.

relationship of electro- and psychoacoustic measures

Paul H. Skinner, Ph.D.

INTRODUCTION

The preceding chapters, "Electroacoustic Characteristics of Hearing Aids," and "Speech Acoustics and Intelligibility," provide a foundation for a discussion of the relationship of electro- and psychoacoustic measures. Successful aural habilitation of hearing-impaired persons through the use of amplification depends largely on these relationships. These relationships, although the subject of considerable research, remain encumbered by serious unresolved problems and conflicting results.

Not the least of these problems is the fact that some laboratory measures of psychoacoustics, particularly speech intelligibility, may lack validity for predicting how one hears and understands in "real life" situations. A notable example is the relationship of laboratory speech discrimination scores for phonetically balanced word lists as predictors of how well one understands conversational speech outside the laboratory. The problem is most apparent when discrimination values deviate from normal.

The relationships are confounded further by poor reliability in laboratory measurements and conflicting results which relate electro- and psychoacoustic measures. A notable example in this case is the relationship between discrimination test results and different frequency response characteristics of hearing aids. Also, the question persists as to whether there is an interaction between certain hearing impairments and certain electro-acoustic characteristics of hearing aids as measured in the laboratory. A confounding factor is that electroacoustic data for hearing aids vary mark-edly between manufacturer specifications and specific hearing aids, and with volume level or gain adjustments (Lotterman, Kasten, and Revoile, 1967; Kasten and Lotterman, 1969). The variable response of one sample group of aids is shown in Figure 7-1. Also, measures typically are reported for the hearing aid suspended in a free field with the acoustic output of the receiver measured in a hard-walled, standard 2 cc coupler (artificial ear). Input at the microphone and output of the receiver change significantly when the hearing aid is placed on the body and sound pressure level (SPL) is measured at the eardrum. These problems will be considered later.

Many of the decisions audiologists have made regarding hearing aid selection and use are based upon clinical procedures and impressions. The purpose of this chapter, given the difficulty of the task, is to discuss the relationship of electro- and psychoacoustic measures on scientific grounds. The physical and electroacoustic characteristics of hearing aids were pre-sented and explained in Chapters Three and Five. I simply shall refer to those characteristics and attempt to relate them to what the hearing aid user can perceive.

GAIN AND COMFORT LEVEL, SATURATION SOUND PRESSURE LEVEL AND DISCOMFORT LEVEL

The gain of the hearing aid has been defined in Chapter Five as the difference in SPL between the input signal and the output signal. It was explained that gain of the hearing aid is regulated by a volume control which is a potentiometer or a variable resistor which adjusts the amount of amplification of the input signal in the hearing aid. Thus, it controls the output intensity of the amplified signal to the listener. The determination

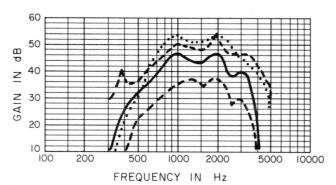

Fig. 7-1. Frequency response characteristics of 15 eye-glass aids of the same model. The *dotted line* represents the full-on gain curve indicated by the manufacturer. The *solid line* is the actual mean response established for the 15 instruments. The area within the lines composed of *dashes* represents the range of response of the 15 aids (data from Kasten, Lotterman, and Revoile, 1967).

of the amount of gain required for a hard-of-hearing person is explained in Chapter Eight. In the context of this chapter, we shall discuss gain as regulated by the volume control switch as it relates to psychoacoustic measures.

The primary criterion for the determination of the amount of gain required by the hearing-impaired individual is based upon a determination of a most comfortable loudness level (MCL) by the patient. The comfort level in a hypothetical sense is assumed to be a loudness level at which the input is amplified to a level approximating the center of the subject's dynamic range; that is a signal level that is "not too soft and not too loud." Dynamic range is defined as the range between the level at which the patient can just perceive the loudness of the signal to a level where the signal becomes uncomfortably loud. MCL is the usual criterion for setting the gain at which hearing aids are evaluated clinically. This is, the gain control is rotated until the patient reports MCL while listening to speech at about 65 dB SPL. Patients also, usually are advised to adjust their gain control for MCL under differing everyday listening situations.

Since MCL is the usual criterion to set gain control, attention needs to be given to the reliability of this determination. Ventry et al. (1971) reported on MCL for pure-tones, noise, and speech determined by normal hearing subjects. They found that MCL can be a relatively stable measure under well controlled test conditions. Similar studies were conducted with hearing-impaired subjects using hearing aids by Carhart (1946c) and Hochberg (1975). These studies indicated that MCL was sufficiently reliable as a loudness criterion in hearing aid gain setting. MCL generally is established at about 25–40 dB sensation level (Hochberg, 1975). In cases of recruitment, however, the MCL setting may be problematically close to a level of discomfort at which the subject cannot tolerate the increased loudness of the amplified signal or the hearing aid gain.

Methods of reporting gain vary among manufacturers. Some provide specifications with the gain control full on, others give measurements made with less than full-on gain. Input varies and may not be reported. Most give the Hearing Aid Industry Conference (HAIC) maximum gain, as discussed in Chapter Five. Regardless, the gain as derived with pure-tones, should not be expected to indicate exactly the gain for speech which the hearing aid wearer will achieve. Lotterman et al. (1967) reported that threshold improvement for speech is about 10 dB less than the gain measured electroacoustically with pure-tones. That is, a hearing aid with a gain of 40 dB, measured electroacoustically, may be expected to change a subject's unaided threshold for speech about 30 dB. The experimenters speculated that differences were related to such factors as body or head baffle effects, and differences in leakage between real and artificial ears.

It was determined by Kasten and Lotterman (1969) that rotation of a typical volume control dial does not provide a gradual and linear increase in the gain of the hearing aid. They reported also that different hearing aids had widely variant gain characteristics and that considerable gain was provided by some aids simply by turning them on. Typically, relatively little gain was available once the volume control was advanced beyond 50% of its total range. Stated otherwise, most of the hearing aid gain was delivered in the first half rotation of the volume control and only a limited amount was available in the second half of the rotation of the control. Taper characteristics of the gain control of several hearing aids are shown in Figure 7-2. Thus, in many cases, using the gain control beyond a 50% rotation setting produces little increase in gain but an increase in harmonic distortion which may negatively affect speech intelligibility. The relationship of speech intelligibility to associated electronic distortion in hearing aids will be discussed later.

Carhart (1946a) recommended that a hearing aid be selected for the patient which provides reserve gain for certain listening situations. Since the study by Kasten and Lotterman (1969) indicated that harmonic distortion often increased significantly when the gain control was rotated about 50% of its range, one should be careful to recommend a hearing aid with adequate gain.

As defined in Chapter Five, the saturation sound pressure level (SSPL) or maximum acoustic output of a hearing aid is the maximum sound pressure level the hearing aid is capable of generating regardless of the

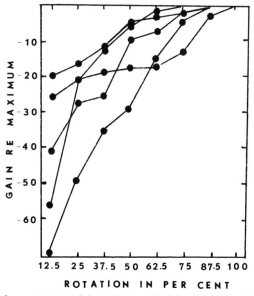

Fig. 7-2. Taper characteristics of the gain control of five hearing aids with more than 45 dB gain (data from Kasten and Lotterman, 1969).

amount of gain or intensity of the input signal. Two limiting factors must be considered. Amplification systems can produce an SSPL limited by the number of amplification stages in the amplifying system. Amplifiers reach a saturation level at which further increases in output will not be linear increases of the input signal. Thus, the output signal of the hearing aid becomes distorted. The problem of hearing aid distortion will be discussed later.

Two psychoacoustic factors must be related to the electroacoustic output limitation of hearing aids. The SSPL of a hearing aid may not exceed the tolerance level of the hearing-impaired person who uses the hearing aid. The intensity level at which an auditory stimulus becomes uncomfortable is referred to as the loudness discomfort level (LDL). A second consideration in SSPL is the risk of producing additional hearing loss as a result of overexposure of the auditory system to very intense stimuli. Thus, the SSPL must be considered in the context of loudness discomfort level and a possibility of increasing hearing loss through permanent threshold shift.

Two techniques have been used to limit SSPL in hearing aids. They are called peak clipping and automatic gain control, and are discussed in Chapter Three. Peak clipping has been the traditional mode of output limiting and this method is used in most hearing aids. This limiting characteristic is commonly used in simple amplifiers and occurs when the output stage of the amplifier is driven beyond its linear amplification level or point of saturation. The physical distortion of the input signal associated with peak clipping degrades the perceived quality of the signal. Nevertheless, a considerable amount of such distortion can occur before intelligibility is reduced. Eventually, as clipping is increased, the resultant distortion causes a decrease in intelligibility.

Compression amplification through automatic gain or volume control (AGC) achieves output limiting without peak clipping and has potential for better speech quality. There are variables, however, which must be considered in AGC that may affect speech intelligibility. Attack time was explained in Chapter Three as the time required for controlling action to take effect after a strong signal is presented at the microphone. Release time was defined as the time required for the amplification stages to return to full amplification after the strong signal is no longer present. Schematic examples of output limiting through peak clipping and AGC are shown in Figure 7-3.

Lynne and Carhart (1963) studied the effects of attack and release time on speech intellibibility and demonstrated that speech discrimination decreased as release time increased beyond a critical period. As mentioned in Chapter Six, vowels carry most intensity in speech signals. The relatively low intensity consonants, however, carry the cues for speech intelligibility. Since compression amplification typically occurs in response to the power

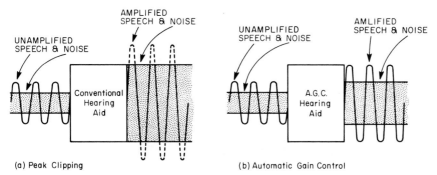

FIG. 7-3. (*a*), waveform disortion that occurs in peak clipping. (*b*), absence of waveform distortion in automatic gain control. Note that the background noise is reduced proportionately when AGC is invoked. This does not occur in peak clipping (after Davis and Silverman, 1960.)

produced by vocalic signals, low intensity consonants may be reproduced too faintly to maintain speech intelligibility if the release period is too long. Release time is typically longer than attack time in order to avoid the effect of acoustic fluttering or rapid modulation of intensity between syllables which constantly raise and lower gain. Liberman et al. (1967) reported that the average phoneme duration is 70–80 msec and vowel duration 200–300 msec. Johansson (1973) indicated that attack times greater than 20 msec will not assure full protection against discomfort. He recommended also that a release time about 150 msec is satisfactory.

Recently AGC has been developed which does not maintain a 1–1 relationship between input and output as the limiting level is approached. For example, some systems maintain a 3–1 ratio, such as a 15 decibel increase in input would produce a corresponding increase in output of only 5 dB. Thus, the more dramatic effects of attack and release time as a part of traditional compression amplification circuit are reduced. Other systems of AGC provide a constant and variable gain adjustment which develops progressively greater compression at higher input levels. Thus, some limiting occurs at all input levels and the specific effects of attack and release time are precluded. These three types of AGC are compared with conventional peak clipping output limiting in Figure 7-4.

All forms of compression amplification offer advantages over peak clipping: (1) compression reduces the amount of distortion of the signal; (2) output is limited at a level below the amplifier saturation through gain reduction over the entire signal. In addition, compression ampification permits an expanded dynamic range for the hearing aid user since it provides a wider range of input level to the ear yet still maintains maximum output levels which can be adjusted to the tolerance levels of the hearing impaired.

Clinically, AGC is used to provide a tolerable output limit without an

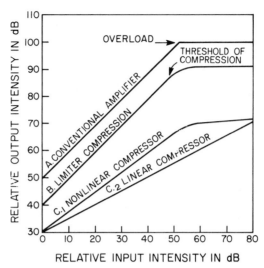

FIG. 7-4. Various types of automatic gain control compared with conventional output limiting. (A) output limiting by peak clipping, (B) peak limiter, (C₁) nonlinear compression, and (C₂) linear compression.

unacceptable amount of distortion resulting for the patient with a narrow dynamic range. For the patient with a wider dynamic range, whose amplification requirements cannot be expected frequently to drive the aid to its SSPL, peak clipping is satisfactory for output limiting.

Several investigators have studied the relationship between intensity level and loudness discomfort level (LDL) for auditory stimuli. Davis et al. (1946) concluded that LDL for normal hearing subjects was about 110 dB SPL for pure-tones and about 117 dB SPL for speech. For hearing-impaired subjects they found higher LDLs. However, Schmitz (1969) reported LDLs for speech to be about 90 dB SPL for hearing-impaired subjects in contrast to 120 dB SPL for normals. Variability in established LDLs probably relates to difference in instructions and measurement procedures, the phenomenon of recruitment, and the variable presence of conductive components. At any rate, in clinical evaluation, individual tolerance limits must be established. This procedure is discussed in Chapter Eight.

As indicated earlier, SSPL should be controlled to minimize a potential risk of producing additional hearing loss as a result of overexposure to intense stimuli. The available evidence suggests the probability that this occurrence is low. However, it is clearly established that threshold shifts associated with hearing aid use do occur. The problem and efforts at solution are discussed in Chapter Twelve.

ELECTROACOUSTIC DISTORTION: SPEECH QUALITY AND PERCEPTION

Different forms of distortion as described in Chapter Five may occur in the electronic amplification of sound. As indicated, distortion occurs when the acoustic output is said to be distorted. Several kinds of distortion may occur in the amplification of sound through wearable hearing aids; however, harmonic distortion has been most closely identified with reduction of clarity and intelligibility of amplified signals. Several studies (Harris et al., 1961; Jerger, Speaks, and Malmquist, 1966; Olsen and Carhart, 1967; Olsen and Wilbur, 1968) revealed that speech intelligibility is inversely proportional to the level of harmonic distortion produced by hearing aids. It is likely that with increased harmonic distortion other forms of distortion were increased which may have affected speech quality and intelligibility.

Harris et al. (1961) indicated that harmonic distortion does not degrade speech appreciably until it exceeds about 20%. The report stated further that while intermodulation distortion also affects speech intelligibility, intermodulation and harmonic distortion (HD) correlate highly and thus effects are confounded.

Jirsa and Hodgson (1970) studied the effects of HD in three groups of subjects: normals, conductive hearing loss, and sensorineural hearing loss, using four speech intelligibility tests with different levels of HD. Their results were consistent with the findings of Harris et al. (1961), and indicated also, in contrast with Jerger (1966), that these measures did not differentiate among hearing aids at levels of HD below about 20%.

Flottorp (1971) proposed a method to study intermodulation (IM) distortion and reported that IM distortion at 500, 750, and 1000 Hz influenced the performance of normal listeners in the perception of phonetically balanced lists. He concluded that excessive IM reduces intelligibility.

Lotterman and Kasten (1967b) reported that body hearing aids with external receivers produced greater distortion generally than ear level aids with internal receivers. Maximum distortion was usually below 1000 Hz for body aids and above 1000 Hz for ear level aids.

Harmonic and other forms of distortion tend to be greatest at maximum gain setting. Therefore, one should exercise care in hearing aid selection to provide hearing aids which may be used below a maximum gain setting, with reserve gain for occasional use.

FREQUENCY RESPONSE AND SPEECH PERCEPTION

Considerable attention has been given to the relationship between frequency response characteristics and psychoacoustic measures with hearing aids. Frequency response has been considered in relationship to the configuration of hearing loss (supplementary response) and without regard to configuration of hearing loss (flat response). In fact, it can be stated that perhaps the significance of frequency response has been overemphasized in view of evidence that flat responses are generally satisfactory.

It should be kept in mind that frequency response characteristics have been related to studies of speech discrimination and speech intelligibility in normals and subjects with various types of hearing loss. Often the comparisons ignore the fact that frequency response is determined in a hard-walled 2 cc coupler and that frequency response might be significantly affected by real ear and body baffle or head diffraction effects.

Since conflicting evidence exists regarding effects of frequency response in hearing aid performance, it is necessary to clarify what frequency response modifications are significant. Existing evidence demonstrates that modification of the frequency response range tends to be of significance but that selective frequency response for specific hearing losses tends to be of dubious significance.

Stated otherwise, the shaping of frequency response to accommodate general classifications of hearing loss or the "mirror imaging" of hearing loss configurations appears dubious. The often quoted study by Davis et al. (1946) provided the first extensive study in this area. They reported that subjects with conductive and sensorineural hearing losses performed best by speech intelligibility measures with an essentially flat frequency response characteristic. Whereas this report perhaps has been ignored by some and overgeneralized by others (the study did not include subjects with precipitous or unusual hearing loss), it does provide a basic reference for hearing aid selection.

Several studies have reported improved speech discrimination for subjects with precipitous high frequency loss through high frequency response emphasis (Reddell and Calvert, 1966) or selective frequency response for different hearing losses (Pascoe, 1975). Although such results were established to have statistical significance, one may question whether any practical significance may be obtained from them.

An interesting report by Jerger and Thelin (1968) indicated that smoothness of frequency response is related to sentence intelligibility. They reported that the best aids for synthetic sentence identification were those with the smoothest frequency response by visual inspection. The poorest performance occurred with jagged and irregular curves.

Limiting or extending frequency response range also has received considerable attention. Extended high frequency hearing aids exist which exceed the "critical range" for speech above the area of 3000 Hz. The study by Jerger and Thelin (1968) reported a negative correlation between synthetic sentence identification (SSI) and band width above 1000 Hz. Conversely, correlations for SSI and band width below 1000 Hz were positive. Perhaps this is understandable since Speaks, Karmen, and Benitez (1967) reported the frequency region important for SSI performance to be well below 1000 Hz. That is, they reported that the high-pass and low-pass filtering functions resulting in equal intelligibility for SSI materials intersect at about 750 Hz. French and Steinberg (1947), however, reported that the analogous intersect for equal monosyllabic word discrimination was 1900 Hz.

Extended low frequency response aids have proved beneficial when used as originally intended. The contribution of aids which have an extended low frequency operating range below that of conventional amplifiers is discussed in Chapters Six and Nine. Also, the dangers are stressed of misapplication of such aids to hearing losses for which they are not appropriate.

MONAURAL AND BINAURAL HEARING AND MONAURAL VERSUS BINAURAL HEARING AID USE

This topic well may be the most intriguing and complex among our concerns in the relationship between electro- and psychoacoustic measures. One understandably may feel overwhelmed with the analysis of material which is pertinent to this problem. Whether the topic can be covered adequately in the context of a chapter of this type is indeed a serious question.

The obvious protrusion of two ears, one from either side of the human head, has lead to the implicit assumption that two ears are better than one. Given this assumption, numerous investigators have sought to demonstrate the specific advantages in hearing by two ears. The validation of such assumptions, of course, requires a comparison of monaural to binaural listening and it is in such a comparison that many assumed advantages of binaural hearing become very elusive. In fact, the problem is sufficiently difficult that one is given cause to reconsider the obvious superiority provided by two ears.

The mobile auricles found in lower animal forms offer significant advantage in efficient and accurate localization of sound, an advantage lost in humans. Also, it is plausible to assume that two ears were provided for protective duplication. In considering the ontogeny of the auditory mechanism, however, it is less compelling to assume that the binaural system was planned to enhance speech perception in noise or to provide auditory perspective for listening to symphonic music. In our fascination with binaural advantages, perhaps we have deluded our students, and ourselves as well, that severe limitations are imposed by a condition of monaural hearing.

Information is provided differently at each of the two ears (interaural differences) of a listener which permits perceptions that are not available otherwise:

1. time or phase differences;
2. intensity differences; and
3. spectral differences. These may result from diffraction and shadow by

the head, reflective properties in the environment, and different angles of incidence of wave fronts (Sayers and Cherry, 1957).

Such differences presumably are used to make judgments which otherwise could not be possible.

Numerous advantages have been postulated: (1) one presumably is able to localize the sources of sound more efficiently and accurately; (2) one presumably benefits from improved speech intelligibility and discrimination, specifically in the presence of noise or competing signals; (3) presumably absolute threshold is lowered by 3 dB (Hirsh, 1950); (4) one may gain an advantage of improved differential thresholds for frequency and intensity; (5) greater tolerance to loud sounds occurs; (6) a squelch effect provides suppression of background sounds (Koenig, 1950); (7) suprathreshold loudness increases; (8) binaural fusion is possible (Cherry, 1959); and (9) better auditory perspective or spatial balance and improved quality of listening are gained. We must examine these relative advantages and consider them in the context of binaural hearing aid use.

Having stated often cited binaural advantages, let us return to the question of their validity which may be tested in a comparison of monaural to binaural listening. First, what can be accomplished in listening with one ear only? The classical study by Angel and Fite (1901) compared the listening abilities between a young adult with a profound unilateral loss to judgments made by a normal binaural listener. They stated several findings which have been reaffirmed often in more recent research publications which will be cited. Angel and Fite reported that the monaural listener was competent in the localization of complex sounds in the horizontal plane. In fact, they indicated that binaural superiority for horizontal plane localization occurred only for pure-tones. Also, they indicated no binaural superiority for localization of sounds in the median plane. Recent research reports support these early findings.

Jongkees and van der Veer (1958) also studied localization in subjects with total unilateral deafness who demonstrated "normal" to good directional hearing. Clearly, interaural differences of time, and intensity were not possible explanations. They indicated that directional hearing was possible in these cases through vestibular reflexes, small movements of the head and neck, and the influence of the auricle. Fisher and Freedman (1968) provided supportive evidence that binaural cues are not necessary for accurate localization of sounds in the horizontal plane, given free head movement. This report, however, was challenged by Belendiuk and Butler (1975), who indicated that monaural localization of complex sounds in the horizontal plane was not possible unless the complex sound carried high frequency information at approximately 5 kHz. In concurrence with Angel and Fite, studies by Plenge (1974) and Hebrank and Wright (1974) indicated that monaural localization in the median plane was as efficient as binaural localization in that condition.

It should be noted that interaural time differences and mean amplitude differences cannot, account for precise localization of a sound image outside the head. These clues alone can give only right or left localization within a sound rotational cone (Wallach, 1939, 1940; Mills, 1972), (see Figure 7-5). In addition, time-intensity differences that occur between the two ears are translated into time information only in the auditory nervous system because of the time-intensity trading which occurs. Stated otherwise, signals of greater intensity are revealed in neural translation by decreases in transmission time.

We must recognize then that increased precision in localization of a sound source is possible only by movement of the head for further calculation of the location of the sound source on either side of the head or in the median plane. In summary, localization of complex sounds (speech) in the external environment can be accomplished monaurally in the median and horizontal planes. Such localization is related essentially to head movement rather than binaural hearing. However, localization of complex sounds may be enhanced through the use of two ears, given free head movement.

The ability to localize sound also depends on "short term" and "long term" memory. The studies by Angel and Fite (1901) and Hebrank and Wright (1974) indicated that subjects can be trained to localize reliably both in binaural and monaural listening modes. Thus, "short term" memory plays a role in the localization of sounds in new or changing acoustic environments. "Long term" memory is involved in the localization of sounds in typical or familiar acoustic environments. We should not assume that all monaural or binaural hearing subjects localize with equal ability.

Other binaural advantages, in addition to localization, commonly are asserted. Of particular interest is the assertion that binaural hearing is advantageous for understanding speech in noise or among competing messages; however, such advantages have not always been readily demon-

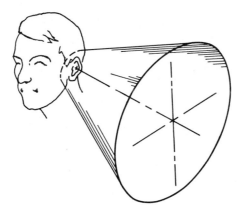

FIG. 7-5. A cone of confusion for a spherical head. The surface of the cone is the locus for sources which produce the same interaural time difference (after Mills, 1972).

strated in the laboratory (Jerger, Carhart, and Dirks, 1961) as well as in real life situations.

In quiet listening, persons who suffer unilateral hearing loss rarely experience disadvantage in understanding speech. Also, one must acknowledge that a corollary of numerous comparisons of monaural and binaural speech perception in noise or competing messages is that a monaural listener also can understand speech in difficult listening situations. These observations, however, do not exclude the possibility of binaural advantages in such situations. For example, fusion and masking level differences, or release from masking, presumably permit the so-called "squelch" and "cocktail party" effects, which of course pertain to binaural advantages in listening to speech in noise.

Fusion, of course, implies a bilateral system and in addition is given credit for the selective attention to a wanted signal and concomitant suppression of unwanted signals. Since interaural differences occur in real life situations, the mechanism and acoustic characteristics of fusion are of interest (Sayers and Cherry, 1957; Cherry and Sayers, 1956; David, Guttman, and Van Bergeijk, 1958). Nevertheless, empirical evidence (observations of monaural listeners in real life situations) reveals that one can selectively attend to or ignore (inhibit) different or competing signals in monaural listening. Moreover, fusion must be considered as a special case in the use of amplification since the effects of unilateral or asymmetric binaural hearing loss and subsequent hearing aid fittings are not known.

Release from masking has been demonstrated to enhance effective signal-to-noise ratios given certain phase relations between signal and noise at the two ears (Hirsh, 1948; Licklider, 1948). Masking level differences (MLD) are reported to be largest when antiphasic conditions exist at the two ears for noise and speech. MLDs for speech intelligibility thresholds for spondaic words have been reported to be about 7 dB for spondees and 4 dB for monosyllables as compared to homophasic conditions (Carhart, Tillman, and Johnson, 1967). It must be noted, however, that these effects are maximized under earphone listening in which phase relationships are manipulated artificially. Whereas release from masking may occur in real life listening situations, Schubert (1956) reported that such situations do not provide conditions that produce large MLDs.

Also it has been reported that binaural listening is superior to monaural in speech discrimination under reverberant conditions. This superiority often has been attributed to the so-called "squelch effect" proposed in an anecdotal account by Koenig (1950) in the absence of any experimental data. Regardless, the concept has received wide acceptance.

Nevertheless, evidence has been presented by several investigators that at least under certain conditions binaural speech discrimination is enhanced at prolonged reverberation times. Moncur and Dirks (1967) demonstrated this phenomenon in normal listeners with monaural occlusion, and Nabelek and Pickett (1974b) in hearing-impaired subjects in monaural and binaural perception through hearing aids.

It has been demonstrated that the effects of sound diffraction and head shadow yield lower speech intelligibility levels for the monaural listener under certain conditions. The head casts a shadow only when the wavelength of the sound is small compared to the dimensions of the head; thus variations in the direction of the source produce greatest intensity differences between the two ears at frequencies above about 2000 Hz. Since the specific relation between the difference in level at the two ears and the azimuth of the source depends on frequency, it is not easy to quantify the intensity differences. Moreover, such intensity differences are changed significantly through head movement by the subject in normal listening. Whereas it can be demonstrated clearly that a loss of intensity for high frequency information occurs as a result of head shadow contingent upon azimuth of the source, it is difficult to assess the effect of head shadow on speech intelligibility or speech discrimination in real life conditions.

Several studies have demonstrated a head shadow effect for speech on the order of 6 dB (Tillman, Kasten, and Horner, 1963; Kasten, Lotterman, and Hinchman, 1967/68). That is, when real or simulated unilaterals listened to spondee words originating from the side of their good versus poor ear, there was a difference of 6 dB in speech threshold. Other studies have shown a significant reduction in speech discrimination scores when subjects listened to speech of low intensity in a "monaural indirect" versus a "monaural direct" situation; that is, when subjects listened under the effect of an acoustic head shadow (Nordlund and Fritzell, 1963; Kasten and Tillman, 1964). Still others have found little difference between "monaural direct" and binaural discrimination scores under conditions wherein "monaural indirect" scores were reduced (Carhart, Pollack, and Lotterman, 1963; Kasten and Tillman, 1964; Olsen and Carhart, 1967). These latter studies suggest that the greatest advantage of binaural over monaural listening is the fact that the binaural condition almost always permits the listener to have one ear favorably situated towards the signal of interest.

Most determinations of the head shadow effect did not permit the subject to move the head. Also, most measures were obtained in a free field. In real life conditions, the listener, of course, relies on head movement to reduce the effect of head shadow. Also, reflected sound may be received by the better ear of the listener. Nevertheless, a common complaint by unilaterals is that when speech originates from the side of the poor ear and is faint, distant, or in the presence of noise, communication problems occur. These complaints substantiate that the deleterious effect of the head shadow is real in many everyday listening situations. Further, it is reasonable to assume that reduction of these problems through use of two hearing aids is the most obvious advantage of binaural amplification. Even so, many people have a successful communication experience in life with hearing in only one ear. Presumably then, special circumstances warrant the use of binaural aids to overcome head shadow effects.

It was stated initially that an analysis of the material on monaural versus binaural hearing is somewhat overwhelming at least in this context. Relatively limited information is available, however, which is directly pertinent to real life situations and a comparison of monaural versus binaural hearing aid use.

Binaural effects or superiority have been demonstrated in studies of precedence or Haas effect (Gardner, 1968), binaural fusion (Cherry and Sayers, 1956), release from masking (Hirsh, 1948); however, these phenomena are most compelling only when stimuli are controlled artificially under earphones.

Many other studies have been conducted to demonstrate binaural advantages (Hirsh, 1950; Nordlund and Fritzell, 1963; Harris, 1965; Olsen and Carhart, 1967; Dirks and Wilson, 1969; Carhart and Tillman, 1972). Most of the information on binaural advantages, however, was developed through research conducted in a free field or anechoic chamber with signal azimuths fixed to maximize a binaural advantage and with the artificial or subject's head fixed to preclude normal movement.

Numerous serious problems arise when extrapolation is made from carefully controlled studies to real life situations regarding binaural hearing. These are complicated further by the effects of hearing loss and amplification.

Considerable confusion remains regarding how one localizes a source in a realistic environment with acoustic reflections, transient signals, head movement, the use of prior knowledge, and the integration of information sampled at different moments in time (Green and Henning, 1969). In the case of the cocktail party effect where one selectively attends to a chosen signal from a number of simultaneous conversations (Kaiser and David, 1960), the listener is not concerned primarily with the localization of the source of sound but rather with how one conversation can be distinguished from another background or competing conversation, which incidentally is not precluded in monarual listening. One must distinguish clearly in an analysis of binaural hearing between sound localization and listening in free fields versus non-free fields or sound fields. Confusion of these two conditions has led to considerable misunderstanding about how sounds are localized in real life or the sound fields which occur in our environment. In such cases and including conditions of sound diffraction and head shadow, the problem of localization is greatly complicated. Intensity differences at the two ears become particularly unreliable since these differences are determined as much by the geometry of the surrounding space as by the localization of the sound source. In a realistic sound field with nodes and antinodes and multiple reflections, reliable judgments of localization often can not be made (Green and Henning, 1969). A most important aspect of localization in real space then is head movement, as Wallach (1939, 1940) has demonstrated in numerous experiments.

Many studies have reported statistically significant differences for speech discrimination or intelligibility in the presence of noise or competing signals which indicate advantages of binaural hearing and binaural hearing aids. One must consider that statistically significant evidence of such differences may reveal no behavioral differences or prediction of social efficiency for communication skills in real life situations.

From this complex and frustrating background, audiologists must deal with decisions whether to recommend monaural or binaural hearing aids for patients. Such recommendations should be based then on objective as well as subjective evidence, and advantages should be weighed in consultation with the patient. It must be stated that very limited conclusive or compelling objective scientific evidence is available to support a recommendation of binaural hearing aids.

Unfortunately, it would appear that decisions regarding monaural or binaural hearing at present rest largely on subjective judgment of clinicians and patients. The subjective response of patients using binaural hearing aids has been reported by Dirks and Carhart (1962), collected from a questionnaire. The authors indicated, however, that such data for numerous reasons must be interpreted with caution. Others have stated that better "acoustic balance" or auditory perspective results as a benefit of binaural hearing aids (Carhart, 1958; Langford, 1970). Wright (1959), however, contested such impressions of better balance in binaural hearing aids. Wright indicated that differences in threshold and suprathreshold loudness balances between ears, particularly in the presence of sensorineural hearing loss, and perhaps significant differences in frequency response and qualitative hearing in the two ears, may preclude "balanced" hearing for many subjects through the use of binaural hearing aids.

Reports of improved sound quality also have been made (Langford, 1970). Judgments in the determination of sound quality are difficult for the clinician to utilize as clinical information. Obviously, such a judgment can be made only by the hearing aid user, and such judgments may differ widely in reliability.

Pseudo-binaural hearing aid fittings or Y-cords might be considered also in this context. Since a Y-cord fitting simply involves the use of a receiver in each ear fed by a common amplifier, such use is limited essentially to bilateral symmetrical hearing loss. Clearly, interaural inhibition or poorest perception in noise (masking level differences) will occur in homophasic signals presented in the two ears. This condition of course results through the use of a pseudo-binaural fitting. Presumably such a fitting would be used only for special reasons which are discussed in Chapter Nine. If a Y-cord is used, care should be taken to insure that the receivers and hearing aid obtained do not result in an impedance mismatch and consequent signal deterioration (Lybarger, 1973).

BODY BAFFLE AND SPEECH PERCEPTION

As mentioned earlier, the frequency response of a hearing aid routinely is determined when the instrument is suspended in a free field and the receiver is placed in a standard 2 cc coupler. It is well known, however, that the frequency response of a hearing aid may be modified considerably when it is placed for use on the human head or torso; that is when the body acts as a baffle, and the receiver is coupled by an earmold to the canal of the ear.

It is recognized then that electroacoustic measurements of a hearing aid in the laboratory will differ from those obtained when the hearing aid is worn by a human. Changes that may occur in psychoacoustic measures as a result have received less attention. It would be expected, of course, that resultant changes would differ significantly when the hearing aid is placed on the torso from when it is placed on the head. Thus each condition must be considered separately.

Several variables may effect the response of a hearing aid worn on the body: sound diffraction, absorption, and reflection (Nichols et al., 1947), position of the microphone and whether it is covered by clothing (Hanson, 1944; Carlisle and Mundel, 1944; Nichols et al., 1947), and the angle of sound incidence (Byrne, 1972). Erber (1973) indicated also that body baffle effects may differ between adults and children. While one should be aware of such effects, presumably their significance for psychoacoustic measures, if demonstrable, can be obtained in trial testing of hearing aids on the patient. Erber (1973) has recommended special procedures to compensate for differences between laboratory and practical measurements in the selection of hearing aids for deaf children.

Placement of a hearing aid on the head (ear level aids) introduces most of the same variables which affect the frequency response of a hearing aid placed on the body. As noted however, the effects of head diffraction and shadow differ significantly from the torso. The data of Sivian and White (1933) and Wiener (1947) revealed differences in monaural pure-tone thresholds for listeners when the sound source was placed at different azimuths. These data are shown in Figure 10-1.

This information gained importance in understanding the effects of ear level hearing aids. Wansdronk (1959) compared the frequency response curves for different ear level aids with different microphone placements when worn by human subjects. He noted that large differences occurred. Lybarger and Barron (1965) and Temby (1965) studied optimal microphone placement in ear level aids to take advantage of head diffraction effects. Both studies indicated that the best microphone placement appeared to be just in front and above the ear since baffle effects were largest and head shadow effects smallest at this microphone location. Conflicting results were reported by Kasten and Lotterman (1967). Olsen and Carhart (1975) studied the problem further and measured head baffle and shadow effects with front- and back-oriented microphones when worn by a human subject and when placed on a dummy head. They reported that their data for the front and back microphone positions were in general in agreement with Lybarger and Barron (1965) and Temby (1965). Olsen and Carhart (1975) indicated further that front microphone placement enhanced the response at higher frequencies from about 1 to 3 kHz by reduction of the head shadow.

Olsen and Wilbur (1967) indicated that a group of persons with sensori-neural hearing loss obtained their best discrimination scores with a hearing aid with a sharp resonance peak at 3 kHz. A reduction in head shadow effects apparently is gained by a front microphone location which presumably would be enhanced further by head movement in localization, but quantitative psychoacoustic information is not available.

DIRECTIONAL MICROPHONES AND SPEECH PERCEPTION

Traditionally, hearing aids have been manufactured with an omnidirectional microphone as a standard component because the microphone receives background sound equally from different directions; however, speech signals, when mixed with background noise, often may be difficult to understand. Since 1970, directional microphones have been used in some hearing aids. A hearing aid with a directional microphone introduces an acoustic delay element in a rear inlet opening. With this delay element, sounds entering from the rear are suppressed, causing reduction in amplification. For most of the directional aids, signals (frequency dependent) coming from the 45° azimuth receive the most amplification whereas sounds coming from the rear are reduced. Directional capability has been reported to improve substantially speech discrimination in the presence of background noise. There is evidence to indicate that speech discrimination scores were influenced by the location and levels of the interfering noise. For example, it was found that the directional microphone was effective only when the background noise is as loud or louder than the speech signal with the noise source at 180° azimuth. Furthermore, differences in discrimination ability in noise between the directional and non-directional hearing aid were not found in a highly reverberant room (Lentz, 1972b).

Lentz (1972a) determined speech reception thresholds and speech discrimination scores using two hearing aids. One type of aid utilized the microphone which had directional sensitivity; the other instrument employed a conventional, non-directional microphone. Discrimination was determined in quiet and in two signal-to-noise ratios, using W-22 monosyllabic word lists. The subject's head was restrained to preclude head movement and signals were presented from speakers located at the 0° azimuth. Results for speech reception thresholds indicated no change in threshold from either the 0 or 180° azimuth with the conventional microphone. The use of a directional microphone, however, provided greater sensitivity for sound arriving from 0° azimuth than from 180° azimuth, whereas the conventional aid was equally sensitive to information arriving from either of these directions. Speech discrimination scores in quiet yielded no significant difference between the directional and non-directional microphones.

However, the average speech discrimination score obtained at different signal-to-noise ratios yielded certain advantages for directional microphones. Results indicated that a directional microphone is superior to a non-directional microphone since it effectively attenuates background sounds (when the source is at 180°) and also improves speech discrimination in a noise background. In addition, subjects used in the investigation indicated that it was far easier to hear and understand words in the presence of background noise using the directional microphone as opposed to the non-directional microphone.

Frank and Gooden (1973) studied speech discrimination measures with different hearing aid microphone types as a function of multitalker noise location. The study was conducted with the use of three loudspeakers which permitted measurements from signals presented at 45 and 180° azimuths. The 45° azimuth was chosen because pilot data indicated the directional microphone hearing aid frequency response at this azimuth to be more linear through the speech range compared to 0° azimuth. "Multitalker" noise consisted of student talkers and was presented at various speech-to-noise ratios either directly in front of the subject or directly behind the subject or from both speakers at 0 and 180° azimuths. When the noise source originated from 0° azimuth, the discrimination scores obtained with the directional hearing aid microphone were not significantly different from scores obtained with non-directional hearing aid microphones. In other words, when the noise was located at 0° azimuth, the directional aid did not reduce the interfering noise. In a second condition, when the noise was presented from the speaker at 180° speech discrimination scores obtained with the directional microphone were approximately 15% better than the discrimination scores obtained with the non-directional microphone at various signal-to-noise ratios. This finding agreed with the previous report by Lentz (1972b). These findings indicate that the directional microphone reduced the background noise when it was located at 180°, thus allowing improved discrimination in a noisy situation.

Sung, Sung, and Angelelli conducted a study of directional microphones in hearing aids (1975). The study was designed to investigate the amount of directionality among three directional microphones of different brands and to compare speech discrimination ability of hearing-impaired persons using directional and non-directional hearing aids in a competing background noise. For each hearing aid, frequency response curves were obtained at 45, 135, 225, and 315° azimuths in an anechoic chamber. Thirty-two hearing aid users served as subjects and discrimination ability was assessed using W-22 word recordings.

The investigators indicated that three directional microphones provided the best averaged discrimination scores in noise as compared to non-directional microphones. Differences were found to be significant, however, in a comparison of the three directional microphones used. It was indicated that the amount of directionality differed significantly among directional hearing aids now available on the market. It was reported further that the best speech discrimination scores were obtained in difficult listening situations with the directional microphones which possess the best qualities in directionality.

TELECOILS AND SPEECH PERCEPTION

The use of an induction coil or telecoil was described in Chapters Three and Five as distinct from a standard microphone pickup. Many hearing aids contain a telecoil so the listener can amplify telephone messages through his hearing aid. As indicated by Hodgson and Sung (1972), relatively little research has been done on the intelligibility of speech produced through hearing aids operating on magnetic signal input. Since school children use the telecoil in conjunction with induction loop amplification systems used with conventional hearing aids, the question of speech intelligibility through such circuits is important.

Vargo et al. (1970) found that speech signals were significantly less intelligible when the hearing aid was operated on the telecoil rather than on the microphone setting. Sung and Hodgson (1971) found that the hearing aid with the better high frequency response produced better intelligibility for monosyllabic words regardless of the mode of signal input. In other words, speech intelligibility transduced by either microphone or telecoil input was dependent upon physical characteristics of the hearing aid. They reported specifically that the configuration of the frequency response in the region of 1.5 to 3 kHz appeared to be associated with the intelligibility of monosyllabic words. Connected discourse is less affected by poor frequency response than are discrete words as indicated by Giolas and Epstein (1963). Thus, Hodgson and Sung (1972) assumed that the relatively better lower frequency responses of telecoil systems would contribute more to the intelligibility of sentences than monosyllabic words. The purpose of their study was to extend investigation of the intelligibility of speech through two hearing aids operating on either microphone or telecoil inputs. Frequency response appeared to determine the performance difference in the hearing aids even with microphone or telecoil input. The better low frequency response below 1 kHz of the telecoil appeared to increase sentence intelligibility over microphone input. Since no other significant difference in physical characteristics was noted other than frequency response, Sung and Hodgson assumed that frequency response through telecoil with low frequency emphasis resulted in superior speech intelligibility for connected discourse but that the poor high frequency response of the hearing aids with telecoil provided poor monosyllabic word intelligibility.

Most importantly, Matkin and Olsen (1970a) found that classroom induction loop amplification systems were often defective in operation. That is, incorrect control setting, defective amplifiers, or impedance mismatches caused faulty signals. Under these conditions a poor signal resulted, regardless of the operating characteristics of the hearing aid. More information on induction loop amplification is given in Chapter Thirteen.

CONCLUSION

The relationship between electro- and psychoacoustic measures is fundamental to the utilization of amplification in aural habilitation. Considerable scientific information has been developed beyond the basic concepts of critical frequency range for speech intelligibility and intensity thresholds for dynamic range. Even so, it is apparent that we lack sufficient scientific basis for many aspects of hearing aid recommendations that must be made. Many questions remain. It often has been stated that our scientific and clinical measures lack the refinement or sensitivity necessary to provide definitive answers to these questions. We should consider, however, that the redundancy in spoken language and the capacity of the human brain to perceive and synthesize perhaps may render insignificant many of the issues that have obsessed us.

Nevertheless, the inadequacy of scientific knowledge makes it more important that we understand the many aspects of electro- and psychoacoustic measures so we may exercise enlightened judgment in recommendations for amplification in audiologic habilitation.

clinical measures of hearing aid performance

William R. Hodgson, Ph.D.

INTRODUCTION

In this section we will discuss the clinical evaluation of hearing aids and individuals being considered for hearing aids. The purposes of the evaluation-selection procedure are (1) to assess the need for amplification, (2) to estimate how well the patient can benefit from amplification, and (3) to determine the characteristics needed for effective amplification. The selection procedure may vary, depending on the philosophy of the evaluating audiologist. Whatever the procedure, these questions should be considered:

1. Is there a medical problem which would either contraindicate hearing aid use or, if corrected, remove the need for a hearing aid? This concern necessitates a medical otologic examination prior to recommendation for hearing aid use.

2. Is the loss of hearing sensitivity amenable to hearing aid use? Or is it too little, or too great?

3. Is discrimination ability adequate for hearing aid use?

4. What are the patient's (or the parents') expectations from an aid? Are they realistic? Must they be revised?

5. What are the demands on the patient's hearing?

6. Are there tolerance problems for intense sound? These may arise from areas of normal hearing within an aid's amplifying range, or from loudness recruitment.

7. What type of aid is needed; body worn or at the ear? Monaural or

binaural, and if monaural, which ear? What should be the maximum gain, the maximum output, and the frequency characteristics? What kind of earmold should be used?

8. What kind of training program will be needed? This training includes orientation to hearing aid use and remediation of prior effects of the hearing loss.

9. Should the aid be used part or full time? If part time, what are the conditions in which it should be used?

10. Does the patient want a hearing aid?

If these questions are answered correctly, enough information should result to ascertain how much the patient needs and can benefit from amplification, and the type of hearing aid he should have.

FACTORS THAT DETERMINE NEED FOR AMPLIFICATION

There are some non-auditory determinants of need. That is, there are factors in addition to the hearing loss which must be considered. One of these relates to how critical are the demands on the patient's hearing. The person who must hear accurately to retain his job has a greater need than the individual with less critical demands on his hearing. The same may be true for the person who is involved in many social activities compared to the person who prefers more solitude.

Need for amplification is also influenced by the acoustic environment in which the patient must listen. Need is greater for people who work in quiet places where people talk softly. Those who must listen at conference tables to speakers on either side and at a distance have a relatively greater need for amplification. In contrast, the industrial worker in a high noise level area should not wear a hearing aid on the job.

Motivation is another non-auditory factor of great importance. Some people seek an evaluation not because they want a hearing aid or are convinced of their need for it, but because of pressure from relatives or other influential persons. Unless such people can be motivated, they may not buy an aid if recommended or use it if they should purchase one.

From an auditory viewpoint the basic determinant of need for amplification is auditory sensitivity. The greater the loss of sensitivity the greater the need for a hearing aid. Table 8-1 shows a general guide to the relationship between hearing loss and need for amplification, based on sensitivity in the better ear. Sensitivity in this case is determined by the appropriate pure-tone average, or by the speech reception threshold. In addition to the non-auditory influences mentioned above, other exceptions must be considered.

First, the guide does not apply to people with normal sensitivity across part of the speech range and a sharply falling high frequency loss. These individuals may have substantially normal overall sensitivity but need

TABLE 8-1. **General guide to relationship between hearing loss and need for amplification, based on PTA* or SRT† in better ear. See text for important qualifications**

Hearing Loss in dB re: 1969 ANSI‡ Norms	Need for Amplification
0–25	No need
25–40	Part time need for special occasions
40–55	Frequent need
55–80	Area of greatest satisfaction
80+	Great need — partial help

* PTA, pure tone average.

† SRT, speech reception threshold.

‡ ANSI, American National Standards Institute.

high frequency amplification to improve audibility for high frequency consonants. For this group the criterion of need is whether or not the person can understand unamplified speech spoken at the levels at which he must often listen.

The guide also excepts unilaterals with normal or near normal hearing on their better ear. Depending on their motivation and demands on their hearing, they may choose amplification. Problems of the head shadow and their resolution with CROS-type hearing aids are discussed in the chapter on hearing aids for special purposes.

With the above limitations in mind, and others that will be mentioned occasionally, the relationship between loss of sensitivity and need for an aid can be considered. Most people with hearing in the better ear between 0 and 25 dB, re: 1969 American National Standards Institute (ANSI) norms, do not report enough difficulty to justify amplification. Obviously a person at the bottom of this range will have more trouble in more situations than someone at the top. Nevertheless, under most conditions the average person in this category gets along well and feels no need for a hearing aid. Exceptions may consist of people with heavy demands on their hearing who are highly motivated toward optimum performance (Ross, Barrett, and Trier, 1966).

People with sensitivity in the better ear between 26 and 40 dB may be part time hearing aid users who need amplification in particular listening situations. Under good listening conditions, characterized by a strong acoustic signal in quiet, they probably will not need an aid. In noisy listening situations, they may do as well without the aid as with it. However when they listen to faint or distant speech signals, they benefit from amplification. Such people wear their aids at a lecture, take them off during the noisy drive home, and may or may not use them during a conversation in the parlor, depending on the vocal intensity of the speakers.

Those with sensitivity in the better ear between 41 and 55 dB are likely to wear aids most of the time. In very difficult or noisy conditions, as when trying to listen in a room full of talking people, they may not wear an aid. In this situation, they will probably communicate poorly with or without an aid, and may remove it to eliminate amplified noise.

The range between 55 and 80 dB has been called the "area of greatest satisfaction" for hearing aid use. The term does not imply that people in this category function better with hearing aids than people with smaller losses. Rather it refers to the extreme need for amplification of those in this range and the handicap they suffer without amplification. These people are likely to be full time hearing aid users. Even in unfavorable listening conditions where their aided performance is likely to be poor, it would be even poorer without amplification.

The final category, made up of losses greater than 80 dB in the better ear, constitutes a group who have great need for amplification, but can expect only partial help. Powerful hearing aids can make many sounds audible to persons in this group. As in all cases, the benefit to be expected from amplification depends on discrimination ability. The poor discrimination expected of those with sensorineural loss in this group limits the benefits of amplification. Individuals in this category who wear an aid are likely to be full time users.

FACTORS THAT DETERMINE BENEFITS OF AMPLIFICATION

As a generalization hearing aids can make sounds louder but not any clearer. Amplification makes sounds audible for the hearing-impaired person. Benefit from the amplified sound is then primarily determined by his auditory discrimination ability. Another factor is dynamic range, the range between the speech reception threshold and threshold of discomfort.

People with conductive hearing loss are ideal hearing aid candidates since they have good discrimination ability and a wide dynamic range. Because of the normal cochlea, they retain good discrimination ability once sound is amplified enough to overcome the conductive blockage. However, since most conductive losses are potentially reversible, relatively few people with such loss elect to wear a hearing aid. Most hearing aid users have sensorineural loss. In these people discrimination ability varies, depending on the magnitude and etiology of the loss. The poorer the discrimination ability, the poorer the hearing aid candidate. Many interrelated factors make it difficult to be specific about the relationship between auditory discrimination ability and successful hearing aid use. Receptive language ability has a strong influence on auditory discrimination scores. Discrimination test scores are not as reliable as desirable, and there is no universal standardized test procedure. In spite of these problems, the following generalizations may be justifiable, when a vehicle such as the recorded W-22 test is used to obtain unaided discrimination scores from an individual with an acquired hearing loss. If the discrimination score on the ear considered for amplification is above 70%, it is a reasonable expectation that amplification should permit understanding of speech. Two clarifying comments are needed. First, within this range, the better the discrimination the better the candidacy for amplification. Second, poor listening conditions may prevent understanding of speech, and have a disproportionate effect on people with discrimination deficit listening through a hearing aid, relative to normal ears. Nevertheless, people with enough loss of hearing sensitivity to need an aid can expect to benefit materially if the discrimination score is above 70%.

Individuals with unaided discrimination scores between 50 and 70% can expect amplification to permit only partial understanding of speech. In quiet, under good listening conditions, they may follow speech fairly well. Under the less ideal circumstances in which they listen much of the time, they cannot expect to understand everything. They should be aware of this limitation before they decide to try an aid, to permit a realistic decision and to prevent unnecessary disappointment.

If the individual's unaided discrimination score is below 50% he cannot expect to follow conversation by listening only under most listening conditions. Benefits from amplification will be primarily associated with assistance in lipreading, monitoring of the person's own voice, and the detection of environmental sounds. These benefits may be considerable, and should be explored (Dodds and Harford, 1968b). However, someone who undertakes use of amplification without understanding these limitations is bound to be disappointed.

Dynamic range is an important determinant of expected benefit in hearing aid use. Again, conductive loss produces the ideal hearing aid candidate in this respect. Because of the conductive blockage, the tolerance threshold will be raised and a wide dynamic range maintained. In sensorineural loss the dynamic range may be greatly reduced. Davis et al. (1947) estimated hearing aid candidacy in this manner: dynamic range greater than 45 dB suggests a good hearing aid candidate in this respect. If the range is between 25 and 45 dB, candidacy is fair. The patient is a poor candidate if the dynamic range is less than 25 dB. The use of hearing aids with automatic gain control, discussed in Chapters Five and Seven, helps to solve the problem.

Trial use of amplification should be considered for anyone, even poor candidates according to the above criteria. Interrelated factors; motivation, critical demand, or others, may combine to produce a successful hearing aid user from the most unlikely candidate. Nevertheless, the prospective hearing aid user deserves to know the level of help that is likely and the problems that can be expected.

TYPE OF AID

There is general agreement that at-the-ear aids are preferable since placing the microphone near the ear simulates some of the acoustic conditions which obtain in unaided listening. However, because of the magnitude of the loss or for other reasons, it is sometimes necessary to recommend body-worn aids. The age of the patient may be a factor. Most audiologists are reluctant to recommend an ear level aid for a child under two-and-one-half to three years of age. Body-worn aids, securely held in a carrier garment, are probably less susceptible to loss or damage. Elderly people, or others with motor problems, may not be capable of the relatively finer movements required to put on and adjust an ear level aid. Recommendation of a body-worn aid may be necessary for this reason. Beyond these factors, the amount of gain necessary determines whether a body-worn or at-the-ear aid should be recommended. For losses up to 60 dB, ear level aids are preferable. To get enough gain without feedback occurring, losses greater than 80 dB usually require a body-worn aid. Traditionally it has been felt that losses between 60 and 80 dB constitute a borderline area in which individual decisions must be made. More powerful ear level aids are available and may, with a well fitting earmold, deliver adequate gain to individuals in this range without feedback. Particularly if the patient has a low tolerance threshold and cannot benefit from the high output usually found in powerful body-worn aids, an ear level aid may be preferable. As discussed in Chapter Ten, greater gain without feedback can be achieved in an ear level aid using the CROS principle.

CHOICE OF AIDED EAR

Except in binaural amplification, a decision must be made regarding which ear to fit. If the ears are not bilaterally equal, the poorer ear should be aided if (1) it is good enough to benefit from hearing aid use and (2) if the better ear is good enough to function partially without amplification. The following guidelines are based on the above criteria and other important considerations:

1. If one ear is in and the other out of the "area of greatest satisfaction," fit the ear that is in.

2. If both ears are in the "area of greatest satisfaction" fit the ear that is closest to 60 dB.

3. Fit the ear with the flatter audiometric configuration.

4. Fit the ear with the better discrimination ability.

5. Fit the ear with the wider dynamic range.

6. Consider the patient's preference, remembering that most people will prefer the aid on their right ear.

HEARING AID SELECTION PROCEDURES AND PHILOSOPHIES

Various procedures are used to determine appropriate amplification for a hearing-impaired individual. Philosophies vary. At one end of the continuum is the belief that a few basic patterns of amplification are sufficient to serve most people who require amplification. At the other end is the belief that specific characteristics must be prescribed for each individual hearing loss. The fact that disagreement exists does not necessarily mean that valid procedures for recommending amplification do not exist. Problems can be solved using different procedures just as the same point on a map can be reached using different routes. Selection procedures are discussed below.

Selective Amplification

Selective amplification means tailoring the frequency response to fit the individual audiogram. This concept arose during the early days of electronic hearing aid development. At that time amplifying power was weak, and broad flat responses were not available. It was necessary to fit peaks of amplification into areas of greatest hearing loss where the available amplification was most needed. As better and more flexible amplifying systems were developed, use of the concept was expanded. Strict adherence to the principle would result in a hearing aid whose response was a mirror image of the patient's audiogram. That is, hearing loss at each frequency would determine the corresponding sound pressure level (SPL) output from the aid. Using such an aid, the wearer's pure-tone thresholds are ostensibly corrected to normal sensitivity. In other words, the gain requirements for optimum response to suprathreshold signals are projected from the patient's threshold performance. A problem with this practice lies in the fact that many hearing aid wearers have loudness recruitment. Therefore, they may experience normal loudness sensations at reduced sensation levels. If the amount of amplification needed is projected solely from unaided thresholds, and the aim is to correct the audiogram, the result will probably be overamplification.

In an early study, Davis and his coworkers (1947) established that subjects with dissimilar hearing loss obtained better discrimination scores with a system which had either a flat response or moderate high frequency emphasis. They did not perform better with responses which tended toward "fitting" their audiograms.

However, some experimenters have found advantages in selective amplification. Reddell and Calvert (1966) evaluated subjects who had fairly sharply sloping sensorineural losses. These subjects obtained better discrimination scores with aids that had frequency responses "custom tailored" to fit their losses than with commercially available aids that were considered appropriate but not specifically adjusted to the subjects' audiometric configurations. The authors cautioned, however, that there may have been differences between aids other than frequency characteristics which could have accounted for the superiority of the experimental aids.

From subjects with high frequency sensorineural loss Thompson and Lassman (1969) obtained better discrimination scores using high frequency emphasis rather than flat amplification. However, the differences were slight and emerged only when testing was done in noise, rather than quiet. In the same study the subjects were divided into three groups, based on the amount of "distortion" indicated in their ears by a group of special auditory tests. The low distortion group benefitted more from selective amplification than the middle or high distortion group. In other words, there was an interaction between condition of the subjects' ears and frequency response characteristics. This finding suggested to the authors that selective amplification, a form of external distortion, may be harmful to ears with high internal distortion but helpful to ears which operate at a low distortion level.

Over the years our concepts of hearing aid candidacy have changed. Today people with sharply falling sensorineural loss or with substantial areas of normal sensitivity may be successful hearing aid candidates. Previously these people would not have been considered for amplification. In these cases it is probably helpful for frequency response to reflect audiometric configuration in at least a general fashion. However, decisions regarding amplification should never be made on the basis of pure-tone threshold testing alone. Such decisions suffer through lack of important information about the patient's ability to benefit from and tolerate amplification.

Hearing Aid Evaluation

Carhart (1946a) reported this procedure and the method often bears his name. The procedure was developed and used when hearing-handicapped veterans of World War II required rehabilitation. It is discussed in some detail in Chapter Twelve. The evaluation aspects are presented below, with the reminder that the procedure often referred to as the Carhart Method represents a considerable abridgement of the original selection procedure.

The goals of the program were (1) to find a hearing aid with optimal efficiency for everyday listening, (2) to orient the user to hearing aids, give him efficient listening habits, and start auditory training, and (3) to instill psychological acceptance of the hearing aid.

Otologic examination and audiologic evaluation were done first. The hearing problem and the nature of hearing aids were then discussed with the patient. An ear impression was taken and an earmold made. General decisions about the type of aid and the aided ear were reached, and a number of promising aids were selected for trial use and evaluation. Practice in aided listening as well as elicitation of the patient's reaction to various aids was interspersed throughout this procedure. Eventually three or four of these aids were selected for clinical evaluation leading to the selection of one aid. The clinical procedure, before and during the selection process, consisted of these steps:

1. Initial audiologic evaluation; pure-tone air and bone conduction thresholds as well as speech thresholds and discrimination scores.

2. A corroborating audiometric retest.

3. With each aid, aided gain for speech and tolerance thresholds.

4. Performance tests in noise and discrimination tests in quiet.

On the basis of these tests and the patient's ratings, an aid was selected.

Certain advantages of the procedure are obvious. It was thorough and intensive. It got the patient involved in decision making regarding the selection procedure, fostering psychological commitment and responsibility. It involved training as a part of the selection procedure. Early amplification experiences were in a structured and controllable acoustic environment. A custom earmold was available for the evaluation; an important consideration according to Konkle and Bess (1974). They reported a difference in aided performance depending on whether a custom or stock earmold was used.

One major disadvantage is obvious. The procedure was time consuming and therefore expensive. Seven to 15 days were required exclusive of rehabilitative training given after the patient received his aid. Over time, the classic procedure was shortened, probably due to time and cost considerations, to consist of the following:

1. Otologic and audiologic assessment.

2. Counseling the patient about the nature of his hearing problem and of hearing aids, realistic expectations of help from amplification, and the nature and importance of other avenues of aural rehabilitation.

3. The measurement of speech gain and intelligibility through various hearing aids in quiet, and the subsequent recommendation of a specific aid.

4. Counseling the patient relative to the care and use of the aid recommended.

Usually all of the above procedures except the otologic examination were done in one session.

The conventional hearing aid evaluation procedure requires a representative stock of hearing aids for clinical evaluation. Traditionally, manufacturers and dealers have placed aids for this purpose in University and other non-profit clinics. Problems have arisen from this consignment system. There have been in some cases poor care and accountability of the aids on the part of the clinics. Dealers have felt, sometimes justifiably, that clinic personnel do not understand some aids or know how to demonstrate them efficiently. There is sometimes antagonism between dealers and clinics because more patients are not "sold" hearing aids. Clinics may put equal emphasis on advantages and limitations of an aid for a particular individual. The patient, not wanting an aid for a number of reasons, may not be "sold." These problems may be alleviated by following a careful system for accounting, maintenance, and reporting; such as that detailed by Harford and Musket (1964b).

Professional criticism of the conventional evaluation procedure soon arose. The conventional procedure assumes that there is an interaction between hearing aids and people with hearing loss. That is, it is felt that the hearing aid that is best for one individual might not be best for another, even if the two persons had similar hearing loss. Further it is believed that auditory tests are sensitive to this interaction and can differentiate the performance of hearing aids. Doubts arose about these assumptions. As already mentioned, Davis et al. (1947) suggested that a complex procedure of evaluation was not necessary in most cases, but should be done when special problems became evident. They reported that most types of loss could benefit from aids with flat response or moderate high frequency emphasis.

Newby (1964) stated that in the early postwar days hearing aids were crude and somewhat unreliable, and he suggested that differences from aid to aid could be demonstrated by clinical tests. He reasoned that, as hearing aids became more refined and their parts standardized, it may have become more difficult to establish differences by clinical tests. He suggested that clinics move from evaluation procedures to "hearing aid consultation," a more generalized process, de-emphasizing comparative hearing aid tests.

In a widely quoted study, Shore, Bilger, and Hirsh (1960) presented evidence which suggests that discrimination test scores, obtained from PB lists may not be sufficiently reliable to differentiate among hearing aids. They obtained aided discrimination scores from 15 adult subjects. An equal number had conductive, sensorineural, and mixed losses. Four body aids were used. For each subject, the most appropriate and least appropriate tone and other control settings were selected (adequate gain was provided for both conditions). These settings were called "good" and "bad." The good setting followed established clinical practice in making the aid's adjustment as appropriate as possible and the bad setting was as much the opposite as could be obtained within the limits of the aids and settings available. The most widely quoted conclusion from this study is that the reliability of discrimination measures is not good enough to warrant the investigation of a large amount of clinical time with them in selecting hearing aids.

There has probably been some overgeneralization from the studies mentioned above. They have been cited as negation for all comparative hearing aid evaluation procedures. Recall, however, that Davis et al. (1947) felt that comparative procedures were unnecessary only for the typical hearing aid candidate and should be utilized for problem cases. The Shore et al. study (1960) found that significant differences attributable to tone settings did occur in those subjects who had sensorineural loss and, for some aids, in about half of the subjects in the other two categories.

Shore et al. (1960) used half-lists rather than full 50 word lists in their study. This practice may have contributed to the observed lack of reliability. Jirsa, Hodgson, and Goetzinger (1975) suggest that the good reliability previously reported for half-lists may result from a statistical artifact which when corrected shows poorer reliability than previously reported.

In summary, it is probable that small difference in discrimination scores obtained with different hearing aids may be more apparent than real. The conventional procedure probably cannot select from a group of similar aids the one best for the typical patient. These probabilities do not preclude comparative procedures in problem cases. Most importantly, doubts about the validity of comparative procedures should not prevent aided evaluation with an appropriate hearing aid to determine the patient's general response to amplification.

Jerger and Hayes (1976) reported a hearing aid evaluation procedure with the underlying philosophy that the evaluation is not an end in itself, but part of the total rehabilitation procedure. They aimed for an evaluation procedure which would (1) systematically differentiate among hearing aids, (2) achieve face validity by using test materials more like conversational speech than PB-lists, and (3) be simple to administer with standard clinical instrumentation. They used "synthetic sentences" (Speaks and Jerger, 1965) in competition consisting of continuous speech from a single talker. The sentences were always delivered at 60 dB SPL, while the competing message intensity was varied. The message-to-competition ratio varied from +20 to −20 dB. Results were obtained unaided, aided, and again unaided. The latter condition was to assess the effect of practice. Based on aided improvement, the authors hoped to determine the most suitable hearing aid arrangement, achieve realistic prognostic information, and make accountable rehabilitative recommendations. A survey of patients who purchased aids recommended by this procedure showed a high percentage of user satisfaction.

Hearing Aid Consultation

Resnick and Becker (1963) suggested an alternative to the conventional evaluation procedure. They were concerned that the conventional procedure may not reliably differentiate between aids, that it was time consuming, and about the difficulty of keeping a representative and operating stock of aids in the clinic. They proposed the following steps to compose a hearing aid consultation:

1. Audiologic assessment; pure-tone air and bone conduction thresholds, speech thresholds, and discrimination scores.

2. The patient is counselled regarding the nature of his hearing loss and of hearing aids. The help he can realistically expect from amplification is explained, as well as the possibilities of other aural rehabilitation.

3. The patient is referred to a participating hearing aid dispenser, to whom the audiometric information is sent. When necessary, particular problems are discussed. The dispenser fits the patient with an aid of his own choice.

4. The patient returns to the clinic where his performance is evaluated with his new aid. He is instructed in the use of the aid and, if deemed necessary, a formal program of auditory training is offered.

This program has the advantage of testing the patient with the aid he will actually wear, which may be important in light of the report of considerable variability from manufacturers' specifications in given hearing aids (Kasten, Lotterman, and Revoile, 1967; Birt and Alberti, 1973). It also provides a custom earmold for the evaluation. Followed exactly, it has the potential disadvantage of never assessing the patient's reaction to amplification before a hearing aid is purchased. Another possible problem, which may be present in other procedures as well, is that the patient may not follow the clinic's recommendation to return for evaluation and orientation after purchase of the aid.

Shapiro (1976) proposed and illustrated a procedure for specifying recommended hearing aid characteristics. Specifications are based on threshold of discomfort and most comfortable loudness for narrow bands of noise centered at 0.25, 0.5, 1, 2, 3, and 4 kHz. These data are given to the hearing aid dispenser who is to provide an aid that matches the prescribed response characteristics.

Master Hearing Aid

Master hearing aids are instruments which simulate some of the operating characteristics of hearing aids. Usually the maximum gain, maximum power output, and some frequency response characteristics can be varied. Thus this flexible instrument can be made to simulate in a general way many different hearing aid characteristics. They have been used for this purpose both in research and clinical situations. Davis and his coworkers (1947) used a master hearing aid to achieve the frequency response and output characteristics they wanted to study. Some advantages of the use of a master hearing aid are presented by Bergman (1959). Critics point out that master hearing aids approximate rather than duplicate characteristics of specific hearing aids, and additional important characteristics, such as harmonic distortion and frequency range, may not even be approximated. Presumably efforts to compare the appropriateness of different master hearing aid settings, using routine clinical procedures, would also have whatever problems these procedures show in conventional hearing aid evaluations.

ELECTROACOUSTIC CHARACTERISTICS AND HEARING AID EVALUATION

Hearing aid assessment must include exploration of the patient's tolerance levels or uncomfortable loudness (UCL). The aid eventually obtained must have a maximum output less than the UCL of the patient. The usual procedure is to tell the patient to respond when loudness reaches a level of definite discomfort, then increase the intensity of a speech signal to the test ear until that level is reached. A maximum output for amplification just less than that level is subsequently recommended. For patients with UCL of 120 dB SPL, or less, the determination is often made under earphones. One hundred twenty dB SPL is the usual maximum earphone output associated with speech audiometers. Therefore, if the patient requires a greater maximum output, it is usual to do the testing with a hearing aid of known Saturation Sound Pressure Level (SSPL) on the patient.

The aid or amplification characteristics recommended must combine adequate gain with an SSPL that is tolerable. The available relationship in aids produced by one company is shown in Table 8-2. Logically, aids with

TABLE 8-2. **Relationships between maximum gain and maximum power output for aids manufactured by one company**

Maximum Gain in dB	Saturation Sound Pressure Level in dB
32	109
38	113
39	98–114
39	113
39	116
44	123
49	120
49	120
49	121
50	118
51	120
52	119
53	116–26
71	135
80	143
87	148

low gain have low SSPLs; high SSPL is associated with high gain. Note that the correlation is not perfect, permitting some latitude based on patient needs, and that two aids have adjustable SSPL.

In my opinion, an adequate aid should provide an aided speech reception threshold between 20 and 30 dB with no more than two-thirds rotation of the gain control. This generalization does not apply to persons with primarily high frequency loss, whose unaided SRT may be no poorer than 30 dB. This person's criterion for adequate high frequency gain is an aid which permits increased audibility of consonant sounds spoken at conversational speech levels. At the same time, the low frequency gain must be sufficiently controlled so that uncomfortable loudness in this area does not occur before the gain control is rotated sufficiently for adequate high frequency amplification.

A wide dynamic range is desirable for undistorted amplification when aids control output by peak clipping, as described in Chapter Seven. This requirement motivates us to recommend an SSPL as high as the patient can tolerate comfortably. However, as is explained in Chapter Twelve, there is on rare occasion record of high output SPLs causing further change in threshold of a hearing aid user. This consideration, plus of course the UCL of the patient, may require use of automatic gain control (AGC). AGC, as explained in Chapter Seven, accomplishes output limitation without the harmonic distortion associated with peak clipping. If the dynamic range is marginal, perhaps up to 50 dB, the use of AGC should be considered. The narrower the dynamic range, the more important the use of AGC.

CONCLUSIONS

Several hearing aid selection procedures have been discussed above. Burney (1972) conducted a survey to determine the procedures audiologists were using at that time. Results are shown in Table 8-3. Of the 191 respondents the majority were using the conventional evaluation procedure, or some adaptation from it, in which patients were evaluated with a hearing aid or aids prior to recommendation. Most of the clinics indicated they spent 1–2 hours on an evaluation but a sizable minority gave the time required as 2–3 hours. A large majority indicated they recommended follow-up evaluations almost all the time.

It is probably helpful to make an initial assessment of the patient wearing an appropriate hearing aid. The purpose may be, not to find out if it is the best aid for the patient, but to assess aided performance and the patient's response to amplification. Sometimes discrimination drops sharply because of the low fidelity characteristics of hearing aids. Sometimes discrimination can be improved with high frequency emphasis amplification over the flat response of the speech audiometer. Stated differ-

TABLE 8-3. **Survey of hearing aid selection procedures (Burney, 1972)**

	Type of Clinic				
	University	Hospital	V.A.*	Others	Total
Type of evaluation performed (%)					
Conventional†	31.4	17.8	11.2	24.3	84.7
Consultation	7.6	1.8	1.2	4.7	15.3
Master H/A‡	0	0	0	0	0
Time allotted					
Less than 1 hour	0.6	0.6	0	1.2	2.4
1–2 hours	21.9	12.1	4.1	19.1	57.2
2–3 hours	12.7	7.5	5.8	8.6	34.6
More than 3 hours	1.7	0	2.9	1.2	5.8
Clinics recommending follow-up evaluations (% of time)					
100–96%	31.1	17.7	5.3	24.7	78.8
95–61%	0	1.2	0.6	0	1.8
60–41%	3.5	0.6	1.2	1.8	7.1
40–6%	2.9	1.2	5.3	1.8	11.2
5–0%	0.6	0	0.6	0	1.2

* Veterans Administration hospital.

† At least to the extent that patients are tested while wearing a hearing aid.

‡ H/A, hearing aid.

ently, one cannot be sure of aided performance without sampling it. It is also helpful to learn the initial reaction of the patient to amplification. Patients are usually surprised at the sound of their voice and the multitude of small unaccustomed sounds they hear with amplification. They sometimes comment that it sounds as if they are listening down in a barrel. They may be enthusiastic or horrified regarding the amplified signal. It is important to learn this information before making a recommendation, and to talk about these phenomena with the patient before a hearing aid is purchased.

The original Carhart method included testing the aid's performance in noise. This procedure was subsequently dropped in many instances, probably because of time considerations. Patients with sensorineural loss suffer a disproportionate drop in auditory discrimination ability between quiet and noise, as compared to normals (Watson, 1961; Olsen and Tillman, 1968). Because hearing aid users listen in noise most of the time, it is no doubt helpful to have a measure of their aided ability to do so, as compared to their performance in quiet. Olsen and Tillman (1968) demonstrated that differences in performance between hearing aids that were not measurable during discrimination testing in quiet were noticeable in noise. They concluded that discrimination tests in noise reliably differentiate among hearing aids, as well as providing a more realistic measure of everyday listening ability.

Aided discrimination testing in noise can be structured to give information about the effect of the head shadow on aided performance and, in binaural evaluation, about the relative efficiency of aided binaural listening in noise. Tillman, Kasten, and Horner (1963) reported a 6.4 dB head shadow effect. The increasing effect of the head shadow for high frequencies was reported by Sivian and White (1933) and Kasten, Lotterman and Hinchman (1967–68). Carhart, Pollack, and Lotterman (1963) studied the comparative aided efficiency of monaural listening when the signal originated on the aided and the unaided side, and of binaural listening. All tests were done in background noise with the same nominal signal-to-noise ratio for each condition. They concluded that binaural advantages were dependent on the elimination of the head shadow effect.

Carhart and Olsen (1967) proposed a test procedure for the evaluation of binaural hearing aids. The patient was seated in a sound-treated room with two loudspeakers equidistant from him and at 45° azimuth to the right and left. Discrimination testing was accomplished with PB lists in the presence of competing speech originating from the other loudspeaker. For monaural testing the non-test ear was masked by white noise originating from the other loudspeaker and also was covered by a circumaural muff. Thus the primary signal could originate from the side of the test ear or the non-test ear. This procedure revealed the effect of the head shadow on performance. There was, moreover, an additional improvement during binaural performance in noise, over the best monaural score. Nabelek and Pickett (1974b) reported superiority of aided binaural discrimination over monaural in quiet as well as in noise when hearing-impaired subjects were tested in a reverberant room. They speculated that the reflected speech energy constituted an interfering noise which was more damaging in the monaural than in the binaural condition.

The considerations mentioned above suggest the importance of evaluating hearing aids in noise. The head shadow effect should also be considered during the hearing aid evaluation procedure, particularly if binaural aids are being contemplated.

Many hearing aid wearers use their aid's telecoil when telephoning. Children enrolled in classes for the hearing impaired may use the telecoil in conjunction with an induction loop as their most important channel of aided listening. Studies have shown that a given aid may operate much differently on telecoil versus microphone setting, and an aid appropriate for a particular loss when receiving acoustic signals may be inappropriate on telecoil operation (Sung and Hodgson, 1971; Hodgson and Sung, 1972; Sung, Sung, and Hodgson, 1974). When an aid with telecoil is recommended its performance characteristics should be known. Consideration should be given appropriateness of the characteristics.

Hearing aids with directional microphones reduce the effective intensity of some sounds originating behind the listener. Their purpose is to limit the effect of competing noise. Lentz (1972a) demonstrated a clinical procedure for evaluating these aids. He presented discrimination tests from various origins around the patient's head, and used various signal-to-noise ratios. Frank and Gooden (1973) evaluated performance of hearing aids with directional microphones by originating noise from either directly in front or in back of the subject. Speech originated from a loudspeaker positioned at 45° azimuth from the midline of the subject's head. Discrimination scores were obtained under each noise condition. These procedures probably should be used when considering the recommendation of an aid with directional microphone, to assess the patient's performance and demonstrate to him the effects of the aid.

The selection procedure should lead logically to a program of hearing aid orientation and training. Institutions which perform hearing aid evaluations should also conduct, or have ready access to, programs for habilitative training to meet all of the patient's auditory needs (Castle, 1967). This training is discussed in Chapters Eleven through Thirteen.

In summary, the considerations above lead to the following conclusions regarding hearing aid evaluation:

1. Otologic evaluation should preclude consideration of amplification.

2. Unaided audiometric evaluation should include pure-tone air and bone conduction thresholds, speech thresholds, and discrimination testing; procedures which inform about the patient's needs and expected benefits regarding amplification.

3. Demands on the patient's hearing and his motivation regarding amplification are important considerations.

4. Evaluation of aided discrimination gives important information about the patient's aided performance, and his reaction to amplification.

5. Comfortable listening levels and thresholds of discomfort should be established.

6. Aided discrimination testing in noise may give a more realistic measure of everyday listening performance and may contribute comparative information about different aids.

7. Additional characteristics, such as telecoil or directional microphone should be evaluated when present.

8. A follow-up evaluation should be conducted with the actual hearing aid the patient is to use.

9. The hearing aid evaluation and selection procedure should be part of a comprehensive program of aural habilitation or rehabilitation.

Successful use of amplification depends on the patient's discrimination ability, his dynamic range, and the signal-to-noise ratio in which he listens. A patient with wide dynamic range and good discrimination ability will do well when he listens in quiet. If one or more of these conditions deteriorate, the patient will not do as well. The task of the audiologist is to decide if a hearing aid is feasible, recommend an appropriate amplification arrangement, and help the patient learn to use it.

chapter *9*

hearing aids for children

Noel D. Matkin, Ph.D.

INTRODUCTION

In recent years audiologists have been confronted with an increasing number of young children referred with suspected hearing impairments. No doubt this trend reflects a growing awareness among physicians, educators, and communicologists of the importance of early identification and habilitation of youngsters having bilateral hearing loss. As a consequence, the audiologist is expected to obtain more definitive audiologic information at an earlier age to enhance the medical management, the selection of appropriate wearable amplification, and the educational placement of preschool hearing-impaired children.

At the outset, it should be kept in mind that the bulk of clinical research has focused upon the adult hearing-impaired population. As a consequence, the audiologist functions on a rather tenuous basis during the selection of suitable amplification for young hearing-impaired children once a hearing loss is identified. As has been previously noted, the selection of an appropriate hearing aid for a particular patient represents a series of measurements, decisions, and compromises (Davis and Silverman, 1960). The comment is still pertinent when discussing wearable amplification for young children. Since there is a paucity of clinical research with the pediatric population, many of the comments and suggestions included in this chapter will be based both on personal clinical experience and upon data collected during a longitudinal study of 253 children completed in the Children's Hearing Clinic at Northwestern University (Matkin, 1971).

Underlying the following discussion is the belief that there are similarities as well as differences in the audiologic management of adults and children. The development of a hearing loss during the adult years essentially imposes limitations upon receptive auditory communicative abilities. In sharp contrast, a hearing impairment during childhood often results in receptive and expressive language deficits which become pervasive in terms of the child's social, emotional, and cognitive functions. Thus, pediatric audiologic management must from the outset be diagnostically oriented with focus on the whole child, not merely upon the auditory function of the youngster. Further, such management including the selection and modification of hearing aids must be viewed as an ongoing process over a relatively long period of time. Finally, as has been pointed out by Grammatico (1975), the selection of a suitable hearing aid for a child should be a team effort involving not only the audiologist but also the child's teacher and parents.

While numerous issues with respect to wearable amplification for children are controversial, there appear to be at least two basic premises upon which there is agreement. First, *maximum utilization of residual hearing should be made regardless of the prevailing educational philosophy*. Therefore, whether a child is to be placed in an acoupedic program, an oral-aural program, or in a total communication program, emphasis should be placed by the educator upon the optimal utilization of aided hearing. With respect to total communication programming, it should be noted that results from a recent investigation indicate that there is a positive relationship between the utilization of aided hearing and the child's emerging skills in sign language (Crandall, 1974). To explain, Crandall points out that early auditory stimulation was an asset in learning a language in the signed mode, even for the profoundly hearing-impaired child.

As mentioned, there has been increased emphasis in recent years upon early identification and education. Early identification in audiologic terms obviously leads to a second premise; that is, *wearable amplification should be provided as early as feasible*. "As early as feasible" in this context is interpreted to mean as soon as medical clearance for hearing aid use has been obtained, as soon as at least a general estimate of the degree and the configuration of the hearing impairment is confirmed and finally, as soon as there is a basic readiness for acceptance of amplification, not only by the child, but also by the parents.

Rationales for Early Hearing Aid Use

There are several rationales for providing amplification as early as feasible. First, it seems important to avoid possible detrimental effects of sensory deprivation. Sensory deprivation refers to both the physiological and psychological aspects of development. While research in this area is limited, there are indications that physiological changes in the visual sensory system may result from early and prolonged sensory deprivation (Barnet, 1965). Since the available research regarding deprivation has been focused upon the visual modality, systematic investigations in the area of audition are needed. Another aspect of early sensory deprivation which should be considered has to do with the psycho-social development of young hearing-impaired children. The theory of Ericson regarding personality development indicates that a basic level of development is related to the emergence of a sense of trust (Maier, 1969). Trust apparently develops as the child's environment becomes more predictable. Predictability in this context must have to do not only with visual but also with auditory monitoring of the environment. Thus the question must be posed, "Does the lack of auditory input during early developmental periods have detrimental effects with respect to the hearing-impaired child's psycho-social development?" Even if a hearing aid brings the profoundly hearing impaired infant into only limited contact with the world of sound, the early use of amplification may be highly desirable as a means of minimizing the possible deleterious effects of sensory deprivation.

A second critical reason for stressing the provision of early amplification for children is the enhancement of language development during critical periods of readiness. As has been pointed out by Lenneberg, among others, the development of speech and language appears to be based upon innate biologically programmed factors (Lenneberg, 1967). Thus, early intervention with respect to language stimulation via aided hearing is essential. Finally, it appears that the provision of wearable amplification during the preschool years fosters hearing aid acceptance. A study by Sortini (1956) in which the utilization of hearing aids was compared between groups of preschool and school-age children clearly highlights the importance, not only of early identification, but of early hearing aid use.

ESSENTIAL STEPS IN PROCURING AN AID

Otologic Management

As with adults, there are five essential steps to consider when procuring a hearing aid for a young child. Step one is to obtain otologic clearance before proceeding with the selection of a hearing aid. Obviously, one would not recommend the purchase of a hearing aid for a child if the hearing loss can be either medically or surgically remediated in the immediate future. Less obvious, however, is the need for continued medical surveillance, especially for preschoolers who may be characterized by frequent upper respiratory infections and associated middle ear problems. Various reports indicate that a substantial number of youngsters with permanent sensori-neural impairments have conductive overlays which result in a significantly greater loss of hearing. For example, a 30 dB conductive hearing loss which goes unrecognized and is superimposed upon a 60 db sensorineural loss can result in inappropriate management of a child with respect both to the selection of a hearing aid and the educational placement. Thus, parents need to understand that periodic otologic care is an essential feature in an ongoing management program for all hearing-impaired children. The younger the child, the more frequent such evaluations should be scheduled.

Audiologic Evaluation

Step two in the sequence of obtaining a hearing aid for a youngster is the completion of a comprehensive audiologic evaluation. As stated earlier, audiologic management especially with preschoolers must be viewed as an ongoing process so that as more detailed audiologic information becomes available the hearing aid as well as the habilitation program can be adjusted accordingly. The goal is to evaluate each youngster's auditory status with greater precision over time as well as to evaluate continually the suitability of the hearing aid initially selected, making whatever electroacoustic modifications that are necessary.

With respect to the audiologic evaluation, a basic premise which should be considered is: *more, not less, testing should be undertaken with children.* In other words, the less a child is able to verbalize his auditory experiences the more important structured observations and formal testing become. For far too long, hearing aids have been selected and classroom placement has been determined for young children on the basis of only a pure-tone audiogram. It is well recognized that two adult patients with identical audiograms may not function the same auditorially. The same difference may be seen among children if extensive audiologic testing is routinely undertaken.

An equally important concept is that one of the basic goals in undertaking a comprehensive assessment is to have extensive baseline data available so that one can compare the aided performance of a child with the unaided findings, thus assuring not only that a suitable instrument is recommended but that a realistic level of expectation from hearing aid utilization is established.

Often the audiologist essentially relies upon one procedure such as conditioned play audiometry to obtain audiologic data with a variety of children irrespective of their maturation and degree of hearing loss. When one considers the range of functional levels encountered in a pediatric population with respect to cognitive and visual-motor abilities, a more insightful approach is to rely upon a pediatric test battery rather than upon a favorite audiometric technique.

In the utilization of a pediatric test battery, there is little reason to encounter numerous clinical records which note "child uncooperative, could not test." In fact, there is evidence with a battery of conditioning techniques from which to choose and with a well calibrated sound field, reliable estimates of auditory sensitivity can be successfully established for the vast majority of preschool children (Matkin, 1973). Since the completion of masked bone conduction audiometry is often not possible at an early age, impedance measurements should also be considered essential in a pediatric audiologic battery.

Measures of auditory sensitivity both for pure-tones and for speech via air and bone conduction are essential. Of prime importance is the determination of the potential for using residual hearing as well as the determination of the degree and type of hearing loss. Therefore, measures of auditory discrimination for speech in quiet as well as in competition are critical. Again, at least an estimate of auditory discrimination can be made provided the clinician utilizes a variety of test materials rather than one set of test materials such as the PBK-50 word lists. Finally, an assessment of tolerance for intense sounds should be undertaken.

While the purpose of this chapter is not to discuss a pediatric test battery, it is well to note that there are several audiometric techniques which have been found worthwhile. While conditioned play audiometry, which can be completed either in an unaided or aided condition, has long been recognized as a worthwhile approach, it should be recognized that various studies indicated limited success in utilizing this technique with many children under the age of 30 months and with children who are found to be difficult to test. Subsequent research investigations, as well as clinical experience, have indicated that tangible reinforcement operant conditioning audiometry (TROCA) is well suited as an alternate approach for use with those children who are difficult to test (Lloyd, 1966). It also should be noted that it is helpful to have available such an alternate technique so that if behavioral conditioning is not maintained until a detailed audiometric evaluation is completed, the clinician can move to a second conditioning technique and subsequently complete the assessment. Finally, a third technique which has been described by a number of writers has been found to be especially valuable when evaluating either youngsters under the age of 30 months or youngsters who are severely developmentally delayed. This technique was described in the early literature as conditioned orienting reflex (COR) audiometry (Suzuki and Ogiba, 1961). Later, the technique was modified by Liden and Kankkunen (1969) so that localization was not required as the response and the technique has become termed VRA or visual reinforcement audiometry. A recent clinical investigation completed with normal hearing children between the ages of 9 months and 36 months indicates that by coupling VRA to sound field audiometry, the vast majority of youngsters in this age range can be successfully tested (Matkin, 1973). Further, minimal response levels to sound field presentations were typically established within 15 dB of those obtained later under earphones for the better ear while using an alternate conditioning technique. In summary, by utilizing a battery of pediatric audiologic measures including conditioned play audiometry, tangible reinforcement operant-conditioning audiometry, and visual reinforcement audiometry, most hearing-impaired youngsters can be successfully tested without resorting to the use of electrophysiological measurements. Obviously, if reliable and valid responses can be obtained in the unaided condition, the same techniques are applicable when evaluating a child's aided sensitivity across frequency while wearing different hearings aids. An example of the sound field findings in such a case is illustrated in Figure 9–1.

Prior to assessment of auditory discrimination for speech it is worthwhile to establish a general estimate of each child's receptive language age either through input from parents and teachers, or through utilization of appropriate screening material. In other words, discrimination testing, both in quiet and in competition, should be undertaken only after it has

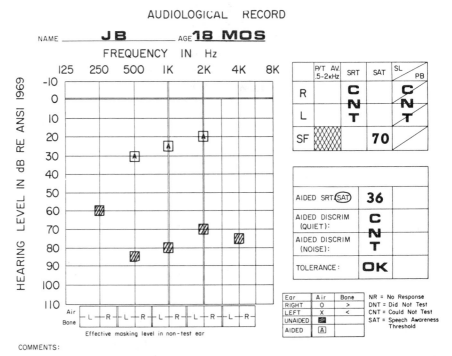

FIG. 9–1. Audiometric results obtained in sound field with visual reinforcement audiometry, for an 18 month old.

TABLE 9-1. **Auditory Discrimination Testing**

A guide based on receptive vocabulary age (RVA) for selecting materials to be utilized during the discrimination testing of children

RVA	Test Material
years	
12 or >	Adult word lists
6 to 12	PBK-50 word lists
4 to 6	WIPI* test
Up to 4	Selected words, or environment sounds
Non-verbal	Phoneme imitation and differentiation

* WIPI, Word intelligibility by picture identification.

been determined that the materials to be utilized for such testing are appropriate with respect to the child's receptive vocabulary. Otherwise, one does not know whether discrimination scores for children reflect auditory discrimination or language deficits. While PBK-50 (phonetically balanced kindergarten) word lists have gained wide clinical acceptance for utilization with children, it is important to keep in mind that a receptive language age of approximately 6 years is necessary before numerous words contained in such lists are within the average child's receptive vocabulary. Since many hearing-impaired children reflect substantial deficits in the area of receptive vocabulary, it again is important to develop a battery of alternate materials rather than relying upon only the PBK-50 word lists. Table 9-1 summarizes the guidelines currently used. In brief, for those children whose receptive language age is 12 years or greater, the use of adult monosyllabic discrimination materials appears to be appropriate. For those youngsters whose receptive language age falls between 6 and 12 years of age, PBK-50 word lists are employed. If receptive vocabulary knowledge falls approximately between 4 and 6 years of age, the word intelligibility by picture identification (WIPI) materials developed by Ross and Lerman (1970) have been found to be useful. This latter test not only incorporates language items which are less complex, but also incorporates a picture pointing response which is ideal for use with many hearing-impaired children whose speech production is less than fully intelligible. Finally, it has been found to be helpful to attempt informal testing of auditory discrimination when receptive language development is limited. In other words, the clinician can choose either pictures or objects which are reflected by the child's spoken language for assessing basic discrimination abilities. An alternate approach with the non-verbal child is to utilize familiar environmental sounds as test stimuli such as those incorporated into the Sound Effects Recognition Test (Hieber et al., 1975). As a precaution, it is preferable to report the performance on such informal tasks as the number of correct responses out of the number of trials rather than as a percentage. In other words, by not recording a percentage score, it is apparent that an informal measure rather than a standardized formal testing procedure was utilized. Obviously, it is difficult to predict how these informal scores compare to subsequent findings when formal test results are available. However, it has been found that not only can one assess the current level of the child's auditory function but often significant differences between the two ears and/or differences in the child's performance with various hearing aids in quiet and in competition can be highlighted. Such information is valuable in determining appropriate educational management. The audiologist should be assisting the teacher when decisions are made about levels of expectation with respect to auditory function. Obviously, as a child matures such prognosis can be refined through ongoing evaluations. There then are several advantages of including receptive language screening during the initial and subsequent audiologic evaluations. Not only can more appropriate selection of discrimination materials be undertaken, but such testing often highlights the possible presence of additional learning problems. If receptive language deficits are noted which far exceed that which would be expected considering the degree of hearing loss, referral for additional psychoeducational testing should be initiated. Finally, the inclusion of receptive vocabulary testing may help with decisions in a controversial area. The adverse effects of a mild bilateral hearing loss during childhood are often underestimated. By highlighting the lag in a child's receptive language development, it is easier to justify a decision to recommend wearable amplification for the youngster who has a mild bilateral loss — either of a sensorineural or of the chronic conductive type.

It is worthwhile not only to establish performance at an optimal listening level but also to evaluate the child's performance at a normal conversational level (50 dB hearing level (HL)) in quiet and against a background of competition if one wishes to demonstrate the impact of milder degrees of hearing loss during childhood. With children the utilization of speech spectrum noise or a babble of voices rather than a second talker as a competing signal is more suitable. Very often asking a young child to listen to a primary speech signal and ignore a secondary speech message appears to create a confusing perceptual listening task. In other words, requiring a preschool youngster to make a complex foreground-background discrimination may not be feasible.

As this discussion of the essentials in a comprehensive pediatric audiological evaluation is concluded, it is important to note that before considering wearable amplification one should determine through an ascending technique the intensity level at which the child begins to manifest tolerance problems while listening to speech. Such information is valuable later when decisions regarding output limiting of the hearing aid must be made.

Again, the reader is reminded that stress has been placed upon the importance of the audiologic evaluation so that whenever feasible the selection of a hearing aid is based upon a comparison of aided and unaided performance data rather than upon clinician opinion and bias. However, if the initial audiologic findings are limited, one must then rely upon competent professional judgment.

Preselection of Hearing Aids

A pressing need in the area of pediatric audiology is the formulation through clinical research of better guidelines for the preselection of hearing aids to be tried during the clinical evaluation. Preselection is a critical, yet little discussed, step in the total procedure when procuring suitable wearable amplification for a child. The term "Preselection of Hearing Aids" as used in this context refers to the process by which the audiologist selects a limited number of hearing aids from the available clinic stock to be tried during the formal clinical evaluation. The factors considered in this preselection process include the findings from the audiologic evaluation, the technical specification data supplied by manufacturers and/or electroacoustic performance data determined in the clinic, as well as past experience in successfully choosing a hearing aid for similar cases. The insight with which the audiologist chooses various hearing aids to try during the actual selection procedure is of paramount importance. Yet, as mentioned earlier, most research regarding wearable amplification has been completed with the adult hearing-impaired population. Consequently, preselection decisions must often be based on past clinical experience with adults or older children. Nevertheless, as with adults, there are four major decisions which should be considered when selecting hearing aids for trial with a youngster. Basic considerations during the preselection of hearing aids include the following: (1) the type of instrument, (2) the frequency response, (3) the arrangement of wearable amplification, and (4) the maximum power output.

Before discussing guidelines for preselecting hearing aids, it should be mentioned that there are two significant trends which influence present day hearing aid recommendation for youngsters. First, children with severe and profound hearing impairments are much younger at the time of initial referral. Secondly, a substantially greater number of children with mild and moderate degrees of hearing loss are being referred for evaluation during the preschool years. As a consequence, hearing aids are being recommended both for younger patients and for children with a good deal of residual hearing. Thus, many of the older concepts regarding wearable amplification for children should continually be re-evaluated and revised.

One major misconception which is still encountered with some regularity is that body aids are best suited for use with all young children regardless of the degree of hearing loss. Yet in the longitudinal study mentioned earlier over one-half of the youngsters were found to be successful users of ear level hearing aids (Matkin, 1971). In most cases behind-the-ear instruments rather than aids in glasses are preferable, especially with younger children. Otherwise, constant problems are encountered with respect to simultaneous adjustment and maintenance of both sensory aids.

There are at least four considerations when making a decision with respect to the preselection of body or ear level aids for trial with children. First, the degree of the hearing loss in the critical frequencies for the perception of speech (250–4000 Hz) should be considered. In recent years, ear level hearing aids have been designed which provide a significantly greater amount of gain than those commercially available in past years. However, at the present time, it is found that if the hearing loss exceeds 75 to 80 dB across the speech frequencies, conventional ear level instruments frequently may not provide optimal gain. With older children who express a strong preference for a head-borne aid despite the severe degree of their impairment, the suitability of a Power CROS (contralateral routing of signals) arrangement should be considered (See Chapter Ten). Finally, in the rare case where a bone conduction vibrator will be recommended due either to the presence of a bilateral atresia or to medical contraindications for ear mold use, the body aid is usually the instrument of choice.

The second consideration when preselecting instruments for clinical trial is the age of the youngster. While there is not agreement with respect to the age at which ear level aids should be considered, it has been our finding that body aids appear most appropriate for most children below the age of 30 months in that parents and teachers are responsible for the manipulation of the instrument. Further, it is often difficult to secure ear level aids on toddlers. Nevertheless, some success in using ear level instruments with moderately hearing-impaired children under 30 months has occurred. When making the initial decision whether to try a body or an ear level aid, another consideration should be the manual dexterity of the youngster under consideration regardless of chronological age. To explain, it is desirable to recommend a body aid for those children with additional motor handicaps so that the child has the opportunity to learn to manipulate the gain control of the instrument at the earliest possible age rather than to promote dependency by having parents or teachers control the hearing aid. Finally, with children for whom the audiologic information is limited, there is a need to choose an instrument which provides maximum flexibility with respect to the electroacoustic response.

To summarize, the degree and configuration of the hearing loss, the age of the child, the manual dexterity of the youngster, and the adequacy of the audiological information and subsequent need for flexibility should all be considered before a basic decision is made whether or not to try body or ear level amplification during the hearing aid evaluation. Thus, the old premise that body-type instruments are most suitable for utilization with all children should be challenged. Both parents and teachers report that, in fact, fewer, not more, problems are encountered in terms of maintenance with ear level instruments.

With respect to the desired frequency response of a hearing aid, contemporary instruments offer a variety of options for electroacoustic modifications of the frequency response. Couple this fact with potential acoustic modifications of the frequency response through earmold changes and the audiologist has a number of alternatives to be considered. Regarding the frequency response, there are at least three major options. First, a conventional frequency response between approximately 350 and 4000 Hz can be provided. Second, extended low frequency amplification can be considered. Finally, a high-pass effect where there is little amplification below 1000 Hz is also a viable option.

One area in which there is a good deal of controversy is with respect to the suitability of selecting an extended low frequency amplifier rather than an instrument with a more limited conventional frequency response. With the development of the electret microphone, it is now possible to provide extended low frequency amplification with ear level as well as with body-type instruments. Certainly a major consideration which merits further research is whether or not providing extended low frequency amplification to those children with a good deal of residual hearing above 1000 Hz results in poorer auditory discrimination of speech due to spread of masking and/or temporal masking effects.

If one reviews the early literature with respect to the development of extended low frequency amplification it will be noted that low frequency emphasis hearing aids were originally designed for those children whose measurable residual hearing was restricted to the lower test frequencies (Ling, 1964). Clinical experience, as well as research investigations, has indicated that extended low frequency amplification often does result in better development of basic receptive and expressive communication skills for such limited hearing children. However, subsequent studies suggest that there may be cases with substantial residual hearing where the use of a hearing aid with an extended low frequency response may result in poorer aided discrimination than would have been obtained with a conventional hearing aid (Danaher and Pickett, 1975); (Sung, Sung, and Angelelli, 1971). Since critical acoustic information below 300 Hz is relatively limited it is this writer's opinion that the utilization of extended low frequency amplification should be restricted to those children with a fragmentary hearing loss, bilaterally. In other words, a more conventional hearing aid response which does not amplify the very low frequencies should be considered for those children with measurable hearing above 1000 Hz.

Obviously, the clinician must also make a decision when selecting an instrument with a conventional frequency response whether it is desirable to set the tone control for a flat response, for high frequency emphasis, or for low frequency emphasis. Such decisions should ultimately be based on aided performance data. To explain, the preferred setting of an instrument tone control can best be determined by considering either a child's optimal discrimination score or, in the case of the very young child, the best aided thresholds across the frequency range from 250 Hz to 3000 Hz.

It should be mentioned that in the past, children manifesting marked bilateral high frequency sensorineural hearing impairments with essentially normal hearing in the lower test frequencies have not been considered as candidates for conventional hearing aid use. In such cases, a hearing aid with a closed earmold often provides an excessive amount of gain in the lower frequencies. However, in recent years, it has been found through the use of open earmolds that a high-pass effect is quite appropriate for such youngsters. Thus, the older misconception that children with so called "ski slope" audiograms such as seen in Figure 9-2 are not candidates for hearing aid use must be re-evaluated since a clinical investigation by Matkin and Thomas (1971a) indicates good success while using HICROS (CROS amplifying system emphasizing high frequencies) instruments with selected cases having such audiometric configurations.*

While successful adjustment to the use of a classic CROS arrangement by pediatric cases having a unilateral loss has been quite disappointing, there are other versions of CROS instruments which merit consideration. With older youngsters having bilateral impairments, both IROS (ipsilateral routing of signals) and BICROS (amplification system made up of one complete hearing aid plus one extra microphone) aids have been found to offer significant benefits in selected cases (See Chapter Ten for further description of such instruments).

A basic premise with respect to the various arrangements of wearable amplification suitable for children is that *any hearing aid arrangement found to be worthwhile with adults should be considered as a possibility for trial use with pediatric cases*. This variety of options is most easily considered by discussing body versus ear level instruments.

With respect to body-type hearing aids, one of three alternatives regarding preselection should be considered. Should the hearing aid initially be

---

* Test results in the example shown in Figure 9-2 and subsequent figures indicated a sensorineural loss. However, bone conduction symbols have been omitted for clarity. In each case, discrimination testing in noise was accomplished at a signal-to-nose ratio of +6 dB.

AUDIOLOGICAL   RECORD

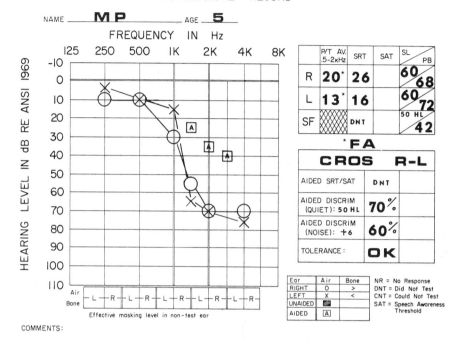

FIG. 9–2. The audiologic data for a 5 year old youngster with a sensorineural hearing impairment who became a successful user of a HICROS (contralateral routing of signals amplifying system emphasizing high frequencies) behind-the-ear instrument. Note the improved aided sensitivity from 1500 to 3000 Hz, as well as improved aided discrimination score at 50 dB HL (decibels hearing level) in quiet. In this audiogram and those which follow, bone conduction thresholds have been omitted for clarity. In each instance when discrimination testing was conducted in noise, the SNR (signal-to-noise ratio) was + 6 dB.

fitted with a single cord, with a Y-cord, or should binaural body aids be used? First, regarding whether to utilize a single cord or a Y-cord, a major decision which merits consideration is the amount of audiologic information that is available for each ear with respect to sensitivity, discrimination, and tolerance. In many very young children where the initial findings are restricted to unaided sound field results it has been found that providing the youngster with a Y-cord is a reasonable approach to minimize the possibility of fitting a single ear with the least potential for responding to amplified sounds. The utilization of the Y-cord is deemed as an appropriate decision only until detailed audiologic information is available for each ear. Another alternative to the use of a Y-cord is to recommend the purchase of two earmolds and to alternate the use of a single cord between ears until parents and teachers perceive either a preference for one ear by the child or improved function with amplified sound directed to a particular ear. Obviously, this latter strategy requires extremely close interaction and communication between the audiologist, teacher, and parents.

In those cases for which substantial audiologic information is available for both ears, the utilization of a single cord seems a reasonable solution. When the initial fitting is to be monaural through the utilization of a body aid with a single receiver, it is most appropriate first to choose the ear in which the hearing loss falls into the so-called area of greatest satisfaction as defined in Chapter Eight. In other words, it is inappropriate always to fit the better ear or always to fit the poorer ear. If both ears fall in the area of greatest satisfaction, consideration should be given to the ear with the better discrimination potential and/or dynamic range. Very often it is worthwhile to initiate hearing aid use for young children with a single instrument until both the youngster and the parents adjust to hearing aid use. After such an adjustment period, a decision must ultimately be made whether or not to evaluate the potential benefits of binaural body aids on at least a trial basis. Unfortunately, solid research data with respect to the formulation of a preselection guideline in this area are lacking. Therefore the decision is often made through a period of trial use with careful observation again by the audiologist, by the teacher or clinician, and by the parents. Ross and associates have developed a rating scale which is useful in systematizing the observations of the child's performance over time with a binaural body aid arrangement (Ross et al., 1974).

It may be far easier to describe the child who will benefit from binaural body aids than it is to describe the hearing loss of children who may not benefit from a binaural fitting. Cases, such as the one illustrated in Figure 9-3, who have measurable hearing through the speech frequencies, who have measurable discrimination in each ear, and who do not manifest a severe tolerance problem do appear to achieve a higher level of auditory development over time when binaural body aids are utilized. In contrast, those youngsters with residual hearing limited to the lower frequencies, who generally function with amplification primarily on a signal/warning level, have not been found to change significantly in aided behavior when a binaural rather than a monaural arrangement is provided. As stated earlier, while both clinicians and parents attest that selected children with severe and profound losses do benefit from two body-borne instruments, guidelines based on objective data are lacking so that these youngsters can be identified and provided with such amplification at the earliest possible age.

With respect to ear level instruments, it is somewhat easier to demonstrate the advantage of binaural instruments. In a noisy environment it is often possible to demonstrate that having an aided ear favorably placed toward the primary speech signal is an advantage to the child. By comparing discrimination scores in noise in the indirect listening situation with a monaural fitting to scores achieved via binaural listening, a substantial improvement in auditory discrimination often can be demonstrated (Olsen

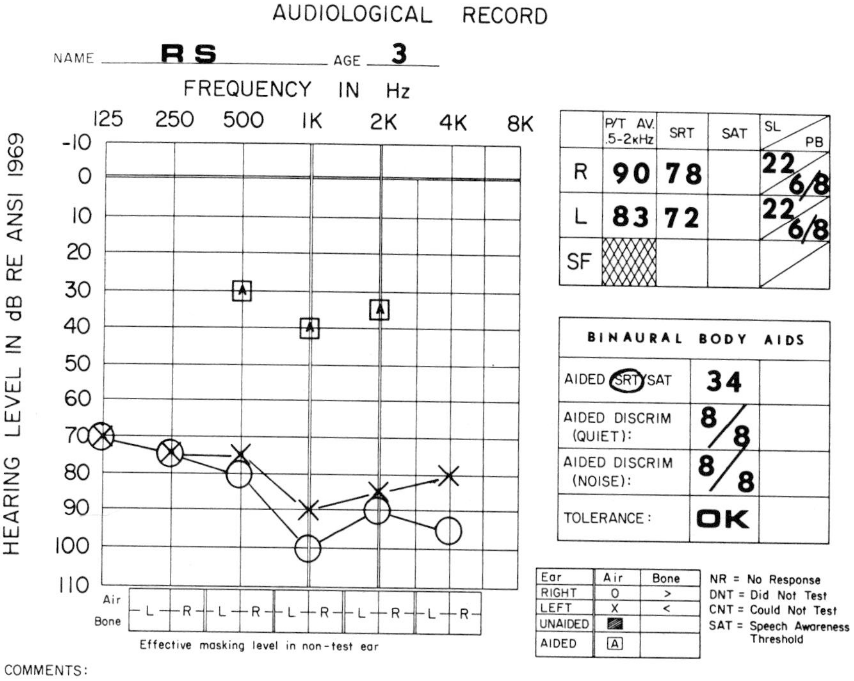

AUDIOLOGICAL   RECORD

NAME ___**R S**___ AGE __**3**__

FIG. 9–3. The audiologic findings for a child who successfully utilized binaural body instruments. Estimated receptive vocabulary age: 20–24 months. Responses were obtained with conditioned play audiometry and TROCA (tangible reinforcement operant conditioning audiometry).

COMMENTS:

and Tillman, 1968). In such cases hearing aid use is often initiated with one ear level instrument during the initial adjustment period before a second hearing aid is provided for trial use. With increased emphasis on integration of hearing-impaired children into the regular classroom it seems important to consider the utilization of binaural ear level amplification wherever possible since such classrooms are typically noisy and highly reverberant. Recent research highlights improved discrimination in noise and reverberant rooms when binaural rather than monaural amplification is available (Nabelek and Pickett, 1974a).

Finally, with respect to children manifesting marked bilateral high frequency impairment, the utilization of open earmolds should be considered. Since acoustic feedback is a major problem encountered with open earmolds in the presence of a marked impairment, the HICROS rather than the IROS arrangement should be considered.

While it is not possible to discuss in detail all of the possible options when selecting various arrangements for hearing aid preselection for children, the guiding premise that has been found useful as previously stated is that any hearing aid arrangement found to be suitable for adults should be considered for use with children. By following such a premise one is not unduly influenced by the prevailing concepts that conventional ear level aids or CROS instruments are not suitable for use with young children.

It is quite important to proceed with caution when considering the maximum power output (MPO) of hearing aids preselected for trial use with children. While neither temporary nor permanent threshold shifts from hearing aid use appear to be common phenomena, there is evidence that the utilization of wearable amplification without regard to MPO can be traumatic in selected cases (Ross and Lerman, 1967). Thus as a general guideline it is strongly recommended that the output of aids be reduced to 130 dB sound pressure level or less, wherever possible. Further, it is imperative, especially when a binaural fitting is to be considered, that provisions be made at the outset for audiologic monitoring during the initial months of hearing aid utilization. In this way, appropriate modifications in hearing aid use can be undertaken immediately if decrements in hearing sensitivity are encountered. For example, after reducing the hearing aid output, the initial strategy may be to revert to a monaural fitting and to alternate hearing aid use between ears on a daily basis with systematic audiologic surveillance.

A further consideration is whether to preselect hearing aids whose output is limited by a peak clipping circuit or through some form of compression amplification. While clinical evidence is lacking upon which to base such a decision, there is good reason to favor the utilization of compression amplification in those cases where a markedly reduced dynamic range was encountered during the audiologic evaluation.

The Hearing Aid Selection

Due to the limited attention span of younger children, it is often necessary to utilize an abbreviated comparison approach to the selection of a suitable hearing aid. In other words, it may only be possible to reliably determine a youngster's performance with two or three different instruments. Ideally, in many pediatric cases, the selection of hearing aids should be scheduled for two appointments rather than for a single clinic visit. In either event, the particular hearing aids preselected from the clinic stock by the audiologist for trial during the hearing aid evaluation become a critical issue. Otherwise, none of the hearing aids tried may yield optimal aided performance. Obviously, the younger the child the more limited will be the performance data upon which to base the final recommendation and the more important ongoing evaluations become. Nevertheless, it is necessary to strive for detailed clinical information in each and every case irrespective of age.

Regarding the actual selection procedure, that is performance tests with the hearing aid, it is desirable to obtain measures of sensitivity, discrimination in quiet, discrimination in competition, and of tolerance before the final decision is made with respect to a hearing aid recommendation. The various behavioral conditioning techniques and discrimination materials discussed above under the section entitled "Audiologic Evaluation" are applicable during the actual selection procedure. It is feasible in many pediatric cases to establish aided thresholds for speech. Also, it has been found extremely valuable, especially in those cases with limited language competence, where discrimination testing is not possible, to establish aided warble tone thresholds across the test frequencies. One can then begin to appreciate the potential advantages and limitation of hearing aid use by considering the aided audiogram in terms of which components of conversational speech will and will not be audible. An overlay transparency upon which the spectrum of conversational speech has been plotted and which can be superimposed upon the aided audiogram has been found useful in understanding which speech sounds will remain inaudible even with the hearing aid.

Again by utilizing a battery of auditory discrimination materials, it is possible in many instances to obtain aided auditory discrimination scores at a normal conversational level (50 dB HL) in a quiet test environment.

By comparing aided sound field results at 50 dB HL with unaided discrimination scores obtained at an optimal listening level, one is better able to determine the adequacy of the particular hearing aid being tried. Furthermore, such data are invaluable when discussing the limitations of hearing aid use with both parents and teachers since the audiologist's primary responsibility should be to set realistic levels of expectation from initial hearing aid use. It must be kept in mind when working with pediatric cases, however, that an unaided discrimination score may, in fact, represent only the child's present developmental level of auditory function, not the ultimate potential for auditory processing. Thus, the importance of ongoing auditory training and teaching cannot be overstressed. Continued audiologic surveillance not only permits the audiologist to assess the effectiveness of such training by monitoring changes in auditory discrimination as the child matures but also provides the opportunity to modify levels of expectation.

The term "level of expectation" refers in this discussion to at least three different levels of auditory function with wearable amplification. Some children when provided with a suitable hearing aid and appropriate training, continue to function primarily as visual learners with auditory input serving the limited purpose of signaling, warning, and self-monitoring. In contrast, other youngsters with amplification essentially come to rely upon a combined visual and auditory input for receptive communicative purposes and language learning. Finally some pediatric cases may function primarily through the aided auditory modality for the understanding of speech with visual input serving a supplemental purpose. By sharing such information with parents, the audiologist provides a more comprehensive overview of the nature and impact of the hearing impairment.

The third essential measure when comparing a youngster's performance with various hearing aids is to establish discrimination scores in the presence of a competing signal. With the contemporary trend in special education of integrating hearing-impaired youngsters into the regular classrooms as early as possible, such performance data becomes critical. The hearing-impaired child with a suitable amplifier may, in fact, function quite adequately in a quiet listening environment. However, the placement of such a youngster in a noisy reverberant classroom may result in inability to adequately process auditory information (Finitzo-Hieber, 1975). It appears that in many cases children with the best potential for auditory learning are placed in educational settings in which they are forced to rely primarily upon visual clues. By citing actual scores when the child attempts to discriminate speech in a noisy listening situation, it is often possible for the audiologist to influence the ultimate placement of the child in terms of the preferred educational setting.

With respect to aided tolerance, it is difficult to establish the level of discomfort in those instances where the child's ability to verbalize auditory experiences is limited. Nevertheless, it becomes important for the audiologist to observe the youngster carefully in terms of overt signs of discomfort, nystagmus, and/or disequilibrium when listening via a hearing aid to speech presented at relatively high levels, such as 80 to 90 dB HL. After a period of hearing aid use, teacher and parent observations in selected cases may be valuable in determining subtle problems of discomfort in that the child reportedly may consistently reduce the recommended gain setting of the aid without any apparent need to do so.

Hearing Aid Recheck

The fifth and final step in the selection of a hearing aid is the hearing aid recheck. The primary purpose of the hearing aid recheck is to assess the adequacy of the child's performance with the actual instrument procured. Secondary considerations during this brief clinic visit include recommendation of the final purchase, if the initial recommendation was for a month's trial-rental period; modification of the initial hearing aid settings, if necessary; assessment of both parent and child attitudes toward hearing aid use; and, ongoing parent education, guidance, and counseling with respect to hearing aid utilization and maintenance. With the cost of commercially available hearing aid test equipment now within the budget of many clinics, the electroacoustic performance of the child's instrument can be determined and recorded for future reference during the hearing aid recheck.

AUDIOLOGIC RE-EVALUATION

Following the hearing aid recheck, periodic audiologic re-evaluations become an important consideration in the total management program. The purpose of such re-evaluations is multifaceted. One apparent reason for evaluating the child over time is to permit the audiologist to maintain surveillance of the hearing aid both in terms of its electroacoustic performance and the child's aided performance. Further, as previously mentioned, it is important to have the opportunity with those youngsters where relatively limited audiologic data were initially available to modify the electroacoustic characteristics and even the type and/or arrangement of the hearing aid as the youngster matures and more precise audiologic measurements can be completed. The findings for such a case are highlighted in Figures 9-4 through 9-7. Another critical reason for scheduling periodic re-evaluations is to monitor and to detect any changes in hearing sensitivity over time. Occasionally, a child is encountered who manifests a

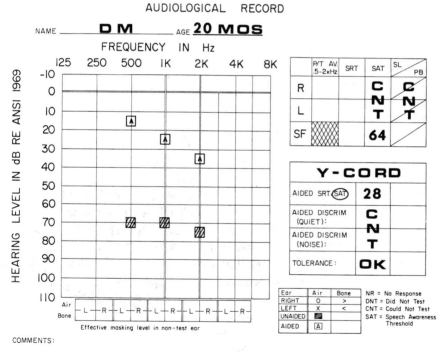

COMMENTS:

FIG. 9-4. Aided and unaided sound field conditioned response data obtained with warble tone audiometry and speech for a 20 month old infant for whom a body instrument with a Y-cord was initially recommended. Responses were obtained with visual reinforcement audiometry.

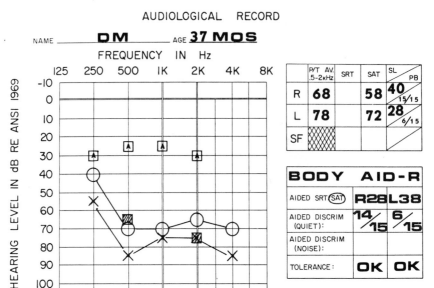

FIG. 9–5. Audiologic findings obtained at 37 months of age, on which the decision was based to modify the hearing aid arrangement from a Y-cord to a single cord to the right ear. Note that both unaided and aided informal testing revealed relatively limited discrimination ability in the left ear. Estimated receptive vocabulary age: 24 months. Responses were obtained with conditioned play audiometry and TROCA (tangible reinforcement operant conditioning audiometry).

significant decrement in auditory function after hearing aid use is initiated even though the MPO of the instrument is restricted (Macrae, 1968). Of equal importance is to permit the audiologist to monitor the child's development after the initiation of hearing aid utilization with respect to the original levels of expectation that were established. Finally, it is critical that the audiologist have the opportunity to assess both the attitude and acceptance of hearing aid utilization by the child and his parents over time. In many cases it is found that repeated sessions with parents are needed before the youngster becomes a successful full time hearing aid user.

Careful attention should be given to the schedule upon which periodic re-evaluations will be maintained. Obviously there are numerous issues which will influence such a schedule including the adequacy of the initial audiologic information, initial parent attitude and, finally, the adequacy of the child's educational and training program. A reasonable approach, especially when hearing aid use is initiated at a very young age, is to schedule re-evaluations every 3 months during the first year of hearing aid use. During the 2nd year, reassessments should be scheduled every 6 months. If all goes well, it is then realistic to schedule re-evaluations on a yearly basis until the child reaches the age of 5 or 6. Thereafter, it is worthwhile to re-evaluate the child in terms of auditory status and hearing aid performance at least every 2 years.

PARENT MANAGEMENT

Before concluding this chapter, a brief consideration of the audiologist's role in dealing with parents of a hearing-impaired child is essential. While it is widely recognized that the involvement and support of the parents in the management of any handicapped child is critical, it is my belief that this essential aspect of audiologic management has not been carefully analyzed. Frequently, parent counseling is used as a generic term to cover a very wide range of professional activities. It is worthwhile to view the audiologist's interaction with parents in terms of parent education, parent guidance, and parent counseling. While it is apparent that such activities are not mutually exclusive, it is helpful to make such a distinction when

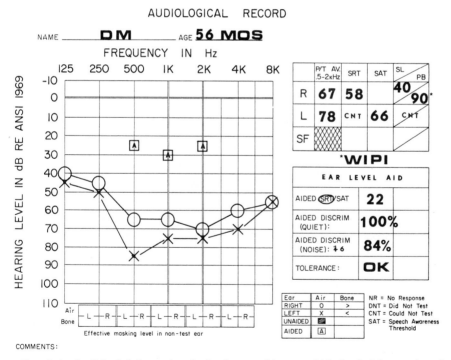

COMMENTS:

FIG. 9–6. Audiologic information obtained at age 4¹/₂ upon which the decision was based to recommend an ear level instrument for the right ear. Note the marked difference in the unaided discrimination ability between the two ears. Responses were obtained with conditioned play audiometry.

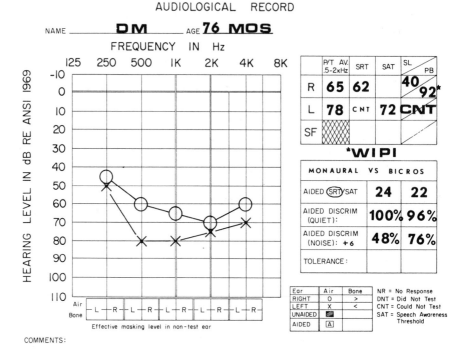

FIG. 9–7. Audiologic findings from which the decision was made to modify the monaural ear level instrument to a BICROS (amplification system made up of one complete hearing aid plus one extra microphone) aid. The discrimination test in noise involved "monaural indirect" listening. That is, the speech originated from the left side, opposite from the side of the aided ear. During the one month trial/rental period, both the teacher and parents noted better receptive auditory communication in certain listening situations which substantiated the improved aided discrimination performance in competition recorded during the audiologic re-evaluation.

attempting to evaluate, modify, and improve the provision of clinical services.

With respect to the topic under consideration, clinical experience has substantiated numerous reports in the literature which indicate that many children are wearing hearing aids that are not functioning properly (Gaeth and Lounsbury, 1966; Porter, 1973; Zink, 1972). In my opinion, the audiologist should assume the primary responsibility for parent education regarding both hearing aid use and maintenance of the instrument. Such orientation is a time-consuming endeavor when undertaken on an individual basis. In other words, a good deal of time is required to teach parents adequately how to troubleshoot a hearing aid and how to complete a daily listening check. In an effort to assure consistency with respect to parent education and yet to utilize time wisely, a clinical investigation was completed in which an automated instructional program of narration and slides was incorporated into the clinic routine (Matkin and Thomas, 1973). In this way, parents were actively involved in learning about the basics of hearing aids and their care during the clinical visit rather than sitting idle in the waiting room. In the majority of families, such an approach has been found to be effective in preparing parents to maintain constant surveillance of their child's instrument. It is apparent that the ultimate success in hearing aid utilization by a child is often directly related to parental attitude and education. Further, it appears that a good deal of basic parent education with regard to such information as an understanding of the advantages and limitations of hearing aid use as well as the troubleshooting of a hearing aid can be effectively conveyed through the utilization of programmed instruction.

By developing programmed materials, the audiologist can then more effectively utilize time to discuss with parents specific audiologic findings and recommendations with respect to the particular child under study. Parental guidance becomes more effective since a basic foundation of information has already been acquired by the parents through the "sound on slides" program. Consequently, the audiologist has a good deal more time to devote to guidance and counseling rather than to basic education.

While parent counseling in the narrow sense of the word has always been considered as one aspect of clinical audiologic endeavors, it has come to be realized that as a profession we have not always been sensitive to the emotional impact on the family that having an impaired youngster creates. Without professional support, many of the audiologic and educational recommendations will not be followed and, as a consequence, primary steps toward habilitation may be delayed during critical periods of growth and development. In brief, the audiologist must not only be willing to undertake parent education and guidance but must also be prepared to deal with parents in terms of their psychologic response when told that their child is permanently hearing impaired and that a hearing aid is needed. At the same time, the audiologist must be aware of his or her own limitations in professional training and be prepared to make appropriate referrals for counseling of those families in crisis or with limited coping behavior.

It is well to keep in mind that a hearing impairment is essentially a hidden handicap only until the time when an individual begins to utilize wearable amplification. Thus, it is not surprising in some instances to find that parents, who seemingly had accepted the fact that their youngster had a hearing handicap, react negatively when the time comes for them to participate actively in a hearing aid orientation and utilization program. In summary, a primary responsibility of the audiologist should be to assure support of the parent by incorporating aspects of parent education, and guidance and counseling activities into ongoing audiologic services.

RECOMMENDED READINGS†

HEARING AIDS FOR CHILDREN

BELLEFLEUR, P., AND VAN DYKE, R., The effects of high gain amplification on children in a residential school for the deaf. *J. Speech Hear. Res.*, 11, 343–347 (1968).

BENDER, R., AND WIIG, E., Binaural hearing aids for young children. *Volta Rev.*, 62, 113–115 (1960).

BLAIR, J., The contributing influences of amplification, speech reading and classroom environments on the ability of hard of hearing children to discriminate sentences. Doctoral Dissertation, Northwestern University (1976).

BOOTHROYD, A., Stereophonic amplification for severely and profoundly deaf children. *Audiology*, 11, 140 (1972).

BRICKER, D., AND BRICKER, W., A programmed approach to operant audiometry for low-functioning children. *J. Speech Hear. Dis.*, 34, 312–320 (1969).

CARHART, R., The advantages and limitations of a hearing aid. *Minn. Med.*, 50, 823–826 (1967).

CASTLE, W. (Ed.), Hearing aid procurement and characteristics: Procedures for children. A conference on hearing aid evaluation procedures. *A.S.H.A Reports*, Number 2, 14–38 (1967).

DOWNS, M., The establishment of hearing aid use: A program for parents. *Maico Audiological Library Series*, 4, Report 5 (1966).

ELLIOT, L., AND ARMBRUSTER, V., Some possible effects of the delay of early treatment of deafness. *J. Speech Hear. Res.*, 10, 209–224 (1967).

ELLIOT, L., AND VEGELY, A., Some possible effects of the delay of early treatment of deafness: A second look. *J. Speech Hear. Res.*, 11, 833–841 (1968).

ERBER, N., Evaluation of special hearing aids for deaf children. *J. Speech Hear. Dis.*, 36, 527–537 (1971).

FISHER, B., An investigation of binaural hearing aids. *J. Laryngol. Otol.*, 78, 658–668 (1964).

JOHANSSON, R., The use of the transposer for the management of the deaf child. *J. Int. Audiol.*, 5, 362–372 (1966).

KOENIG, W., Subjective effects in binaural hearing. *J. Acoust. Soc. Am.*, 22, 61–62 (1950).

KUYPER, P., AND DE BOER, E., Evaluation of stereophonic fitting of hearing aids to hard of hearing children. *J. Int. Audiol.*, 9, 524–528 (1969).

LECKIE, D., AND LING, D., Audibility with hearing aids having low frequency characteristics. *Volta Rev.*, 70, 83–85 (1968).

LEWIS, D., AND GREEN, R., Value of binaural hearing aids for hearing impaired children in elementary schools. *Volta Rev.*, 64, 537–542 (1962).

LING, D., Conventional hearing aids: An overview. *Audecibel*, 21, 80–93 (1972).

LUTERMAN, D., Binaural hearing aids for pre-school deaf children. *Maico Audiological Library Series*, 8, Report 3 (1969).

MATKIN, N., AND THOMAS, J., A longitudinal study of visual reinforcement audiometry. Presentation: American Speech and Hearing Association (1974).

McDONALD, E., *Understand Those Feelings*. Pittsburgh, Stanwix House (1962).

ROSS, M., Hearing aid selection for young hearing impaired children: A point of view. *Maico Audiological Library Series*, 9, Report 1 (1970).

ROSS, M., Classroom acoustics and speech intelligibility. *Handbook of Clinical Audiology*. Baltimore: Williams & Wilkins, Chapter 40, pp. 756–777 (1972).

ROSS, M., Hearing aid selection for the preverbal hearing impaired child. *Amplification for the Hearing-Impaired*. New York: Grune and Stratton, Chapter 6, 207–242 (1975).

ROSS, M., AND LERMAN, J., A picture identification test for hearing impaired children. *J. Speech Hear. Dis.*, 13, 44–53 (1970).

---

† References cited in this chapter are included in the Bibliography at the end of the book.

SANDERS, D., Noise conditions in normal school classrooms. *Except. Child*, 31, 344–353 (1965).

SORTINI, A., Importance of individual hearing aids and early therapy for preschool children. *J. Speech Hear. Dis.*, 24, 346–353 (1959).

STAAB, W., Warble tone audiometry. *Maico Audiological Library Series*, 11, Report 1 (1972).

WHETNALL, E., Binaural hearing. *J. Laryngol.*, 78, 1079–1089 (1964).

WHETNALL, E., The question of the critical period. *Acta. Otolaryngol.*, Supplement 206 (1965).

special cases of hearing aid assessment: CROS aids

William R. Hodgson, Ph.D.

INTRODUCTION

The initials, CROS, stand for "contralateral routing of signals." Initially, CROS referred to an amplification system in which signals picked up on one side of the head were routed to the ear on the other side. The original purpose was to afford hearing from both sides of the head for those with unilateral loss. Currently, CROS may refer either to such a system or be used generically to refer to a family of hearing aid types. This family includes aids which route signals contralaterally for reasons other than unilateral loss, and others which amplify ipsilaterally but use the open (non-occluding) earmold popularized by CROS.

CROS aids were first recommended by astute clinicians who were concerned about the problems of people with unilateral hearing loss. Historically, the hearing difficulty experienced by unilaterals has been underestimated. This error resulted because clinical tests and observations are usually done in quiet, under good listening conditions, where unilaterals perform well. As a result, authorities reported that people with unilateral loss are not seriously handicapped (Newby, 1958; Carson, 1960).

Nevertheless, unilaterals kept complaining. They said they had trouble locating the source of sounds. They reported trouble understanding speech in noise. Sometimes they complained that their acoustic environment was unbalanced; that they had the sensation of a live side and a dead side. They indicated they had trouble, under poor listening conditions, when head movement was restricted and they were forced to listen with their head between their good ear and the signal source. A common example of the latter problem occurs when a unilateral is in a noisy restaurant sitting at a table between two friends. The unilateral will always place the speaker he cares less about hearing on the side of his poor ear.

THE HEAD SHADOW

Many of the unilateral's problems result from the head shadow. This effect arises whenever the head is more or less interposed between the good ear and the signal source. Chance dictates that this condition will obtain about half the time, unless the unilateral takes pains to prevent it. Indeed, unilaterals attempt to orient themselves favorably, but when they cannot, the head shadow effect may reduce their listening ability.

The magnitude of the head shadow is determined by the azimuth and the frequency of the signal to which the unilateral is listening. Figure 10-1 shows the effect of the head shadow on pure-tone threshold. The data points represent monaural threshold relative to the threshold at 0° azimuth. For a low frequency tone, 300 Hz, there is little difference in threshold as the sound source moves around the head. For progressively higher frequencies the head shadow grows, and is greater than 15 dB at 3200 Hz. At the same time an enhancement, or head baffle, effect grows when the tone is on the side of the good ear, reaching a maximum of just less than 5 dB.

The effect of the head shadow on speech threshold was established by Tillman, Kasten, and Horner (1963). They found a mean difference of 6.4 dB in thresholds for spondees of 24 subjects, between monaural direct and indirect conditions. In the latter condition, the subject's head was between the sound source and the functioning ear. Thus, the overall reduction in the intensity of speech caused by the head shadow is approximately 6 dB. Kasten, Lotterman, and Hinchman (1967–68) measured the effect of the head on ear level hearing aids. They reported that both shadow and baffle effect increase with an increase in frequency, but that the magnitude of the baffle effect was negligible. They concluded that the position of the hearing aid microphone contributed differentially to the head shadow effect.

The head shadow can have a considerable effect on the intelligibility of low intensity speech. A monaural listener, with his good ear unfavorably situated, may suffer substantially because of the reduction in effective sensation level or the degradation of signal-to-noise ratio. For example, Tillman and Carhart (1966) found that the articulation curve of the Northwestern University no. 6 discrimination test was linear up to a sensation level of 9 dB, and rose at a slope of 5.6% per decibel. If the magnitude of the

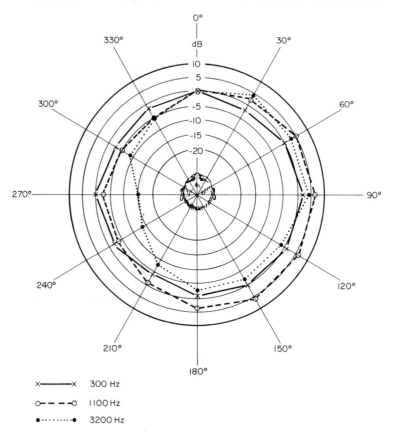

Fig. 10-1. The head shadow effect. At 0° the subject faces the sound source. At 90° the open ear faces the sound source. Data from Sivian and White (1933).

head shadow is 6.4 dB then in theory the difference between listening directly and indirectly to very soft speech could be as much as 5.6 × 6.4, or 35.84%. In the above example, "listening directly" means with the good ear toward the sound source, and "listening indirectly" means with the good ear away from it. Experimental evidence is available regarding this subject; experimenters have simulated the conditions mentioned above. Nordlund and Fritzell (1963) reported a decrease in intelligibility of 21 to 23% between direct and indirect listening. Kasten and Tillman (1964) found a maximum difference of 29% for subjects with sensorineural hearing loss under conditions simulating aided direct and indirect listening. Of course, these differences would not obtain if the subject were able to move his head at will.

HEARING AIDS THAT REDUCE THE EFFECT OF THE HEAD SHADOW

In spite of the prevailing opinion that unilaterals did not experience much hearing difficulty, and that they could not benefit from amplification, their continued complaints led to experimentation. At first these efforts explored the use of amplification directly on the impaired ear.

Binaural Hearing with One Hearing Aid

Bergman (1957) and Haskins and Hardy (1960) suggested that unilaterals might benefit from a hearing aid to restore presumed benefits of binaural hearing. Malles (1963) reported improved discrimination in noise for 8 unilaterals when they wore hearing aids. He did not indicate, however, whether the head shadow was considered in the placement of his subjects during the aided versus the unaided condition, or in calculation of the signal-to-noise ratio.

Harford and Musket (1964a) coined the acronym, BOHA: binaural hearing with one hearing aid. They reported improved discrimination in 3 of 8 aided unilaterals when PB lists were directed toward their aided ears, in comparison with an identical unaided condition. The intensity of the speech was 70 dB SPL (sound pressure level). In spite of the fact that a clear improvement in aided discrimination did not occur for the other 5 subjects, all 8 were regular hearing aid wearers. The authors attribute their findings to restoration of binaural hearing. Kasten and Tillman (1964), investigating the effects of azimuth on monaural and binaural speech discrimination, concluded that binaural superiority was primarily attributable to the reduction of the head shadow effect afforded by that condition as opposed to monaural listening. Stated differently, the listener with two ears seldom has to listen with his head in the way, and this advantage results in a substantial improvement in discrimination. An example of a case who benefited from BOHA is shown in Figure 10-2.

In spite of the favorable results reported in some instances, not many people with unilateral loss wear an aid directly on their impaired ear, since the causes of many unilateral losses render the poor ear unfit for hearing aid use. Another method had to be found to help the majority of unilaterals.

Contralateral Routing of Signals

Many unilaterals have an unaidable ear. That is, either the ear is dead or auditory discrimination ability is too poor for hearing aid use. To reduce the effect of the head shadow, such individuals may utilize the principle shown in Figure 10-3. With this arrangement, the microphone is placed on the side of the poor ear, usually in the temple bar of eyeglasses. The signal from the microphone is carried electrically to the good ear. There it is amplified slightly and changed back to sound energy. In routine fashion, a tube carries the sound into the good ear. Instead of a standard earmold, which occludes the ear canal, an open—non-occluding—mold is used. Sometimes, no earmold is used at all; the polyethylene sound tube being

AUDIOLOGICAL RECORD

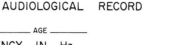

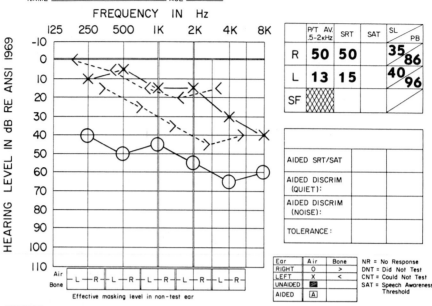

COMMENTS:

FIG. 10-2. An example of Binaural Hearing with one hearing aid (BOHA). In sound field testing, with the good ear covered, the SRT (speech reception threshold) unaided was 45 dB; aided, 25 dB. Discrimination scores, at a presentation level of 70 dB SPL (sound pressure level), were 32% unaided, 76% aided.

shaped to fit into the ear canal. Either way, the canal remains open. Thus the listener hears sound from the side of his poor ear via the hearing aid, and from the side of his good ear unamplified sound enters directly. He hears sound from both sides of his head although in only one ear. The undesirable effects of the head shadow are circumvented.

The term CROS — contralateral routing of signals — was first used by Harford and Barry (1965). Actually, the CROS principle was first utilized for purposes unrelated to the wearer's hearing loss. The first ear level aids were large in size and were also prone to feedback. To alleviate these problems, a CROS arrangement was sometimes used, placing the microphone on one side of the head and the receiver on the other. There are other reports in the early literature describing some of the principles of CROS. Fowler (1960) was concerned with restoring binaural hearing to those with bilateral loss and one ear too poor to benefit from a hearing aid. He suggested adding a microphone on the side of the unaidable ear to carry a signal to a conventional hearing aid. This principle was later termed BICROS. Wullenstein and Wigand (1962) adapted Fowler's device to use for unilaterals by removing the microphone on the side of the good ear.

Schaudinischky (1965) described a CROS-type aid in which the microphone was placed in the ear canal of the wearer's poor ear. He felt this placement was important to utilize the sound collecting and the orienting properties of the outer ear. From the microphone, signals were transmitted electrically across the head to feed a bone conduction receiver on the side of the good ear. This arrangement left the good ear open to receive unamplified signals. Schaudinischky reported improved localization ability in 8 subjects with unilateral loss. Miller (1965a) reported successful use of an aid worn on the poor ear with plastic tubing carrying the signal across the head to a vented earmold on the good ear. There are two reports of CROS aids improving localizing ability in blind individuals with unilateral loss (Conkey and Schneiderman, 1968; Rintelmann, Harford, and Burchfield, 1970).

A series of reports from Northwestern University explored the practicality of the CROS aid. In the germinal article, Harford and Barry (1965) reported the experiences of two groups of unilaterals. Group I had normal hearing in the good ear and group II had a slight hearing loss in the good ear. As a generalization, improvement in aided threshold and discrimination could be demonstrated clinically for subjects in group II, but not in group I. Nevertheless, after a period of trial use, 17 of the 20 subjects making up the two groups indicated improved performance with the CROS aid. On their own initiative, 7 of the 20 bought and successfully used CROS

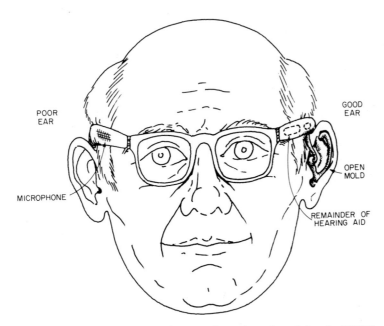

FIG. 10-3. Typical arrangement for contralateral routing of signals (CROS).

aids (2 from group I and 5 from group II). The following conclusions were reached regarding the candidacy of a unilateral for a CROS aid.

Motivation of the patient is crucial, as are the demands on his hearing, and his listening environment. An individual with only moderate demands on his hearing, or one who functions mostly in easy listening situations needs a hearing aid less and is less likely to tolerate the nuisance of an aid. Conversely, unilaterals with critical demands on their hearing, or those who must listen under more adverse conditions, are more likely to need and use a CROS aid. However, there is a point of diminishing returns. That is, if the person functions most of the time under *really* difficult listening conditions, benefit from the aid may be so minimal that acceptance is not likely. Further, the authors concluded that the better the hearing is in the individual's good ear, the less likely he is to need and use a CROS aid. Finally, they indicated that formal tests cannot evaluate improvement in some cases, and that a period of trial use is always indicated. Figure 10-4 shows the audiogram of an ideal CROS user.

A followup study by Harford and Dodds (1966) corroborated the conclu-

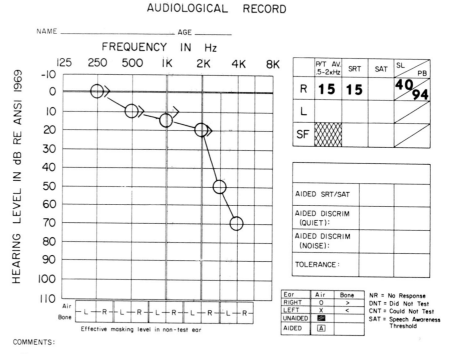

FIG. 10-4. An example of CROS. There is no audiometric response on the left ear. In sound field testing, monaural indirect for the unaided condition — the signal originating from the patient's left side — the SRT (speech reception threshold) unaided was 20 dB; aided 15 dB. Discrimination scores at a presentation level of 60 dB SPL (sound pressure level) were 70% unaided; 90% aided.

sions related above. In this report, the authors also considered the use of CROS aids by children with unilateral loss. They were not optimistic, feeling that motivation might often be a problem and that the child's most demanding listening environment—school—constitutes a structured listening situation in which the effects of unilateral loss can be mitigated by preferential seating. Subsequent clinical experience has confirmed that children with unilateral loss are not likely to be satisfied CROS users, as did a report by Matkin and Thomas (1971b).

The practicality of CROS amplification was assessed by Aufricht (1972), who sent a questionnaire to 60 male veterans who had been issued CROS aids because of unilateral loss. Of the 54 who replied, 85% wore the CROS aid and liked it. Fifteen per cent neither liked it nor wore it. The subjects' comments were reminiscent of those made by wearers of conventional aids. CROS amplification was reported most helpful in conversational speech, least helpful in noise.

The CROS aid need not be built into eyeglasses. Figure 10-5 shows two

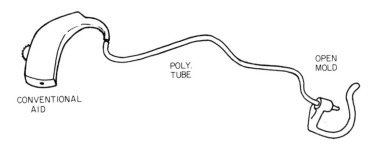

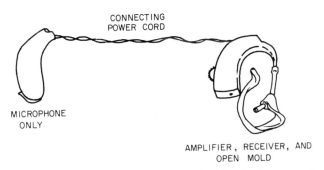

Fig. 10-5. Two alternative arrangements for CROS aids. *Top*, acoustic CROS. *Bottom*, electric CROS.

alternatives. In an acoustic CROS, the tube transmits sound from the aid to the good ear, where it is held in place by an open earmold. This arrangement may have acoustic and cosmetic penalties. A preferable alternative is to house the microphone in a hearing aid case which rests on the poor ear and to transmit the signal electrically via a cord which passes behind the head to the other hearing aid components in a case on the good ear.

Bilateral Amplification with One Hearing Aid

Harford (1966) used BICROS to refer to an amplification system made up of one complete hearing aid plus one extra microphone. BICROS is intended for individuals with loss in both ears, but with one ear unaidable. The extra microphone is placed on the side of the unaidable ear, and transmits a signal from that side of the head to the aidable ear. At the same time amplification is provided in routine fashion for sounds reaching the aidable ear directly. Thus one system provides amplification and reduces the effect of the head shadow as well. Harford classifies unaidable ears as follows: (1) an ear with complete loss or loss of such magnitude that amplification is not feasible, (2) an ear with speech discrimination ability too poor to benefit from amplification, (3) an ear in which medical problems contraindicate use of an earmold, or (4) an ear with a tolerance problem so marked as to preclude normal amplification.

BICROS is usually built into eyeglasses, with the off-side microphone located in the temple bar on the side of the unaidable ear. An arrangement such as that shown in Fig. 10-5 (*bottom*) may also be used, with the addition of a microphone to the apparatus on the side of the aidable ear. Because of the ipsilateral microphone, use of a standard earmold is usually necessary to avoid feedback. The audiogram of a typical candidate for BICROS is shown in Figure 10-6.

EFFECT OF THE OPEN EARMOLD

The original purpose of the non-occluding earmold used with CROS was to allow unamplified sound to enter the unilateral's normal ear. The open earmold alters the electroacoustic characteristics of the hearing aid, and this fact has provided a considerable dividend. The use of the open earmold has expanded beyond its original purpose and led to a series of innovative amplifying systems.

On Electroacoustic Characteristics

Feeding the hearing aid signal into an open ear canal causes loss of low frequency energy. Lybarger (1967) estimates that amplification below 1000 Hz is almost eliminated, whereas frequencies above 2000 Hz are enhanced. Lybarger's measurements were made with a coupler simulating an open

AUDIOLOGICAL   RECORD

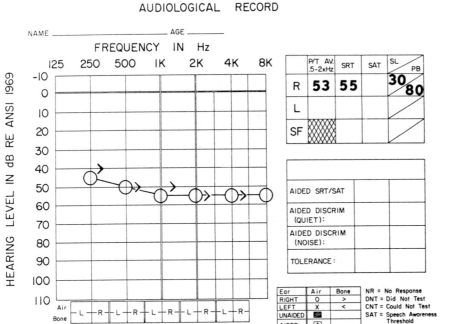

COMMENTS:

FIG. 10-6. Example of bilateral amplification with one hearing aid (BICROS). There is no audiometric response on the left ear.

ear canal. Green and Ross (1968) obtained aided sound field Bekesy threshold tracings on a subject using a standard and an open earmold. With the open mold, thresholds were markedly poorer for all frequencies below 2000 Hz.

Two studies looked at the effect of the open earmold in more detail. McDonald and Studebaker (1970) inserted a probe-tube microphone assembly into the ear canals of 8 subjects. They then measured the effects of different earmolds upon SPL in the canal at selected discrete frequencies. Weatherton and Goetzinger (1971) required 5 normal hearing subjects to trace discrete frequency Bekesy thresholds, using a hearing aid receiver coupled to different earmolds. Results of these studies are shown in Table 10-1. Clearly, the effect of the open earmold, in addition to permitting audition of unamplified sound, is to reduce low frequency amplification.

On Speech Threshold

Regardless of the altered frequency response, studies indicate that there are only small differences between aided thresholds obtained from subjects using standard and open earmolds. Dodds and Harford (1968a) reported average thresholds 3.4 dB poorer for sensorineural subjects with high

TABLE 10-1. **The effect of an open earmold**

	Frequency in HZ				
Mean attenuation in dB, relative to response with standard earmold	250	500	1000	2000	4000
McDonald and Studebaker	40	24	22	0	3
Weatherton and Goetzinger	28	23	11	7	8

TABLE 10-2. **Comparison of discrimination scores obtained unaided and aided using standard and open earmolds**

Study	Type of Loss	Unaided under Phones	Aided	
			Standard	Open
Dodds and Harford (1968)	Sloping S/N*	67.7%	71.4%	81.4%
Hodgson and Murdock (1970)	Sloping S/N	71.89%	79.33%	84.66%
Jetty and Rintelmann (1970)	Flat conductive	95%	92.6%	93.6%
	Sharply falling S/N	69.4%	76.8%	87.0%
	Gradually falling S/N	79.6%	75.0%	80.0%

* S/N, sensorineural.

frequency loss and an average slope of 20 dB per octave across the speech range. Hodgson and Murdock (1970) found a 3 dB difference in the same direction for a similar group of subjects. Jetty and Rintelmann (1970) found the following differences: For subjects with flat conductive loss, the average speech threshold was 1.7 dB poorer with use of open earmolds. However, for subjects with sharply sloping sensorineural loss (25 dB per octave across the speech range), the average threshold was 2.0 dB better with the open mold. For subjects with gradually sloping sensorineural loss (about 7 dB per octave), thresholds obtained with the use of standard molds averaged 2.0 dB better. These studies indicate that the deterioration in aided speech threshold resulting from use of an open earmold does not pose a significant problem.

On Speech Discrimination

The greatest dividend obtained from the open earmold is enhancement of auditory discrimination ability. Several studies have compared aided intelligibility using the open mold with unaided discrimination and with scores obtained using standard earmolds. The results from these studies are summarized in Table 10-2. In general, subjects with high frequency loss performed better with open earmolds than with standard molds, or when unaided. Subjects with flat loss performed about the same for all three conditions. Presumably, the superiority of the open mold for subjects with high frequency loss is related to two conditions. First, the open mold affords more comfortable listening to those with high frequency loss because of its attenuation of low frequency amplification. The subject can, therefore, without discomfort increase the gain of his hearing aid and obtain greater amplification of high frequency signals, where his need is greatest. Second, unaided audition of low frequency signals afforded by the unoccluded ear canal results in better fidelity and greater intelligibility.

Subjective Effects

It has been widely reported that subjects with high frequency loss prefer open earmolds to standard. A survey by Dodds and Harford (1970), resulted in the conclusion that, for people with high frequency loss, those who use open earmolds are more likely to wear their aids full time than those with standard earmolds. Of 18 subjects evaluated by Hodgson and Murdock (1970) in a study using open and standard earmolds, 12 preferred the open, and none preferred the standard mold. In general, these subjects with high frequency sensorineural loss indicated that speech was more comfortable, clearer, or more natural when using the open mold. Bresson (1971) reported that 200 patients nearly unanimously stated that their situation had improved when they changed from standard to open earmolds. These individuals were mostly presbycusics or had noise-induced loss. They indicated that with open earmolds, they could hear and understand better in meetings, became less tired than previously, and were less troubled with canal humidity and irritation.

HEARING AIDS THAT UTILIZE THE HEAD SHADOW

The advantages listed above that accrue from use of the open earmold justify its use in patients with high frequency loss. Except for those with the mildest of losses, however, feedback becomes a problem when a regular at-the-ear aid is used with an open mold. CROS aids place the head between microphone and receiver and reduce the feedback problem. CROS aids used for this purpose are called HICROS.

Historically, individuals with normal hearing sensitivity to 500 or 1000 Hz, and sharply falling bilateral high frequency loss, have been considered poor hearing aid candidates. Representing the classic example of the person who "hears but does not always understand," these cases have complained of discomfort and excessive noise resulting from amplification. Use of the open earmold has sharply modified their reaction to amplification. Patients have reported more comfortable amplification and better practical discrimination ability mediated by increased high frequency gain without tolerance problems. They also experience clearer, more natural sounding speech. Successful clinical application of HICROS with adult patients has been reported by Green (1969), Dodds and Harford (1970), and Bresson (1971); and by Matkin and Thomas (1971b) with children.

The following case history illustrates the unique problems of the person with high frequency loss, and the benefits obtainable from HICROS. The patient, a priest, had a precipitous loss above 750 Hz, and very poor auditory discrimination ability. His audiogram is shown in Figure 10-7. His speech was good except for a severe /s/ distortion. He was a good speech reader, and reported an overwhelming communication handicap only in the confessional, where soft speech and lack of visual clues incapacitated him. He was fitted with a high frequency emphasis CROS aid utilizing an open earmold. The microphone was placed on the right side and the signal fed to the left ear. He did not require vision correction, and elected not to use eyeglass frames for housing the hearing aid. He selected the arrangement shown in Figure 10-5 (*bottom*). He anticipated wearing the aid only in the confessional.

A week after acquiring the aid he returned to the clinic reporting little if any help. It was found that, in the process of putting the aid on, he had

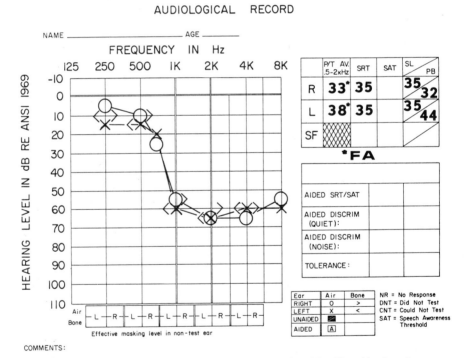

FIG. 10-7. Example of a high frequency CROS aid (HICROS). The aid microphone was located on the right side of the head, sending a signal to the left ear. Aided, with the signal originating on the right at a presentation level of 70 dB SPL (sound pressure level), the discrimination score was 64%.

bent backward the portion of the sound tube that extended beyond the open earmold. Thus, instead of extending into the ear canal, the tube had been permanently crimped backward into the concha. The result was little or no amplification. The problem was corrected and the patient given practice in replacing and removing the aid. When seen again in 2 weeks, he was enthusiastic. He had expanded use of the aid to general listening situations. He reported that, in addition to better intelligibility of the speech of others, he could monitor his own speech better. He was particularly happy about the increased audibility of the /s/ sound, which he knew he did not articulate well. He reported no tolerance problems and required no further orientation to the use of the aid. This individual, who almost certainly would have had extreme problems adjusting to a conventional hearing aid, quickly became a satisfied and effective HICROS user.

CLINICAL EVALUATION OF CROS-TYPE HEARING AIDS

In their original CROS article, Harford and Barry (1965) reported the following procedure for clinical evaluation. Sound field speech thresholds and discrimination scores were obtained unaided and aided. For both conditions, speech signals originated from a loudspeaker located on the side of the subject's poor ear and at an azimuth of 45° from midline of the subject's head. For discrimination testing presentation level was 70 dB SPL. For subjects with normal hearing in the good ear, aided threshold was better than unaided, but there was no difference in discrimination scores. The effective sensation level of speech reaching the poor ear was sufficient for maximum discrimination ability in spite of the head shadow. For subjects with slight hearing loss in the good ear, the aided condition resulted in significantly improved speech thresholds and discrimination scores. Even so, the authors concluded that whether or not clinical evaluation indicated improvement, the most meaningful approach to recommendation regarding a CROS aid is an actual period of trial use. Such trial is influenced by the user's needs and motivations, critical determinants of successful CROS use.

Lotterman and Kasten (1971) conducted a study aimed at developing procedures for evaluation of the CROS aid. They assessed sound field discrimination in noise for 20 unilaterals, unaided and wearing a CROS aid. Conditions varied from most favorable for unaided listening (speech directed toward the good ear; noise toward the poor) to most favorable for aided listening (speech directed toward the poor ear, where the aid's microphone is located; noise directed toward the good ear). They found an inverse relationship between unaided and aided listening. That is, under those conditions where the unilaterals did well unaided they did poorly aided, and vice versa. Because of the location of the CROS aid's microphone, the unilateral finds when listening in noise that the situation which is relatively good unaided becomes relatively poor aided. Stated differently, the CROS-aided unilateral has no effective head shadow, and noise originating from the side of his poor ear is amplified and directed into his good ear, reducing the intelligibility of speech entering his good ear directly.

Navarro and Vogelson (1974) reported the clinical assessment of a CROS aid with one 9 year old subject who had a unilateral loss. The subject's poor ear was directed toward the loudspeaker, and low intensity speech was presented. The unaided discrimination score was 64%, and the aided score was 96%. These studies indicate the practicality of clinical evaluation of CROS, and also emphasize the potential disadvantage of CROS amplification under certain listening conditions.

Clinical hearing aid evaluation of CROS should serve two purposes; to assess improvement with the hearing aid, and to demonstrate that improvement to the patient. The following procedure should accomplish those purposes, by measuring auditory behavior under extremes of acoustic conditions and comparing unaided versus aided performance. It should work equally well for evaluation of CROS or HICROS. First, unaided versus aided discrimination in quiet should be measured. The speech should originate from a loud-speaker located on the side of the head where the hearing aid microphone will be placed. That would be the side of the poor ear in the case of the unilateral. The presentation level should be sufficiently low to render the head shadow a hazard to intelligibility. For unilaterals, under the unaided condition, speech should reach the far ear at a sensation level less than 25 dB, an intensity which approximates PB Max for normals. For patients with high frequency loss, where the effect of the head shadow is not being assessed, the speech in the unaided condition should be audible but not maximally intelligible. A sensation level of 30 dB re: SRT (speech reception threshold) of the better ear would probably be appropriate in most cases. Comparison of unaided and aided discrimination ability will measure and demonstrate for unilaterals the effect of removing the head shadow. For those with high frequency loss, it will measure and demonstrate the added intelligibility afforded by high frequency amplification.

A second clinical procedure should assess unaided and aided discrimination in noise, with speech originating on the side where the aid's microphone will be placed, and the noise on the side of the aid's receiver. This condition will result in amplified speech and unamplified noise, or at least the amplification of the noise will be reduced by the magnitude of the head shadow. For both unilaterals and those with high frequency loss, this condition measures and demonstrates the effect of the aid under a listening condition that is unfavorable for unaided listening and favorable for aided listening.

A third clinical condition should measure unaided and aided discrimination in noise, with the noise originating on the side of the aid's microphone and speech on the side of the aid's receiver. Noise will thereby be amplified and speech unamplified, or at least its amplification will be reduced by the magnitude of the head shadow. For both unilaterals and those with high frequency loss, this situation will measure and demonstrate the effect of the aid under a condition that is unfavorable for aided listening, favorable unaided for the unilateral, and relatively neutral unaided for the patient with high frequency loss. This condition may not be necessary for clinical evaluation since it is fairly certain that aided discrimination will deteriorate. However, it should be demonstrated to the patient as part of his training in the use of CROS.

Many non-auditory factors play a role in the need and benefit associated with use of a CROS aid. As mentioned earlier, these include motivation, demands on hearing, and the environment in which the user listens. Because these factors can be only grossly evaluated in the clinic, a period of trial use should precede the final recommendation for a CROS aid.

VARIATIONS OF CROS-TYPE AIDS

There are many innovations that utilize either or both the CROS principle and the open earmold in addition to those already discussed (Harford and Dodds, 1974). Some of these are considered below.

POWERCROS

CROS used to achieve the benefits of ear level amplification, instead of a body-worn aid, is called POWERCROS. This principle is utilized by people with moderate or severe loss, who cannot get enough amplification with a conventional ear level instrument without feedback. A standard earmold is used, and a sizable increase in practical amplification results from putting the head between the microphone and receiver. Usually POWERCROS is built into eyeglasses, but the same effect can be achieved using a behind-the-ear aid with an external receiver attached to a power cord and delivering a signal to the contralateral ear.

CRISCROS

CRISCROS is the name for a binaural POWERCROS. It is used for the same reason as POWERCROS, but by those who want binaural amplification. The microphone located on the left side of the head feeds a receiver on the right while the microphone on the right side routes its signal to the left ear. Once upon a time CRISCROS was called DOUBLECROS, but, conceivably because of a poor image, the name was changed.

IROS

IROS stands for ipsilateral routing of signals. The principle exploits the benefits of an open earmold by coupling a conventional at-the-ear hearing aid to the ear with the open mold. It can be used only for mild losses that require little amplification; otherwise feedback becomes a problem.

FROS

FROS (front routing of signals) places the microphone on the eyeglasses somewhere near the midline of the patient's head or at least near the front of the temple bar on the same side as the hearing aid. Thereby, some separation of the microphone and receiver is achieved. This principle may be used with the patient who requires a little more amplification than can be afforded without feedback using IROS, without placing the microphone pickup completely on the other side of the head.

Open BICROS

This principle utilizes a BICROS aid, but with an open instead of a standard earmold. It may be useful to the patient who has an unaidable ear on one side, but only a mild loss—probably high frequency in nature—on the other. Open BICROS can be used whenever the demands for amplification on the good ear are not great enough to cause a feedback problem.

MINICROS

MINICROS consists of a CROS aid without earmold or sound tube, or with a shortened sound tube that travels only part way to the good ear. As reported earlier, CROS aids are often not accepted by unilaterals who have completely normal hearing in their good ear. Apparently one of the reasons for rejection is the fact that even with mild gain and an open earmold, too much amplified sound comes into the good ear. MINICROS alleviates this overamplification (and the head shadow) by more or less spraying some sound of contralateral origin in the direction of the good ear.

FOCALCROS

Some believe that placing the effective sound pickup inside the concha of the unaidable ear affords additional benefit to the unilateral CROS user. This idea, FOCALCROS, is reminiscent of the original apparatus reported by Schaudinischky (1965), described earlier in this chapter.

MULTICROS

MULTICROS is CROS for the sophisticated user. It is achieved by putting an off-on switch on each microphone of a BICROS aid. By manipulating these switches, the user can change his aid from CROS to BICROS to conventional monaural aid at will. For example, MULTICROS might be used by a person with unaidable hearing on one side and a moderate loss on the other. In quiet, and in most listening conditions, he would use the aid as a BICROS, with both microphones operating. However, if so situated that noise was originating primarily from the side of his good ear, and speech from the unaidable side, he might turn off the microphone on the side of the noise. He would thus use the aid as a simple CROS and achieve a better signal-to-noise ratio. If the noise and speech origin were reversed he would use the aid as a conventional monaural system. With training, a perceptive hearing aid user should be able to improve his listening situations appreciably by utilizing or eliminating the head shadow at will.

CONCLUSION

The CROS concept, in its various applications, has grown from what some considered a gimmick, to account for a sizable portion of hearing aid sales. It has sometimes been applied injudiciously, but it has often solved problems for people who otherwise could not have been hearing aid users. The application of the open earmold, originating with CROS, has been of real benefit to those with high frequency loss. If the potential CROS user has sufficient need and motivation, and if he has adequate training in use of the aid, he can benefit.

learning to use the hearing aid

Roger N. Kasten, Ph.D.

Marilyn P. Warren, Ph.D.

INTRODUCTION

Even before the first battery runs dead, the new hearing aid wearer's success with amplification will be influenced by his knowledge or ignorance of proper hearing aid use. Many persons with impaired hearing abandon the use of amplification because they have not learned to cope with apparent inadequacies or malfunctions of the instrument. To reduce the number of clients who fail to benefit from properly chosen amplification, the audiologist must provide careful postfitting services, bridging the difficult period during which hearing aid use becomes established.

For the adult, inadequate hearing aid orientation services all too frequently result in an unused aid. Surely every audiologic clinic has seen the client who resists amplification because he once purchased a hearing aid, used it unsuccessfully, wrapped it (corroding battery, cerumen-clogged earmold, and all) in a bit of tissue, and relegated it to a drawer. Although the etiology of the "dresser drawer syndrome" is seldom straightforward, ignorance of proper hearing aid use may be at fault at least as often as inappropriate fitting of the instrument's amplification characteristics.

For the child, inadequate hearing aid orientation services are more likely to result in an aid which is worn, but used improperly. The young child, lacking the awareness and resources to seek help on his own, relies on adult attention to ensure that amplification yields benefits. Many parents and teachers fail to maintain proper hearing aid function for their children. Gaeth and Lounsbury (1966) studied adequacy of hearing aid use in 134 school children, the majority of whom were enrolled in regular classrooms rather than in classes for the hearing impaired. Only 44 (33%) of the children came to the clinic wearing their aids, with all parts functioning, and with the gain control set at less than full on (except in two cases where full gain appeared justified). The percentage of adequate hearing aid use rose to 55% only by overlooking cases in which the aid was not worn, was worn inappropriately at full gain, or needed live batteries. Nearly half (45%) of the children used aids with broken or malfunctioning parts, or with feedback problems. Fourteen percent of the parents had no idea how long their child's batteries lasted, and 9% reported that the batteries lasted a year or more.

The results of the Gaeth and Lounsbury study were particularly significant in that 83% of the children had been fitted with their hearing aids at one of two audiological clinics. The inadequacy of hearing aid orientation services was underscored by further questioning of the parents:

> . . . the parents repeatedly reported that no one had told them how to care for the earmold or judge its adequacy, how to help the child adjust the gain or determine whether the aid was working properly, or what to watch for in its ultimate breakdown. Actually, the parents said that the audiologist had told them which hearing aid to buy and the hearing aid dealers how to pay for it and put it on. The fact that these reports are in contrast to the information that was given to them is really irrelevant. The information was not given at the right time or often enough. Clinical centers and hearing aid dealers share responsibility. (Gaeth and Lounsbury, 1966, pp. 287–288. Quoted with permission.)

Even a child enrolled in a school for the hearing impaired is not guaranteed adequate day-to-day surveillance over the functioning of his hearing aid. Porter (1973) examined 82 aids worn by children in the first five grade levels of a state school for the deaf. Forty-two (51%) of the aids were not in good operating condition at the time of evaluation. Of the malfunctioning aids, 77% had problems which could be detected by simple visual inspection or listening checks such as a parent or teacher could perform. Aids worn by day students, which could have been inspected by both parents and teachers, fared no better than aids worn by residential students.

One antidote for inadequate use of hearing aids by children seen in a particular facility may be having someone study their use. Zink (1972) found a 13% rise in the percentage of acceptably used children's aids during the second year of a longitudinal study. He attributed the improvement to increased teacher awareness of their role in hearing aid maintenance.

The audiologist's goal should be prevention rather than cure of inadequate hearing aid use. Helping a client adjust to amplification is a complex task. The audiologist must teach the client a sizable number of cold, hard facts about the care and feeding of hearing aids. He also must help the client to express, accept, and cope with the feelings of apprehension and resentment which so often accompany the prospect of wearing a hearing aid.

Stated differently, learning to use the hearing aid involves more than simply learning about the hearing aid. The most technically competent parents, as an example, may master the care and use of their child's amplification system with ease. However, they may resent dreadfully the use of an aid and the child who must use an aid. As a counselor, the audiologist must be prepared to give the parent the opportunity to show these feelings. Such feelings on the part of the client rarely are modified without first being vented. The audiologist, then, strives to create a situation in which the client can learn facts efficiently while still feeling free to express doubts and questions. At the beginning of this complex process of hearing aid orientation, the audiologist should reflect upon his own priorities and his own responsibilities to the client.

STEP ONE: EXAMINING THE AUDIOLOGIST'S ROLE

Mere recognition of the need for full-scale hearing aid orientation services is worthless without the commitment of the audiologist to provide these services. An early and essential step in the process is to define the roles of the various members of the hearing aid delivery system in instructing the client in the use of his new hearing aid. Definition of responsibilities is particularly important when the aid is recommended and delivered through a multi-facility system such as otologist, audiologist, and hearing aid dealer. The audiologist, pressed for time at the end of a long evaluation, may assume that the dealer will teach the client to work the aid, while the dealer assumes that the audiologist has already done so. As a result, the client may go home in a fog, wondering whether he will be able to insert the aid in his ear. Also to be avoided are conflicting instructions from the audiologist and the dealer. Imagine the client's loss of confidence when the audiologist tells him to wear the aid only a few hours at first and should wash his earmold in warm soapy water, while the dealer tells him that he will never get used to the aid unless he wears it all day long, and that he should not get his earmold wet! Good communication and sharing of experiences between audiologist and hearing aid dealer can help to prevent such confusion, to the benefit of all parties concerned.

When it is time to instruct the client in the use and care of his hearing aid, the audiologist can smooth the flow of information by removing barricades to effective communication. Of course, the client must be able to hear the clinician as clearly as possible, with amplification when necessary and with full view of the clinician's face. Distracting noises from another room, or from a child playing on the floor, can be minimized when adequate facilities and personnel are available.

The audiologist must be convinced in his own mind that the recommended aid functions properly, that it provides adequate amplification with minimal risk of acoustic trauma, and that the client is capable of manipulating the controls of the instrument as it is designed. The audiologist also must have familiarized himself thoroughly with the instrument. A quick review of the manufacturer's specifications prepares the clinician to answer questions and provide descriptions about battery life, compression, or telecoil function with confidence.

It is essential to allot sufficient time for instructing the client in the operation of his hearing aid. Absolutely no less than 30 minutes should be saved in the schedule to impart this information, which should be reviewed with the client during subsequent follow-up sessions. Failure to schedule enough time results in rushed, hit-and-run explanations with little opportunity to determine whether the client has learned or even understood the instructions. Also, the client must understand that the purpose of the conversation for that given period of time is to discuss the use and care of the hearing aid. The client must be ready to listen and to learn the information, with minimal distraction from other worries generated by the hearing loss. The mother who is preoccupied with denial of her child's newly diagnosed hearing loss may not be ready to absorb the fact that poor earmold fit causes feedback! When the parent blurts, "Can Johnny still go to college?" in the middle of your careful demonstration of battery insertion, it is past time to lay the hearing aid aside to demonstrate later when the parent is ready. The audiologist must remain alert to the client's feelings, because they may need to be expressed and because they may be interfering with the flow of information.

The manner in which the clinician delivers the information will determine whether the client regards it as being trivial or important. For case history and counseling sessions, some clinicians prefer an authoritarian approach (Rosenberg, 1972) while others use a more client-centered approach (Kodman, 1967). Regardless of the interviewing style which the clinician uses for other purposes, instructions on the operation of hearing aids should be delivered in a straightforward, pedagogical manner befitting the factual nature of the information to be taught. Of course, the clinician must remain sensitive to the client's state of mind, open to his questions, and flexible in the order of presentation.

STEP TWO: INTRODUCING THE CLIENT TO THE HEARING AID

The specific instructions which the audiologist gives regarding use and care of the hearing aid vary from client to client, and from hearing aid to hearing aid. The choice of instructions depends upon such factors as the type of hearing aid, the complexity of the controls, and the age, physical activity, and manual dexterity of the client. The apparent level of intelligence of the client should not limit the amount of training he receives in proper hearing aid use. All instructions can be simplified to the most rudimentary level and repeatedly demonstrated until learned. Even preschool children and severely retarded adults have learned respect for their hearing aids and have mastered the basic steps in hearing aid insertion, battery changing, and earmold cleaning. Of course, when there is any doubt about the client's ability to assume complete responsibility for the functioning of his aid, family members, teachers, and/or attendants also must be trained.

The listing contained in the paragraphs below includes most of the information which typically would be conveyed to the client regarding the operation of the hearing aid. Not all of the items below would be appropriate for any one hearing aid or for any one client. The clinician needs to choose those items which fit the case, and to eliminate irrelevant material. It is highly recommended that the client be given a written version of the instructions to take home for future study and reference. Such instructions can be printed in each clinic or can be procured from other sources. Good examples of such brochures are Dodds and Harford's *Helpful Hearing Aid Hints* (available from A. G. Bell Association for the Deaf, Inc., 3417 Volta Place, N.W., Washington, D.C. 20007) and Zenith's *Caring for a Child's Hearing Aid* (Zenith Hearing Instrument Corp., 6501 W. Grand Ave., Chicago, Ill. 60653). The clinician should go through the written version with the client, crossing out irrelevant portions, underlining important items, and rewording the instructions to suit the client's understanding.

Hearing Aid Components

The hearing aid user should learn the name, location, and function of each basic part of his hearing aid.

1. The *microphone* changes sounds into electrical energy. Its location on the hearing aid is important, because the sounds closest to the microphone will be picked up most readily.

2. The *amplifier* boosts the electrical signal coming from the microphone.

3. The *receiver* changes the amplified electrical signal back into sound.

4. The *battery* supplies power to the hearing aid.

5. The *earmold* carries the sound into the ear canal, holds the hearing aid in place, and (when properly fitted) prevents acoustic feedback or squealing by not allowing the amplified sound to get back to the microphone.

6. The *tubing* (in the case of an ear level hearing aid) carries the sound from the receiver outlet through the earmold.

7. The *cord* (in the case of a body level hearing aid) carries the electrical signal from the amplifier to the receiver.

When a client learns to use the names of the hearing aid components aloud and with confidence early in the orientation process, he is more likely to be specific in his questions. He will learn troubleshooting more easily. Most important, his appreciation of hearing aid function will help him to understand what the instrument can do to sound and what it can not.

Switches and Controls

The client should learn the location and function of all switches and controls which he will need to manipulate.

1. Some hearing aids have an *on-off switch* which is separate from the volume control. Others have an on-off switch which is part of the volume control. Some aids, however, can be turned off only by removing the battery from the battery contacts.

2. The *input selection switch* (if present) should be set to the "M" (microphone) position for normal usage, and to the "T" (telephone coil) for using the telephone. If the input selection switch has an "MT" position, then both the sounds in the room and the telephone conversation can be amplified at once.

3. The *volume control* is a rotating wheel which can be adjusted for comfortable listening in different situations.

4. The *tone control* is set by the audiologist to de-emphasize certain pitch ranges of the amplified sound, to suit the individual hearing loss.

5. Some hearing aids have an *output control* which is set by the audiologist to ensure that the amplified sound never surpasses the maximum intensity which the ear can use and tolerate.

If there are controls which the client should not adjust, he should be told not to touch them or should not be told about them, depending upon the client. An occasional hearing aid user may benefit from learning to adjust a tone control for different listening situations, using reduced low frequency amplification in crowds or other noisy situations.

Inserting the Hearing Aid

No beginning hearing aid user should be sent home from the orientation session without having assembled and inserted the aid himself, with the clinician's guidance. It is helpful for the client to look in a mirror as he learns to insert his hearing aid.

1. For a body level hearing aid, connect one end of the cord to the receiver and the other end to the hearing aid. Snap the earmold and the receiver together. Note whether plastic washers are in place between the receiver and the cord. Position the plastic "receiver saver" (if used) to

provide an extra connection between cord and receiver in case the receiver is pulled from the ear. (The hearing aid may be stored with all these parts assembled.) Put the hearing aid in the carrier pocket of a hearing aid garment, or in some snugly fitting pocket with the microphone not covered by bulky, loose, or starched clothing.

2. For an ear level hearing aid, one end of the tubing usually is connected permanently to the earmold. Slide the other end onto the plastic sound outlet of the aid, making sure that the earmold is oriented in the proper direction. Be sure the tubing is firmly attached to the aid.

3. For either type of hearing aid, now make sure the volume control is turned down. Insert the battery into the battery compartment, with the positive (+) terminal of the battery against the battery contact marked +. If polarity is reversed, the aid will not function. Click the battery compartment firmly shut.

4. Put the canal portion of the earmold down into the ear. Rotate the earmold back and forth, using both hands if necessary, until it is firmly seated. Now turn the volume control up to the desired setting.

5. When removing the hearing aid, always turn the volume down or turn the hearing aid off before pulling the earmold out of the ear, in order to avoid acoustic feedback.

Batteries

The prospective hearing aid user nearly always asks questions about batteries and their expected life span. The parent of an aided child particularly needs a thorough explanation regarding batteries since the child may be too young to communicate that his battery is wearing down.

1. Learn the type and size of battery which was recommended for use with the aid.

2. Don't be caught without a fresh battery. Buy enough batteries at one time to ensure continued use of the aid between purchases. Carry a spare fresh battery. A school-aged child should either carry a fresh spare or keep one in the teacher's desk.

3. Store batteries in a cool, dry place, preferably in an airtight container.

4. Battery life depends upon the model of hearing aid. If batteries wear down long before the period of time suggested by the manufacturer, the audiologist or dealer should be consulted. The higher the volume control setting used, the more rapidly batteries wear down. For some hearing aids, sound input levels also influence battery life.

5. Rechargeable nickel cadmium batteries can be used with some hearing aids. Before trying rechargeable batteries, however, determine whether the cost of the charger and the rechargeable cells, as well as the necessity for remembering to recharge the batteries, will provide any real savings.

6. When the battery is wearing down, the volume control will need to be turned higher in order to get the needed amount of amplification, and distortion may increase dramatically (Lotterman, Kasten, and Majerus, 1967). You may buy an inexpensive battery tester to check the voltage of your batteries. A nearly dead battery may "recover" to some extent overnight, appear to have sufficient voltage in the morning, and then wear out completely after 30 minutes of use.

7. When the hearing aid is not in use, remove the battery or swing the battery compartment completely open. This removal enables the batteries to last longer and prevents corrosion from extended contact with the metal battery contacts.

8. The battery should be at room temperature and completely dry when inserted. Rubbing both surfaces of the battery on a piece of paper removes any moisture or slight corrosion which would damage the inside of the aid. A dead battery, or one which shows any visible sign of leakage or corrosion, should be set aside immediately and not used again. To preserve both resources and environment, take used batteries to the nearest clinic or dealership which accumulates bulk quantities for recycling.

9. Be aware that hearing aid performance can vary markedly as a result of battery performance. You can expect tremendous variability in battery life even among batteries of the same type. Whether you purchase batteries from a hearing aid dealer, a drug store, or a discount department store, you may find differences in battery life as great as 100 hours or more among batteries of one type (Smith, 1972).

10. If a mercury battery has been recommended for use with your hearing aid, you should be aware that mercury batteries discharge slowly. As the battery gradually weakens, you will have to turn the hearing aid volume higher and you may hear increased distortion. If a silver oxide battery has been recommended, however, you will find that its strength remains nearly constant until it suddenly collapses (See above, Chapter 4). This sudden change in performance will alert you that the battery should be changed.

Earmolds

New hearing aid users must learn the importance of keeping the earmold channel unclogged. It is also essential that they understand the relationship between poor earmold fit and feedback.

1. Detach the earmold from the aid to wash it. Use warm soapy water and make sure that water will pass freely through the channel in the earmold. Use a pipe cleaner or earmold brush to remove any ear wax or moisture stuck in the channel. Dry the earmold completely before reattaching it to the aid. It is a good idea to wash the mold in the morning. Do not wash earmolds with alcohol, because it dries and cracks some earmold materials.

2. In order to detach the earmold from an ear level aid, it may be difficult to pull the tubing off the plastic ear hook. If you need to exert pressure, grasp the ear hook rather than the body of the aid.

3. Repeated removal of the tubing from the ear hook of an ear level aid may cause the tube opening to stretch, resulting in feedback. When this occurs, get the tubing replaced.

4. The most common cause of acoustic feedback or "squeal" is an earmold which is too loose. The earmold should fit snugly, to prevent amplified sound from escaping out of the ear canal and getting back to the microphone. Until the age of 6 years, a child may outgrow his earmolds up to three or four times per year; between 6 and 10, he may need new molds once or twice each year. Adults may need new earmolds on occasion, because earmolds may shrink slightly or the ear may change shape or size just enough to allow feedback.

5. If any part of the earmold causes soreness in your ear, take it to the audiologist (or dealer) to have the part smoothed down. It may be necessary to make a new earmold.

6. A little petroleum jelly or baby oil rubbed onto the earmold may serve as a *temporary* cure for either a too small earmold or one which causes irritation.

7. If the earmold is moist when you remove it, your ear canal may be draining. See a physician.

Care of the Hearing Aid

A list of clear-cut do's and don'ts may help to prolong hearing aid life considerably. As is true for all instructions regarding hearing aid use, the client may remember a rule best when it is accompanied by a reason.

1. Excessive heat and cold may very well damage a hearing aid. Never leave it on a radiator, near a stove, in a sunny window, or in any other hot place. Do not wear the aid when using a hair dryer, or near a sun lamp, heat lamp, or diathermy instrument. In extremely cold or wet weather, do not wear the aid outside unless absolutely necessary.

2. Do not drop the hearing aid on a hard surface. As a precautionary measure, hold the aid over a table or bed, rather than over the floor, when changing batteries or performing maintenance.

3. Moisture damages a hearing aid. Never wear it in the rain or to take a bath. If you perspire excessively and you have a behind-the-ear eyeglass aid, avoid wearing it during strenuous activity in hot weather. If the climate is humid or if you perspire, store the hearing aid overnight in a tightly closed container with a silica gel packet to absorb the moisture.

4. Don't apply hair spray when wearing the aid. It may damage the microphone.

5. Clean the battery contacts occasionally to remove corrosion, by scraping very gently with a sharpened pencil eraser. Battery contacts may be dried with a cotton swab in cases of humid weather or heavy perspiration.

6. Never attempt to open the case of the hearing aid. You may cause more damage and will likely void the manufacturer's warranty.

Using the Telephone

Some persons with impaired hearing report that they use the telephone easily without amplification; others have great difficulty using the telephone. The hearing aid orientation should include a discussion and demonstration regarding the best way for the new hearing aid user to receive a telephone conversation. If the use of a telephone coil is recommended, the clinician should "call" the client, using clinic phones, for demonstration.

1. You may not be able to use the telephone with your hearing aid in its usual mode of operation. That is, few persons can hear clearly over the telephone when using the hearing aid microphone to pick up the acoustic signal from the telephone receiver. If your hearing aid has no telephone coil, you may need to either remove the aid to use the phone, or use the unaided ear.

2. To use your hearing aid with the telephone, set the input selection switch to the "T" position so that the telephone coil of the aid will pick up electromagnetic radiation from the telephone receiver and send it to the amplifier.

3. The telephone receiver must be placed as close as possible to the telephone coil of the aid. For a behind-the-ear aid, hold the receiver slightly behind the ear, over the hearing aid. For a body level aid worn on the chest, invert the receiver so that the "listening" end covers the aid while you hold the "speaking" end to your mouth.

4. Remember that noises around you will not be amplified in the "T" position. If the aid has an "MT" position, and is set on that position, both telephone and room sounds will be amplified. At the end of the conversation, return the input selection switch to "M."

5. Most new telephones are not compatible with the telephone coils of hearing aids. If you frequently use such a phone, or if you often need to use pay phones, you may obtain an adaptor from the telephone company. The adaptor, nicknamed "hockey puck" for its size and shape, can be carried in pocket or purse and fits over the telephone receiver.

It is helpful for the clinic to have one of the telephone adaptors to show new hearing aid users. In addition, one of the clinic phones can be supplied with a telephone amplifier, to show those clients who need help on the phone but do not use an aid with a telephone coil.

Use of Other Communication Aids

With or without a hearing aid, certain special communication situations create inconveniences for the hearing-impaired person and his family. He may have difficulty hearing the telephone or doorbell ring, hearing a baby cry, or listening to TV or radio at the family's comfortable listening level. The clinician should make concrete suggestions to solve these problems.

1. An alarm clock can be obtained which either emits a flashing light or vibrates a bed, instead of emitting an audio signal.

2. A "sound lamp," turned on by a sound-activated switch with a variable sensitivity control, can be used to signal such sounds as the doorbell, telephone, baby's cry, etc. Alternatively, a sound-activated switch is available which can be used to turn on any lamp or other electrical device in the house or office.

3. An induction loop kit can be obtained for TV listening. The loop is connected to the TV, radio, or stereo. A hearing aid which has a telephone coil, set on "T," will pick up electromagnetic radiation from the loop, amplify it, and deliver it to the ear. The person wearing the aid can move about freely within the loop. In this way, the hearing-impaired person can hear amplified TV without disturbing the family or neighbors. In addition, he will hear the signal at a favorable signal-to-noise ratio, because the hearing aid on "T" will amplify the signal without amplifying background room noise.

The above-mentioned devices can be built from components, or can be obtained by the clinic or hearing aid dealership for the client from Hal-Hen Company (36–14 Eleventh St., Long Island City, N.Y. 11106). Helpful devices for the hearing-impaired are also available from the local telephone company.

Checking the Hearing Aid

Each common hearing aid malfunction (dead, weak, squealing, intermittent, or scratchy sound) may have several different causes. If the client learns a systematic "listening check" procedure, he can unearth the cause of many simple malfunctions. The parent of a young hearing-impaired child *must* learn how to listen to the child's aid on a regular basis. The clinician might keep a set of used aids rigged with various malfunctions such as dead or reversed battery, clogged earmold, cracked tubing, internal feedback, etc., to test the parent's grasp of the listening check procedure.

1. First look at the aid carefully. Is the on-off switch "on"? Is the input selection switch on "M," not "T"? Is the tone control setting (if movable) in its correct position?

2. Are the battery contacts clean? Use a fresh battery for the hearing aid check. Is the battery inserted properly and the compartment clicked shut all the way?

3. For an ear level aid, is the tubing free of cracks or holes? Does it fit snugly onto the aid? Is the earmold channel free of wax or moisture?

4. For a body level aid, look at the receiver and cord carefully. Is the insulation worn? Do both plugs fit firmly into the receiver and the aid? Is the receiver cracked or its casing loose? Is the earmold clean, and does it have a metal ring which snaps tightly to the receiver (with plastic washer if used)?

5. Put the aid to your ear, using an earmold if possible, and cover your ear tightly with your fingers to prevent feedback. Now turn the volume up and down slowly. Are there any sudden jumps in loudness as you turn the wheel? Does the wheel itself turn smoothly? Is the sound scratchy as you turn the wheel, as though dust has entered the control? Leaving the volume at one level, listen for gross distortion of the sound and for the level of background noise from the aid itself. A hearing aid stethoscope, if available, may be used for easier listening.

6. For a body-level aid, roll the cord in your fingers at several places as you listen, to check for scratchiness or "cut-outs" due to worn insulation. Wiggle the connections of the cord at both ends; the sound should not cut out.

7. Check the source of any whistling by removing the aid and holding a thumb firmly over the canal opening of the earmold, with the aid full on. If you hear whistling, remove the tubing from the aid (for an ear level aid) or the earmold from the receiver (for a body level aid) and now hold the thumb over the sound outlet (or receiver). If there is no whistling now, the cause was a leak in the tubing or its connection (for an ear level aid) or between the earmold and receiver (for a body level aid). If whistling persists, and the receiver is not cracked, then the aid probably has internal feedback and must be serviced by a repair facility.

8. With the aid on its wearer and adjusted to its customary volume setting, is there feedback as the wearer moves his head back and forth and moves his jaw? If so, and earlier steps have yielded no problems, then the earmold is too small. The wearer should be able to turn the volume up at least somewhat beyond the customary volume setting without feedback, so that the volume setting is never dictated by the feedback level.

Repairs

Not uncommonly during the learning period, inappropriate actions on the part of the hearing aid user may cause the instrument to malfunction. For whatever reason, a large percentage of hearing aids require repair during their usable life span (Ewertsen, 1972; Porter, 1973; Zink, 1972). In the typical situation, the user would return the instrument to the appropriate dealer, who would either repair it or send it to the manufacturer's repair facility. The hearing aid orientation process should include a discussion of long-term service and repair for the instrument.

In a recent investigation conducted by the authors (Warren and Kasten, 1976), the accuracy of hearing aid repair was evaluated. The electroacoustic characteristics of 41 hearing aids were measured following repair in either a manufacturer's repair facility, a hearing aid dealer's office, or two different independent repair laboratories. The investigation was based on the assumption that the performance characteristics of a repaired instrument should at least approximate those of a new instrument of the same model. Therefore, for the purposes of the investigation, an instrument was considered to be appropriately repaired if HAIC gain was within ±6 dB of the manufacturer's specifications, and saturation sound pressure level was within ±6 dB of the manufacturer's specifications. In addition, low and high frequency cutoffs on the HAIC frequency response curve were required to be within 100 Hz and 500 Hz respectively. No attempt was made to evaluate characteristics other than the three previously mentioned.

Only 37% of the aids managed to meet the repair criteria after one trip to the repair facility. Interestingly, the low percentage of acceptable repair was identical whether the instrument had been serviced by the manufacturer's facility or by an alternative repair facility. The two characteristics most responsible for the failure rate were gain and frequency response cutoffs. Six of the 41 aids had been sent to the repair facility more than once in a short period of time because of gross malfunctions that prohibited any kind of subsequent usage after the first repair.

The findings of this investigation have serious implications for all hearing aid users, but particularly for those who are attempting to learn successful hearing aid usage for the first time. One can easily speculate on the effect that large changes in performance characteristics would have on the new hearing aid user. The new instrument, selected because it was "just right" for the user, suddenly could become quite different from what it originally had been.

Whether the apparent lack of quality repair is the fault of the repair facilities or the United States mail is of only academic concern at the moment. The hearing aid user, and particularly the new hearing aid user, stands as the ultimate loser. The finding that less than half of the repaired aids approximated manufacturer's specifications, and that several aids required repeated trips to achieve operational condition, suggests that hearing aid owners must seek verification for the quality of repairs regardless of the type of repair facility used. Hearing aid repairs can be costly, slow, and inadequate. The first encounter between the new hearing aid user and the hearing aid repair system may be still another causative agent for the "dresser drawer syndrome."

STEP THREE: INTRODUCING THE CLIENT TO AMPLIFIED SOUND

As part of the orientation process, the new hearing aid owner should come to master hearing aid use without being overwhelmed by its complexities. Mastery of the "rules" of hearing aid operation, as outlined in the previous section, will help him to determine which of his difficulties are caused by mechanical problems and which ones are part of the adjustment process. However, learning the "do's and don'ts" about hearing aids is only a start. The new hearing aid user must learn to accept the cosmetic appearance of the instrument, which for the first time makes his hidden handicap visible. Most important of all, he must learn to tolerate and use the amplified sound which the instrument delivers to his ear.

Certain basic principles are common to the various approaches used to help children, young adults, and elderly persons adjust to amplified sound. The process of adjustment should begin with an understanding of the purpose of amplification, as well as its limitations. New listening situations should be introduced according to their hierarchy of difficulty, beginning with the easiest situations and saving the more complex ones for later. Family cooperation is almost essential during the adjustment to amplified sound. The recommended aid should be used on a trial or rental basis for roughly 30 days, during which time those difficulties which were not unearthed in the clinical environment may come to light. Finally, the hearing aid orientation session should be left open-ended so that the client feels free to contact the audiologist as new problems arise. Yearly re-evaluations of unaided and aided hearing should be encouraged for adults, with more frequent rechecks for young children.

The Young Child

For the child with impaired hearing, orientation to amplified sound takes place as part of an ongoing habilitative process. Parental enthusiasm is the single most important factor in a child's adjustment to hearing aid use, but it is the responsibility of audiologists and educators of the hearing impaired to kindle that enthusiasm. It is only natural for the child, whether infant or adolescent, to resist hearing aid use until he learns the importance of sounds in his world. Downs (1967) suggests that parents approach the child's period of adjustment to amplification with the same attitude they would use toward administering a prescribed medication; both must be done, although the child resists the short term effects. Thus, the parents must become believers in the use of residual hearing and its beneficial effects.

At first, the child should use the hearing aid only for brief periods and only in quiet, pleasant listening environments. In this manner the child comes to associate hearing aid use with good family attention and interesting sounds. An excellent week-by-week program for initiating hearing aid use in the child is outlined in Northern and Downs (1974). Each week, both the amount of daily hearing aid usage and the complexity of auditory stimulation are increased until the child wears the aid as routinely as he wears his clothes. When such a program is followed, both parents and audiologist can monitor progress by having the parents keep a chart or diary of the number of hours the aid is worn each day, the child's responses to sound, and the improvement in the number or meaningfulness of his vocalizations.

The parents should be prepared not to be discouraged with slow speech development. They should understand the steps which the child must take in developing awareness of the presence or absence of sound, attention to the communicative purposes of sound, and differentiation among sounds. They should be encouraged to play games in which the child's action must depend on his awareness of the onset or cessation of sound, or its pitch, loudness, or rhythmic content. The only limitation to the possible number of such games is the imagination of the parents and the audiologist; specific suggestions can be found in Pollack (1970).

Special problems confront the child who uses a hearing aid in a regular public school classroom. He must endure misunderstanding by his peers. His teacher may not be aware of the effects of classroom noise on his ability to hear with the aid. An audiologist, or a speech or hearing clinician, can help by going into the classroom to give a brief talk about hearing aids and to allow classmates and teachers to listen with the aid. The hearing aid user might go home from school that day feeling as though he is the most fortunate child in the class.

Parents should be reminded of the long-term rechecks which will be required to maintain good hearing aid use for their child. New earmolds, re-evaluation of unaided and aided hearing, and measurement of the electroacoustic characteristics of the instrument should be at least yearly events. They should also become aware that the child with a sensorineural loss is at least as prone to outer and middle ear problems as the normally hearing child, and perhaps more so because of the occlusion of the canal by the earmold. If parents learn when to suspect conductive overlay, and to seek medical attention for it, the child with a sensorineural loss may be spared weeks of poorer hearing or even draining ears.

The hearing aid orientation process for a young child can be an exciting challenge for the child's family. Each family member can make a special contribution depending upon his age or interests. For example, one parent or a teen-aged sibling with a mechanical bent might take on the responsibility of checking the function of the aid, while another sibling might enjoy dancing or clapping in time to music with the child. Ideally, the parents should have an opportunity to share ideas and problems with other parents of hearing-impaired children during the difficult adjustment period.

The Adult

Hearing aid orientation for the adventitiously impaired adult can be handled in several different ways. The "call us when you have problems" approach is not likely to result in good adjustment to amplification unless *intensive* counseling and demonstration have taken place before the aid was obtained. A more safe and reasonable approach is to schedule one to four orientation sessions, on a group or individual basis, after the hearing aid fitting. These sessions have several important purposes. Aided auditory function should be rechecked, and the use and care of the instrument should be reviewed with the client. Special problems encountered by the new hearing aid user, such as wind noise, head shadow effects, or noise conditions on the job, can be pinpointed and sometimes resolved. Basic suggestions to maximize visual and auditory cues during conversation can be taught. A decision can be reached regarding the advisability of long term aural rehabilitation or speech conservation therapy for the client. Most important of all, these sessions provide a chance for the client to discuss his evolving concept of himself as a hearing aid user, as well as the reactions of his family and friends.

The new hearing aid owner is curious to try his aid in his most difficult listening situation. However, he should be urged to start by using the aid at home, alone or with one other person. He can learn to adjust the gain by listening to radio or television or by talking with one other person at a normal level. He can tour the house to relearn the background sounds, such as heating system noises, clocks ticking, and clothes rubbing, which form part of our "unconscious hearing." Gradually he can try the aid in more complex situations, such as in small groups, at work, or in outdoor settings, churches, theaters, and parties.

Two model hearing aid orientation programs are those conducted by the Army Audiology and Speech Center in this country and by the State Hearing Centers in Denmark. The U. S. Army aural rehabilitation program (Northern et al., 1969) includes orientation to amplification, speechreading, and auditory training. A serviceman is required to enroll in the course for 2 to 3 weeks following a hearing aid fitting. Information is conveyed primarily by means of classroom instruction and practice sessions. Follow-up questionnaires showed that roughly 88% of course participants were satisfied with their aids and felt that they had learned enough about its care and use. It was interesting that 53% of those returning the questionnaire would have liked more training in speechreading.

Ewertsen (1974) reports that any resident of Denmark can receive free audiologic testing and free monaural or binaural hearing aid fittings. The basic assumption of the Danish program is that the fitting of hearing aids is only the beginning of aural rehabilitation. All new clients of the State Hearing Centers must attend a free orientation course for 4 weeks, 2 hours per week. In addition, longer speechreading courses are available when necessary. After the initial orientation, the client is referred to a "hearing pedagogue," or teacher of the hard-of-hearing, in his local area. The pedagogue reports back to the Center regarding the success of pedagogical aftercare.

The Severely Impaired Adult

The orientation process is particularly challenging when the prospective hearing aid user is a teenager or adult with severely or profoundly impaired hearing. Many such persons have never experienced amplified sound on a regular basis, or have rejected amplification during elementary school. They are often thought to be poor prospects for hearing aid use because of their earlier rejection of amplification and because of their many years of auditory deprivation. At the National Technical Institute for the Deaf, those students who do not use amplification, but who are willing to try, are encouraged to enroll in a 10 week Orientation to Hearing Aids course. Classroom lecture material (Galloway and Gauger, 1975) includes information on sound and speech, residual hearing, hearing aid components, earmolds, maintenance, and consumer aspects of hearing aid ownership. Students also meet with audiologists for individual counseling sessions. They start the program with their own earmolds and undergo three or more hearing aid evaluations during the course. Each evaluation results in the trial use of a new loaner aid, during which time students record their use of the aid and its advantages and disadvantages.

The results of the program (Galloway, 1974) suggest that persons with severely to profoundly impaired hearing can indeed learn to benefit from amplification in adulthood. Eighty-seven percent of the students served by the program over a 21 month period requested their own hearing aids at the end of the course. Pre- and posttesting showed gains in speechreading and speech discrimination associated with the trial use of amplification over the 10 weeks. The key to the success of the program seems to lie in intensive counseling and trial use *before* amplification is purchased. It is interesting that 90% of the fittings resulting from the program were ear level aids. At the start of the course, 90% of those who had once used aids had said that they had stopped using them because the aids made sounds uncomfortably loud or caused dizziness or headaches.

The Older Person

Another group for whom intensive counseling should take place before the hearing aid fitting, as well as after, is the geriatric population (Alpiner, 1967). Prior counseling helps to remove false expectations about the restoration of "normal hearing" through amplification. Many factors work against the elderly person's adjustment to amplification, but these problems sometimes can be overcome through counseling. Family members, as well as the client himself, may have confused the hearing loss with senility. The family may want the hearing aid more than the client does.

The client may be more concerned about the other problems associated with aging which he is experiencing. Other negative factors include poor understanding of speech in noise with presbycusis, and the conflict between cosmetic interests and stiff fingers.

Hearing aid orientation sessions for the elderly may be held on an individual or group basis. Group sessions provide a chance for the clients to share problems; however, much time can be lost ironing out one person's difficulties while the rest of the group waits. A combination of individual and group sessions maximizes the advantages of both approaches. Fransson (1968) finds that older clients benefit most from practical training with no emphasis on theoretical or engineering aspects of hearing aid use. Training in proper use of the telephone, for example, is valuable for the elderly because the telephone may be their primary means of contact with relatives. Orwall (1968) advises that elderly clients learn the value of induction loops for hearing aid users. In Sweden, many churches, theaters, and nursing homes are equipped with loops, and a hearing aid user can get a state subsidy to have one installed at home for radio and TV listening.

It is vital to orient family members or nursing home attendants to the problems of amplification when the client is elderly. They should learn to speak slowly and clearly and to face the hearing aid user. It is helpful to say the elderly person's name to call his attention before beginning to convey information. Such simple practices help to keep the older person in touch with the world of spoken communication.

SUMMARY

It is a rare individual indeed who is able to put on his first hearing aid and wear it happily and successfully. Learning to use a hearing aid, like any other prosthetic device, requires time and effort. Individual successes are frequently interspersed with difficulties, frustrations, and disappointments. It is critical that the hearing aid user and his family be fully aware of all aspects of the care and feeding of amplification systems. Just imagine what would happen if the well meaning child takes off the hearing aid when it starts to rain and well meaning but uninformed parent tells the child to "put that hearing aid back on because we paid a lot of money for it and you're going to use it." Just imagine the well meaning adult who takes off his hearing aid in the very noisy cafeteria and the well meaning but uninformed spouse insists that he put it back on so that communication with him will be easier. Learning to use a hearing aid is a family affair which can be made entertaining, and which can provide great insight into the dynamics of a family that has within it an individual with impaired hearing.

aural rehabilitation through amplification

Herbert J. Oyer, Ph.D.

William R. Hodgson, Ph.D.

INTRODUCTION

There are approximately 8,500,000 persons of all ages in the United States with hearing loss less severe than deafness and about 236,000 who are deaf (NINDS, 1970). Only a small fraction of these persons wear hearing aids. Of those who do, many do not learn to use their aids to best advantage. The role of amplification in aural rehabilitation involves these basic questions: Why do many hearing-impaired persons not use amplification? Why do many who buy a hearing aid not participate in an aural rehabilitation program to maximize their communication ability?

Some hearing-impaired persons have losses too mild to warrant amplification. Others have losses so great that the limited help associated with amplification is not obvious. For the remainder — the most viable hearing aid candidates — several factors may help to answer the questions we've asked. First, consider the incidence and nature of hearing disorders. In most cases hearing loss is a gradually acquired problem. Presbycusis and noise-induced loss are examples. The insidious onset causes many people to be unaware of the problem or poorly prepared to evaluate it. Additionally, the problem is most prevalent in old age, at a time when more pressing health problems may take precedence.

Second, informed professional assistance is not always available to the hearing-impaired person. The hypoacusic may be told that hearing aids are not useful in cases of sensorineural loss. Conversely, he may be led to unrealistic expectations regarding the correction of hearing loss through amplification.

Third, many hearing impaired cannot easily afford a hearing aid. Financial considerations, interacting with the other problems under discussion, may prevent the individual from trying a hearing aid.

Finally, there are problems with the present delivery system. It is fragmented, with competing components. Its evolution resulted from needs of the groups involved rather than a structured plan to help the hearing impaired. As a result, the role of amplification in an overall rehabilitation program may not be clear to the potential hearing aid user. Furthermore, prospective hearing aid candidates may still feel a stigma associated with hearing loss and hearing aids. Professional groups have not worked to inform the public about the nature of hearing and hearing loss in a way designed to remove the stigma. Advertising has continued to promote the concept of cosmetic penalty associated with visible hearing aids.

To summarize, lack of information or misinformation may prevent a hypoacusic from purchasing a hearing aid, or from participating in a training program to learn effective use of the aid. Logistic problems — scheduling, transportation, etc. — complicate the issue. These problems are related to finance, lack of professional assistance, and a well coordinated delivery system. Additionally, insufficient commitment on the part of the patient to hear well again may defeat the program. Some individuals with severe loss perform remarkably well with amplification. They understand the problem, the advantages and limitations of amplification, how to use the hearing aid, the acoustic and visual conditions they must promote in order to communicate. They have participated successfully in an effective rehabilitation program, in which amplification plays a critical role.

CONCEPTUALIZATION OF THE AURAL REHABILITATION PROCESS

Unfortunately aural rehabilitation has been thought of too often as limited to auditory training and speechreading. Although these are two basic ingredients, they constitute but a part of the process. We need to view aural rehabilitation in proper perspective and carry out systematic research on all the facets, for the rehabilitation of the hearing handicapped is the principal concern of audiology.

Only recently was there publication of a conceptualization of the aural rehabilitation process (Oyer and Frankmann, 1975), in which six major concepts were identified, each with supporting constructs. The concepts are (1) handicap deficit recognition, (2) motivational aspects, (3) identification and acquisition of professional assistance, (4) measurement and evaluation of auditory deficit and handicap, (5) rehabilitative sessions, and (6) measuring effects of training and counseling. Unfortunately there is too little scientific research in the area of auditory training and speechreading. The area with the most substantial research data base is that of measurement and evaluation of hearing.

AMPLIFICATION AND AURAL REHABILITATION

The habilitative-rehabilitative needs associated with amplification may generally be differentiated in three groups of hearing handicapped: children with congenital loss, presbycusics, and adults with other forms of acquired loss. The child with congenital loss must adapt to a complex instrument with which he learns to distinguish sounds and develops speech. Parents must be oriented to realistic expectations regarding hearing aid use and the fact that listening behavior will emerge only through an extended program of training in hearing aid use.

Adults with acquired loss must learn hearing aid use consistent with their social and occupational needs. For example, those with unilateral or slight bilateral loss may or may not require amplification, depending on whether they have critical demands on their hearing. Adults with more severe loss must accept the need to change their behavior and structure their listening situations in a way favorable for hearing aid use. Aural rehabilitation can play an important role in this retraining process.

The typical presbycusic has a slight or mild high frequency loss of sensitivity, reduced discrimination ability, and often impaired attending processes. This combination is far from ideal for hearing aid candidacy. The presbycusic must learn to adapt to a hearing aid and accept the limited help it will offer. He must learn to work hard to utilize all available clues to communication. Acceptance of these facts and the development of a positive mental attitude, absent in many presbycusics, is a critical contribution of aural rehabilitation.

For all who must learn to use a hearing aid, success is associated with the following factors:

1. The patient (or the parents) must learn about hearing and hearing loss.

2. The patient (or the parents) must be taught realistic expectations regarding hearing aid use.

3. There is need for goal-oriented training before hearing aid use is undertaken. In children with severe or profound loss, this training involves teaching the child to respond to sound, the utility of sound, and how sound can give him information about the environment. In adults, the training involves counseling and demonstration, psychological preparation for problems with amplified noise, and for cosmetic concerns. It includes

positive reinforcement; emphasis on what a hearing aid *can* do. It involves training in listening. Patients must learn how to put the aid on, remove it, and how to operate the controls correctly while wearing the aid. They must learn effective procedures with batteries — their selection, testing, insertion, and use.

4. The new hearing aid owner must then learn to wear the device correctly and use it effectively. He must learn to set the gain at a comfort level for maximum discrimination in different acoustic environments. He requires training in the identification of sounds, moving from listening to simple acoustic signals in quiet to complex signals in noise. He must be assisted to decide intelligently whether to be a full or part time hearing aid user. These procedures are considered in detail in Chapter Eleven.

5. In children, the training discussed above is preparatory to language, speech, and educational training. In adults, such instruction should precede other rehabilitative procedures as needed; speechreading instruction, training in listening in specific acoustic circumstances that are important to the patient, and speech conservation.

6. Additional counseling as needed should be available for specific problems.

Rehabilitation is the basic process, amplification is one of the components. Just as amputees are never handed an artificial limb to use without instruction, the hearing impaired should not be expected to use a hearing aid efficiently without training. The material presented in this chapter does not address the multiplicity of problems associated with aural rehabilitation but focuses more specifically upon the use of amplification in the aural rehabilitation process.

Early Attempts

Through past centuries many attempts have been made to use intense sounds as stimuli for training the hearing handicapped. In 1802, Itard, a French physician, used hand bells to train the hearing of six hearing-handicapped pupils. He gradually progressed from bells to drum beats, sound of a flute, sustained vowels, and on to consonants. He registered success with his method and it spread to other parts of Europe (Goldstein, 1939).

A. G. Bell suggested that hearing-handicapped pupils be given telephones directly connected to that of the teacher. Actually, he was suggesting the first group auditory training unit. It was not until the early 1920's, with the advent of electronic amplifying devices, that units for auditory training were made available to schools. Some 20 to 25 years later auditory training through amplifying devices experienced growth as Deshon, Borden, and Hoff General Hospitals provided aural rehabilitation services for returning veterans of World War II. Following the closing of these units, clinics supported by universities and by community enterprises undertook auditory training. Today most audiology clinics throughout the country possess the appropriate equipment for auditory training sessions.

Research Efforts

Auditory Training. When analyzing speechreading and auditory training one should consider the (1) speaker, (2) code, (3) transmission link, and (4) receiver. The studies of Wright (1917), Forester (1928), Ballenger (1936), and Goodfellow (1942) were all aimed at determining the improvement in auditory reception brought about by auditory training. Unfortunately none provided results as clear cut and conclusive as might have been desired. Johnson (1939, 1948) did demonstrate that auditory training was beneficial in helping to retain vocabulary used in the exercises.

Palmer (1955) measured subject response as a function of sex of the speaker. Three adult males, three adult females, and three 12 year old girls served as speakers. Sex of speaker and age differences between females had no significant effect on listener responses. The test material consisted of phonetically balanced word lists and these results may not generalize to continuous discourse.

A number of studies have provided basic data about the relationships of code and auditory training procedures. Miller and Nicely (1955) presented an articulatory analysis which yielded five dimensions that characterize consonants: (1) voicing, (2) nasality, (3) affrication, (4) duration, and (5) place of articulation. They found that noise and low-pass filtering had very little effect on voicing or nasality, but severely affected perception of place of articulation. Oyer and Doudna (1959) studied the discrimination performance of hard of hearing subjects who listened to two repetitions of the Central Institute for the Deaf W-22 lists. They found that errors were primarily those of substitution rather than of omission. In a further study (1960) they found that errors of substitution increased slightly and that errors of omission decreased as word familiarity decreased.

With reference to the effects of word context, Rubenstein and Pickett (1957) asked normal hearing subjects to listen to pairs of complete declarative sentences each of which had the same test noun placed in the initial, medial, or final positions. The principal finding was that the initial sentence position had highest intelligibility. Also, O'Neill (1957) compared the intelligibility of words presented in sentences and in isolation. His finding was that the subjects recognized words placed in context much more easily than the isolated words. These studies were carried out with normal hearing subjects. However, it would appear that the findings would be applicable to the hearing impaired as well, provided language had developed normally.

As regards the transmission link there are also some studies relating to auditory training. Boyd and Jamroz (1963) compared three different group hearing aid systems. In the first sound was delivered diotically through only one microphone, one amplifier, and one attenuator. In the second system there was a separate attenuator control for each ear, and the third incorporated individual microphones, amplifiers, and attenuator controls for each ear. The third system was truly a binaural system. No significant differences between test systems were found. In other words, binaural amplification showed no advantages over monaural amplification. It should be mentioned that the effect of the head shadow and competing signals were not considered in this study.

Regarding the receiver, Siegenthaler (1949) looked at the relationship between ability to perceive differences in voicing, pressure pattern, and influence of consonants on vowels as a function of type of hearing loss. His findings support the contention that losses of high frequency interfere significantly in the word discrimination task.

Carhart (1946a) developed a procedure for selection of and orientation to hearing aids, the clinical details of which are given in Chapter Eight. In the associated training program, attention to speaker, code, transmission, and receiver variables was integrated. The goals were (1) to secure for the patient a hearing aid with optimal efficiency for everyday situations, (2) to give each patient an understanding of hearing aids as well as to establish habits of efficient use and initiate acoustic training, and (3) to help the patient to a full psychological acceptance of hearing aids. Here are the training aspects of the program: An initial conference covered hearing problems and hearing aids, and the patient was oriented to the steps to follow. There was then additional orientation to hearing aids conducted in small groups. Patients listened through a group hearing aid. The use of a hearing aid rating scale to play a role in future steps was explained.

Next, several promising hearing aids were selected. The patient tried each for 24 hours, during which he engaged in a listening hour. This group activity of 25–30 people consisted of listening to sound experiences at levels similar to those encountered in everyday life. It included speech, music, and environmental noise; with practice in sound localization, speech discrimination, and using the telephone. The patient rated the hearing aids he used. There were additional sessions concentrating on care and maintenance of the aid. On the basis of clinical measures and consultation with the patient, a hearing aid was selected. Auditory training, lipreading instruction, and speech correction procedures were continued as deemed necessary.

The procedures described above were derived judgmentally, not experimentally. As discussed in Chapter Eight, subsequent research has caused doubt about some of the assumptions associated with the clinical selection procedure.

Regardless, the rehabilitative aspects of the program were valuable. Hearing, hearing loss, and hearing aids were thoroughly explained to the patient. He learned how to use the aid. He was given varied experiences in aided listening in a controllable and structured environment. Perhaps most important of all, he was involved in the selection process; his opinion was solicited. This procedure must have fostered psychological acceptance of amplification and responsibility for successful hearing aid use.

DiCarlo (1948) made a comprehensive appraisal of a program of auditory training he had developed for 472 servicemen, all of whom had been provided hearing aids. He was able to demonstrate improvement in consonant recognition through training. Other researchers have pointed to the fact that auditory training has a beneficial effect on sound discrimination, pure-tone discrimination, and speech perception (Hudgins, 1954; Miller, 1952; Silverman, 1947). One of the greatest problems of the early research effort was in the lack of reliable tests with alternate forms that could be used to measure the several variables associated with auditory training.

Much later, Northern et al. (1969) conducted a survey of attitudes of military patients regarding the current version of the military amplification and rehabilitation program. The course at that time consisted of 2 to 3 weeks training in hearing aid orientation, speechreading, and auditory training. The survey indicated strong approval of the program and a high percentage of successful adjustment to hearing aid use.

Financial considerations are frequently a barrier outside of government programs. However, one audiologist has designed a hearing aid orientation program at reasonable cost (Carmel, 1975). The fee schedule and associated services are shown in Table 12-1. Looking at amplification as part of a comprehensive rehabilitation program, Carmel states that his approach includes medical ear, nose, and throat examination, audiologic evaluation, and counseling in addition to the services shown in Table 12-1. As indicated, all aids are provided for a trial period of 1 month.

It has been shown that emphasis on amplification with the very young hearing-handicapped child is justifiable. McCroskey (1967) studied early home auditory training programs for infants. He found that children entering nursery school who had been through the training programs as infants had spectrographic tracings of speech sounds more like those of normal hearing children than did children with hearing loss not exposed to amplified sound early in their lives. Lach et al. (1970) demonstrated how voice quality can be improved through early training of hearing-handicapped children fitted with hearing aids.

Many accomplished teachers stress the importance of an aural habilitation program of early, appropriate, and consistent amplification (Horton, 1973; Ling, 1973; Stewart, 1973; Pollack, 1974; Grammatico, 1975). How-

TABLE 12-1. **Fee schedule for a comprehensive hearing aid program***

Services and Other Expenses†	Fee
Services	
Hearing aid evaluation	$25.00
Hearing aid delivery and counseling	50.00
3 visits 1st month @ $15.00 each	45.00
2 additional visits 1st year	30.00
Other Expenses	
Hearing aid ($90.00 to $200.00)	
Earmold	20.00
Overhead factor	75.00
Total average cost of hearing aid program	$380.00
If binaural aids are recommended, average cost would be	$610.00
Fee if aid is returned†	$75.00

* Data from Carmel, 1975.

† A hearing aid is purchased as part of the comprehensive hearing rehabilitation program. If the aid is returned at the end of the evaluation month, the patient is billed for the hearing aid evaluation ($25.00) and the hearing aid delivery ($50.00).

ever, not all authorities believe in the universal application of the aural method to all hearing impaired children. Referring to profoundly deaf children, Vernon (1972) states, "Amplification will help some of these children hear thunder, firecrackers, and other kinds of gross sounds." However, he continues that children " . . . who have losses of 85 dB or greater are not going to learn language through speech or through amplification regardless of how intense the amplification is" (Vernon, 1972, p. 531).

The implications of these statements are twofold. First, more research and less emotionalism are needed to determine the relationship of magnitude of congenital loss and successful learning of language and speech through amplification. There are unquestionably exceptional profoundly deaf individuals who achieve remarkable verbal communication through auditory-visual channels. However, the high probability of success has not been demonstrated with congenitally impaired children who have profound loss, fragmented audiogram, and no response above 500 or 1000 Hz. Kleffner (1973) presents an insightful viewpoint on the relation between hearing-impaired children, hearing aids, language disorders, and the need for training in learning to use amplified sound. He emphasizes that the pure-tone audiogram should serve as a basis for determining whether amplification is needed, and that no amount of information about response to environmental sounds or voice is an adequate substitute.

Second, there is an extreme need for predictors of educational success in one or another type of training program. Valid predictors would identify the kind of program in which a child would perform best and eliminate the tragedy of finding out only by trial and error. Some prognostic tools are available and are discussed below.

Downs (1974) has prepared a Deafness Management Quotient which aims to predict whether a hearing-impaired child would be more successful in an auditory-oral or a total communication educational program. The quotient is derived from (1) magnitude of hearing loss, (2) neurological status (central intactness), (3) intelligence, (4) socioeconomic level, and (5) family considerations. Figure 12-1 shows how each of these factors is weighted and how the Deafness Quotient is derived. A score of 81 or

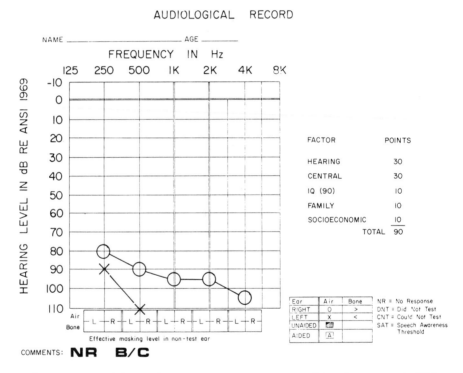

FIG. 12-1. Use of the Deafness Management Quotient (DMQ), (Downs, 1974). With a DMQ of 90, as obtained from the criteria below, this child would be recommended for an auditory-oral program. The criteria are: (1) Residual hearing, 30 points. Zero points (pts) = no true hearing; 10 pts = thresholds at 250 and 500 Hz better than 100 dB; 20 pts = thresholds at 250, 500, and 1000 Hz better than 100 dB; 30 pts = thresholds at 250, 500, 1000 and 2000 Hz better than 100 dB. Ten points are added if a conductive component is present. (2) Central intactness, 30 points. Zero pts = diagnosis of brain damage; 10 pts = positive history of events associated with birth defects other than hearing loss; 20 pts = perceptual dysfunction, 30 pts = intact central processing. (3) Intelligence (determined by appropriate non-verbal tests), 20 points. Zero pts = mental retardation (IQ below 85); 10 pts = average (IQ between 85 and 100); 20 pts = above average (IQ above 100). (4) Support from family, 10 points. Zero pts = no support; 10 pts = completely supporting family. (5) Socioecoeconomic status, 10 points. Zero pts = substandard; 10 pts = completely adequate.

greater was suggested as an indicator of likely success in an auditory-oral program. Based on appealing and reasonable concepts, the validity of the Deafness Management Quotient awaits experimental verification.

Robinson and Gaeth (1975) proposed a program which relates audiometric evaluation, educational training, and prognostic procedures. Their objectives were the acquisition of valid audiometric information, initiation of auditory language development, selection of correct amplification, and determination of appropriate educational placement. They felt the primary importance of their procedure was the integration of auditory testing and amplification selection into a training format.

Far less research has been accomplished in auditory training for adults than with children. Bode and Oyer (1970) compared a number of procedures to determine which was best for improving speech discrimination of hard of hearing adults. The two variables under study were type of response required of subjects and type of noise background in which speech stimuli were placed. Two types of responses were elicited, write-down and selection of multiple-choice answers. The noise (speech babble) was made more intense as the practice session progressed. It was found that 3 hours of practice on monosyllabic words improved the performance of subjects on the CID W-22 words and Fairbanks Rhyme Test words, but not for Semi-Diagnostic Test material. A varied signal-to-noise ratio had a tendency to produce better results with the multiple-choice response. However, the steady state and varied noise yielded highly similar results with the write-down response.

Lundborg et al. (1973) assessed the relationship between amplification and need for training and use of other rehabilitation devices, all as a function of magnitude of hearing loss. They reported on 3,850 Swedish patients, making recommendations as follows:

1. Forty to sixty dB loss (50% of the group): (a) ear level amplification, (b) acoustic amplifiers for telephone, doorbell, and television, and (c) an instruction course in use of the hearing aid and other amplifiers; with lipreading and auditory training needed only occasionally in cases with steeply falling audiometric configurations.

2. Sixty to eighty dB loss (40% of the group): (a) body-worn amplification (ear level if the patient insisted — many more cases in this category in the United States would probably use ear level amplification), (b) optical and acoustic devices, and (c) instruction programs in the use of amplification, with lipreading instruction and auditory training for those judged able to benefit (about 10% of this group).

3. Pure-tone average greater than 80 dB: (a) body-worn aid, (b) optical and vibrotactile warning devices, and (c) full rehabilitative program needed, but of benefit in only about 40% of this group because of age and other factors.

Attempts to modify the characteristics of the amplified signal have included frequency transposition. Mainly there have been attempts towards a downward frequency transposition. The thought is that in so doing the information is provided at those frequencies for sensorineural cases where there is greatest sensitivity. Those involved in this effort have reported some successes (Bennett and Byers, 1967; Oeken, 1963; Johansson, 1966; Ling and Doehring, 1969; Ling and Druz, 1967). However, it can be said fairly that frequency transposition has not yet shown consistent positive results.

It would be a mistake to terminate a discussion of amplification without commenting about the possible deleterious effect of amplification on some hearing loss. Threshold shift can result from applying an aid with too much power. Macrae and Farrant (1965) compared the effect of two hearing aids on 87 children. All had bilateral sensorineural losses. The investigators concluded that a high-powered aid can cause deterioration of hearing. The damage is a function of the power of the aid, the number of hours it is used, the gain setting, and the extent of the hearing loss. Ross and Lerman (1967) concluded that auditory deterioration can be caused by hearing aids and suggested limiting output to about 130 dB sound pressure level. Bellefleur and Van Dyke (1968) found no effect of high gain amplification on hearing of 58 children enrolled in a school for the deaf, but agreed with Ross and Lerman certain individuals, particularly if hard of hearing rather than in the deaf classification, might suffer some shift. Other studies have reported threshold shift as a function of amplification (Macrae, 1968; Roberts, 1970).

Harford and Markle (1955) described a case which is summarized in Table 12-2. A substantial threshold shift was apparent on the aided ear after the child had worn an aid for 3 years. The aid was moved to the other ear. Two changes then resulted. There was partial recovery of sensitivity on the previously aided ear, and the right ear, now aided, suffered a decrease in sensitivity. When no aid was used on either ear for a short trial period, some threshold improvement occurred. While this case had a substantial temporary component in the threshold shift, Jerger and Lewis (1975) have cited a case in which threshold shift associated with use of powerful amplification was apparently permanent.

The picture seems to be this: additional hearing loss from amplification is not likely but possible. Therefore, it is important to watch for change of auditory function in children who use amplification, and, as suggested in Chapter Nine, have audiologic evaluations at 3 month intervals during the 1st year of hearing aid use. A reasonable schedule thereafter is semi-annually for the 2nd year, and then yearly.

If threshold shift is noted, the following steps should be taken. If two aids are being worn, binaural use should be discontinued. An aid with maxi-

TABLE 12-2. **Threshold change associated with hearing aid use***

| Condition | Auditory Thresholds | | | | | | | | | |
| | 250 Hz | | 500 Hz | | 1000 Hz | | 2000 Hz | | 4000 Hz | |
	LE†	RE	LE	RE	LE	RE	LE	RE	LE	RE
Before hearing aid use	60	60	55	60	60	65	55	55	60	60
After wearing aid on left ear for three years	70	60	80	70	90	65	75	60	80	60
2½ months after changing aid to right ear	65	70	70	90	75	100	70	90	65	80
After 1 week of no hearing aid use	70	70	75	80	80	80	75	70	65	65

* Harford and Markle, 1955.
† LE, left ear; RE, right ear.

mum output as low as feasible should be obtained. The use of automatic gain control may be necessary to achieve a low output without excessive distortion. If there are two aidable ears, hearing aid use should alternate daily between ears. Reasonable precautions should be taken against unduly high gain settings, excessive noise exposure, and continuous use of the aid for unnecessarily long intervals. Clinical experience has shown this program to be useful in combatting threshold shift associated with amplification.

Speechreading

To link speechreading instruction with amplification and auditory learning presumes advocacy of a multisensory rather than unisensory approach. As will be discussed later in this chapter, there is some argument against a multi-sensory approach. However, some research suggests the usefulness of such an approach. O'Neill (1954) was among the first to attempt to determine the contributions of visual cues on reception of auditory stimuli. He found that when sensory information from vision and audition were combined, the scores achieved by subjects were consistently higher than when either mode was employed independently. The same general findings were reported by others (Sumby and Pollack, 1954; Sedge, 1965; Erber, 1969; Sanders and Goodrich, 1971). It has generally been found that visual cues have greater influence when the listening situation is at low sensation levels or against a background of noise.

Prall (1957) presented Phonetically Balanced Kindergarten word lists to eight hearing-impaired students. They received one list with only visual clues, another with only auditory stimulation, and a third with combined auditory-visual input. In each case the score for the combined condition was substantially greater than either of the other two conditions.

Ross, et al. (1972) gave the Word Intelligibility by Picture Identification discrimination test to 29 hearing-impaired children. Conditions of presentation were the same as in the Prall study. Twenty subjects obtained scores during the combined condition better than either of the other two conditions. Six had combined scores inferior or equal to one or both single modality conditions. Three subjects could not be tested under all modes.

There was a systematic appraisal of the interaction between auditory and visual systems in the work of Brown and Hopkins (1967). They studied separate visual and auditory threshold functions and a combined threshold function in order to determine more accurately the interaction of the two modalities. They drew a curve for the bisensory condition based on the probable adding of responses to the separate unisensory stimulus conditions. Their experimentation showed that the bisensory function agreed with their predictions. Karlovich (1968), through Alternate Binaural Loudness Balance Test matches for a 1000 Hz tone, concluded that introduction of a visual stimulus had a positive effect on the perception of loudness.

Erber (1972) reported that normal and hard-of-hearing children identified consonants better with simultaneous auditory-visual stimulation than with auditory input alone. However, the performance of profoundly deaf children was similar under both conditions.

Walden, Prosek, and Worthington (1975) examined the differences between auditory and auditory-visual presentation of speech on the performance of hearing-impaired adults. Specifically, they evaluated perception of several articulatory features. They found that adding visual clues substantially enhanced transmission of duration, place of articulation, frication, and nasality features; but helped less to perceive intervowel glide and voicing features.

Not all studies have shown an improvement with combined auditory-visual stimulation, however. Gaeth (1963, 1967) determined through a series of experiments with normal and hearing-impaired children in a paired-associate learning situation that when hearing loss was between 61 and 75 dB, visual perception was significantly better than the combined condition. He never found the combined presentation superior to the single mode presentation. Sometimes the learning curves for the combined procedure coincided with those of the unisensory procedure and at other times were not as high as the learning curves generated by unisensory stimulation.

Ritsma (1974) presented auditory stimuli to hearing-impaired children with and without visual clues. He concluded that, if the hearing aid does not permit discrimination of speech without visual clues, it will not increase speech intelligibility when visual clues are present.

Still other evidence of the interaction between visual and auditory stimuli has been shown by studies of distractions brought into the speechreading situation. Leonard (1962) found that selected auditory distractions led to a significant lowering of lipreading scores. He employed running speech, background music, and white noise as distractors. Ciliax (1973) examined further the effect of auditory distractions on speechreading performance. He found that when he pretrained his subjects in various sound backgrounds that they performed comparably regardless of the kind of noise background in which they received their training.

Miller (1965b) found that a flashing light, a spinning disk, and nonpurposeful hand movements had no real deleterious effect on lipreading scores. He found no significant differences between his control condition and the experimental conditions. Keil (1968) also explored the effects of peripheral visual stimuli on lipreading performance. She also found that visual distractors had no significant effect on lipreading performance.

Dodds and Harford (1968b) illustrated the utility of a lipreading test in hearing aid evaluation. They used the Utley Lip Reading Sentence Test to gain information supplementary to regular evaluation procedures. The test was presented with and without amplification. In each case the patient and examiner were face to face and both auditory and visual clues were available. Comparison of scores determined the improvement in lipreading associated with amplification. They thereby obtained information useful in making a decision about the feasibility of amplification in three types of patients for whom auditory tests were not conclusive: (1) those with poor speech discrimination, (2) patients with mild hearing loss and borderline need for amplification, and (3) patients who needed amplification, but were poorly motivated.

The studies reviewed above generally suggest a positive relationship between amplification and lipreading. However, in some instances, especially in very severely impaired children, amplification may reduce lipreading performance. As Erber (1972) suggests, the audiologist should assess combined auditory-visual aided performance. The results may be useful in justifying hearing aid use or in demonstrating to the patient the merits of amplification. If combined performance is poorer than the visual-only score, perhaps the audiologist can determine if the aid used is entirely appropriate, or if training will improve the patient's ability to utilize both senses.

The conflicting indications of the studies discussed above have not been resolved. One cause of differences probably relates to the heterogeneity of subjects between studies in magnitude of hearing loss. That is, subjects with good hearing who score near 100% on an auditory test may not benefit much from addition of visual clues. Profoundly deaf subjects, on the other hand, may not find their visually-obtained scores enhanced much by the addition of an auditory signal. Additionally, it is probable that the various studies explored different kinds of perceptual tasks, some of which may have been more amenable to combined stimulation than others.

In summary, while it has not been established definitively whether unisensory or bisensory stimulation is superior in training, there is no question that utilization of both auditory and visual information has potential for improving the speech perception of the hearing-impaired individual. Even if he cannot attend to both inputs simultaneously, as theorists believe, he can rapidly alternate sampling of information from both sensory channels, and achieve superior performance.

The results of studies are yet too few to make firm conclusions as to the efficacy of a multisensory or unisensory training approach. There is a growing argument that a unisensory approach is probably superior at least during some phases of development. Our own opinion is to suggest the use of a unisensory approach during the early phases of aural rehabilitation with children or adults. This can be followed with bisensory reinforcement later on. Real life situations are multisensory in nature for those with residual hearing amplified through a hearing aid.

RESEARCH NEEDS

A number of areas deserve further study in the amplification-aural rehabilitation process. There is a great need for further development of stable and valid test materials to assess hearing handicap as well as improvement associated with training. Some researchers feel that valid speech tests must reflect in their content the essential features of everyday conversation, and have developed such tests (Byman, 1974; Ludvigsen, 1974). While it is not usually possible to assess aspects of behavior under entirely "life-like" situations, more complex and sensitive tests are needed to help answer the questions detailed below.

First, there should be a thoroughgoing extensive analysis of the merits of unisensory, bisensory, and total communication approaches to rehabilitation. This should include sequential age groups and a variety of sensory stimuli. Second, there should be more research into the general area of spectral modification in amplifying devices. Third, it would be beneficial to explore the usefulness of visual cues that are available to hearing-handicapped persons. Fourth, it would be worthwhile to develop the training materials necessary for a more prescriptive approach to aural rehabilitation, in both auditory and visual areas. Fifth, there is a need for further study of the potentially harmful effects of hearing aids in some instances.

classroom amplification

Mark Ross, Ph.D.

INTRODUCTION

The traditional distinction between the topics of "classroom amplification" and "hearing aids" in this book reflects the separate, though related, development in each of these areas. While both ultimately depended upon advances in electronics, the hearing aid was developed mainly in response to the needs of adventitiously hearing-impaired adults, while the development of classroom auditory training systems reflected the impact of an educational philosophy espousing exploitation of residual hearing for "deaf" children (Goldstein, 1939). Both devices are hearing aids in that their main function is to amplify sounds and deliver them to the ear of the hearing-impaired person. Because portability was not a factor in the initial design of classroom auditory trainers, they could be engineered to provide the best possible acoustic signal without the regard for size limitations which constrained the electroacoustic possibilities of early hearing aids (Watson and Tolan, 1949).

As it happens, the quality of the auditory signal that each of these devices could provide made sense in terms of the population for which they were intended. Children with severe congential hearing losses, on the one hand, required a high fidelity signal for the optimum development of speech and language. The adventitiously hearing-impaired adult could, as Fletcher (1929) showed 50 years ago, understand spoken messages with a much lower fidelity signal. Much of the confusion regarding the relative merits of classroom auditory trainers versus hearing aids stems from a misunderstanding of the initially separate (but equal) purposes of these two devices, leading to the "consistent" versus the "inconsistent" amplification debate, which is discussed below.

Because the electroacoustic performance of classroom auditory trainers and personal hearing aids may be very different, many teachers and clinicians became concerned that we were, in effect, exposing our hearing-impaired children to two disparate variations of English speech and language. Our children, the reasoning went, have enough difficulty learning speech and language as it is; why make it even more difficult by shifting them between two different amplified versions of our language? Wouldn't the children be better off if a consistently patterned amplified signal were provided at all times? In effect, this meant the full time use of lower quality personal hearing aids instead of the higher quality classroom auditory trainers. The merits of the arguments have been examined in some detail elsewhere (Ross, 1972a, p. 22; and Sanders, 1971, p. 227). In brief, it seems that the proponents of "consistent" amplification have not sufficiently considered the difference between the learning of new verbal material and the recognition of material already learned. What is acoustically redundant for adults with a good knowledge of the language will not be so for a child attempting to learn the language. Although concrete empirical data bearing on this question are not available, it nevertheless seems more desirable that a child use a high quality instrument for as long as possible – that is, an auditory training system – in order to maximize his speech and language development. Once learned through a high quality classroom auditory trainer, the probabilities of recognizing this material through a lower quality personal hearing aid appears higher than if we had attempted initially to teach the new material through the personal hearing aid.

This debate and the continuation of the traditional treatment of classroom amplification systems as a separate entity is being made irrelevant by technical developments. In the past few years, advances in electronic circuitory and design have created a convergence in the development of hearing aids and classroom amplification systems. The newest generation of classroom amplification systems is essentially monaural or binaural hearing aids with the added capacity to receive a frequency-modulated (FM) radio frequency (RF) transmission, and they can be worn both in and out of the classroom. Therefore, we are now able to overcome the deleterious implications of treating hearing aids and classroom amplifiers as different systems.

Because of the emphasis on "classroom amplification," the exploitation of residual hearing in many special programs evolved into an academic topic, with formally structured, sequential "lessons" inadvertently communicating to the children that "hearing" was an academic exercise limited to classroom activities. The out-of-class use of personal hearing aids was often ignored, since "auditory training" was a regularly scheduled classroom activity which presumably took care of the child's auditory needs. The problem was compounded by the lack of supervision of after school use of personal hearing aids and their negative associations for many of the children and staff. In short, the "classroom amplification systems" orientation did not appear to be sympathetic to, and served to impede, the natural approach to speech and language development through an auditory modality.

Classroom amplification systems must permit the reception of a high quality auditory signal under the adverse acoustic conditions usually obtaining in classroom settings (Ross, 1972a). By the time the child has entered school, however, he should have a background of natural auditory language which he can draw on when first exposed to the teacher's speech. Certainly, then, at this stage, refinements and expansions of auditory language can occur as an integral component of the academic material being presented. This optimum condition occurs only when the hearing problem is detected early, permitting suitable parent-infant and preschool programs. Conceptually, there does not appear to be any justification in considering the amplified signal provided by a classroom system any differently from that provided by a wearable hearing aid. Practically, however, at the present time, there are some separate features which have to be considered. I would predict, however, that in the very near future, units will be available which will incorporate all the advantages of both personal hearing aids and classroom auditory trainers.

The organization of this chapter will emphasize a "current needs" approach. Some space and analysis will be devoted to the older classroom systems, but the primary focus will devolve upon contemporary requirements and the kind of systems which can best meet these requirements. The education of hearing-impaired children will more and more be taking place in "mainstream" settings, for good or ill (Northcutt, 1973; Nix, 1976); and the discussion and analysis of classroom amplification systems will be related to this trend.

GENERAL PRINCIPLES

The general principles enumerated below are meant to convey a framework to the reader by means of which he can critically analyze any existing classroom auditory training system. We are concerned with function, with what the unit is supposed to do. If we know this, we can evaluate the performance and utilization of any unit to determine if these requirements are met.

Signal-to-Noise Ratio

The first, and perhaps the most important factor, is that the unit must ensure the deliverance of the teacher's speech at a high signal-to-noise (S/

N) ratio. This factor is critically important. The child must be able to distinguish clearly the speech signal from the noise if he is to make the necessary associations between auditory and experiential events; if he is, in other words, to develop speech and language skills in a naturalistic manner through an auditory approach. Unfortunately, hearing-impaired listeners require S/N ratios on the order of +20 to +30 dB in order to reach maximum intelligibility (Gengel, 1971; Gengel and Foust, 1975), which is higher than normal hearing listeners require. In other words, noise levels which have only a moderate effect upon a normal hearing person can severely disrupt speech intelligibility for the hearing-impaired individual listening to speech through a hearing aid (Tillman, Carhart, and Olsen, 1970).

In judging the adequacy of the classroom S/N ratio, it is important that teachers and clinicians not rely overly on evidence of their own unaided ears (and sometimes their own eyes). That is, a classroom which appears moderately quiet in terms of the ambient noise and activities of the children may in reality be very noisy for the hearing-impaired children if a microphone is located near a noisy radiator, air conditioner, child, etc. A useful check is for the teacher to listen through the child's unit under normal use conditions. In so doing, one can often find "hidden" sources of noise which greatly degrade the S/N ratio. Another procedure is to measure the S/N ratio at the location of the teacher's microphone which should be within 4 to 12 inches of her mouth. Generally speaking, the S/N ratio can be improved by decreasing the distance between the teacher's mouth and the microphone. Some of the acoustic circumstances of inappropriate microphone location will be explored more fully below.

Auditory Self-Monitoring

The child's own speech output must be clearly audible to him, or at least as audible as his hearing loss permits. Speech is normally and naturally developed and best monitored by the auditory consequences of the vocal output (Fry, 1973). Kinesthetic, tactile, and proprioceptive feedback mechanisms are less effective mediators of speech output. The evidence relating degree of hearing loss to intelligibility of the child's speech is clear and emphasizes the contribution of audition in the development of intelligible speech for hearing-impaired children (Montgomery, 1967; Boothroyd, 1970; Smith, 1973). Without the most effective monitoring of his speech output, it is highly questionable that a hearing-impaired child will develop to his fullest potential aesthetically acceptable and intelligible speech. Even the existence of a profound hearing loss does not necessarily preclude the auditory monitoring of the prosodic components of the speech signal (Ross, Duffy, Cooker, and Sergeant, 1973).

For adequate monitoring, it is necessary that the child have an open microphone proximate to his mouth when he is talking. This condition does not obtain when the only open microphone in the classroom auditory training system is the one fastened around the teacher's neck or suspended from the ceiling. Moving the child's microphone just a few inches closer to his mouth can make the difference between adequate and inadequate auditory self-monitoring.

Child-to-Child Communication

In today's educational setting, it is not sufficient for a unit to optimize teacher transmission and auditory self-monitoring. The amplification system must also permit child-to-child communication in a natural and routine fashion. The method a growing child uses in communicating with his peers is apt to reflect his primary communication preference; if the amplification system does not permit an effective auditory-verbal link between the children, then it is not likely that residual hearing will play an important role in the developing communication mode. Children should be able to hear each other with the same efficiency with which they can hear the teachers and themselves.

Except for certain hard-wire arrangements discussed below, optimum child-to-child communication is not possible with existing auditory training systems. The children hear each other directly through the same microphones, located in the unit on their body, that they use to hear themselves. The teacher's microphone is ordinarily located around her neck, and thus does not make a major contribution to child-to-child communication. The units, in other words, function as personal hearing aids and the perceived speech signal depends primarily upon the intensity level of the speech, the distance between the children, and the level of the background noise. These three factors are at least partially under the control of the teacher. That is, the children can be encouraged and taught to increase their speech intensity level, they can be brought closer to one another, and the noise level can usually be diminished somewhat. Thus, some improvement in child-to-child communication is usually possible.

An examination of Figure 13-1 can clarify the three general principles discussed so far, S/N ratio, auditory self-monitoring, and child-to-child communication. In this example, the talker's speech intensity level is assumed to be 84 dB at 6 inches. Applying the inverse square law, in which the SPL (sound pressure level re 20 μPa) decreases by 6 dB with every doubling of distance, we can see that the SPL at 1 foot is 78 dB, at 2 feet it is 72 dB, at 4 feet it is 66 dB, at 8 feet it is 60 dB and at 16 feet it is 54 dB. At the greater talker-microphone distances, these figures are likely to be only rough approximations, since the inverse square law will not apply in classrooms in which sound energy is reflected back into the room. However, we can still get a fairly good idea of the signal-to-noise ratios

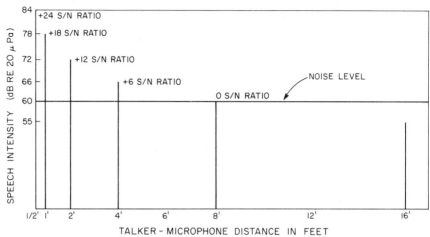

FIG. 13-1. The effect of distance on the signal-to-noise ratio.

pertaining under different conditions. Let us assume that the ambient noise level is 60 dB SPL, a fairly common figure. We then see that our attempts to achieve a high S/N ratio can only be met at the 6 inch distance, with the 1 foot distance a possibly acceptable compromise. Normal hearing listeners can function very well at the 2 and 4 foot distances, but our hearing impaired-students require at least a 20 dB S/N for optimal auditory reception (Gengel, 1971; Gengel and Foust, 1975). The talker-microphone distance should be evaluated for each of the three general principles discussed: Is the teacher's mouth within a foot from the microphone? Is the child's self-monitoring microphone less than 6 inches from his mouth? Is the distance between the children the least possible permitted by the classroom setting?

Electroacoustic Considerations

Some of the older classroom amplification systems made little provision for altering the amplification pattern in accordance with the needs of different children. A child is not receiving an optimum signal if the amplified signal delivered to his ear offers little possibility of individualized variations.

Some group systems offer an acceptable degree of electroacoustic flexibility, while others do not. One must be able to adjust the amplification characteristics of the group system to the same degree possible with a high quality personal hearing aid. At a minimum, it must permit flexible modifications in the gain, output, frequency response, and frequency range for each ear separately. Children differ in respect to their threshold of discomfort and the configuration of their hearing loss. We must therefore be able to adjust the acoustic output and the frequency response, and extend or lower the frequency range of the amplified signal to reflect and maximally exploit these individual differences (Ross, 1976).

Even if a classroom system permits flexible electroacoustic modifications, it does not follow that the possible modifications are desirable. For example, certain units may provide for a maximum power output in excess of 146 dB SPL, while others limit their maximum output to 132 dB or less. In terms of how the ear works and what sound it can tolerate, the 146 dB output figure is dangerously and ridiculously high. As another example, consider the possible variation in adjustments of the frequency range between two different instruments. Both may advertize "low frequency extension," but in actuality the low frequency limits of one may be 100 Hz (and we wouldn't want to go much lower than this), and the other may be 350 Hz. For most hearing-impaired children, who possess residual hearing at 2000 Hz and higher, the differences between these two instruments are trivial. As a matter of fact, it would be desirable to further limit low frequency response so as to optimize perception of the higher frequencies (Danaher and Pickett, 1975). For the minority of hearing-impaired children whose residual hearing is concentrated in the low frequencies, the instrument providing a low frequency cut-off of 100 Hz instead of 350 Hz has the capability of transmitting some potentially valuable acoustic information to the child (Ross, Duffy, Cooker, and Sergeant, 1973).

Other electroacoustic considerations, equally applicable to hearing aids and auditory trainers, are such factors as low internal noise, low harmonic distortion, sturdy construction, and a long battery life. Briefly, sales puffery aside, what we are looking for is the highest quality electroacoustic system consistent with current technology and the needs of children.

Binaural Reception

At first glance, binaural amplification may not appear to be an appropriate general principle, since the teacher transmission in all the current classroom amplification systems is received by the children in a diotic, rather than binaural, mode. That is, the "ear" of a child is represented by the single microphone the teacher uses and this signal is transmitted to the child's wearable instrument where it is fed to one or both ears. If both, the situation is comparable to a child wearing a hearing aid with a Y-cord.

We are concerned, however, not only with how the child receives the teacher transmission, but his capacity to hear himself (auditory self-monitoring) and other children (child-to-child communication). There is no direct evidence supporting the advantages of binaural as opposed to monaural auditory self-monitoring for a hearing-impaired child. The psychoacoustics of the situation, however, suggest a binaural loudness enhancement of the self-monitored suprathreshold signal on the order of 6 dB.

Binaural use is also supported by occasional clinical observations in which a child's vocal output appears negatively influenced when one aid of a binaural system becomes inoperable.

A binaural receiver unit is most advisable in those educational settings which place a great deal of stress upon individualized instruction and child-to-child communication. The recent evidence supporting binaural amplification clearly supports the notion of binaural superiority for most hearing-impaired individuals (Ross et al., 1974; Yonovitz and Campbell, 1974; Nabelek and Pickett, 1974b). In any situation in which the receiver unit of the classroom amplification system must function as a hearing aid (in other words, when the teacher microphone is turned off), the binaural signal reception offers a greater possibility of increasing the child's perception of an auditory signal. Binaural advantage may be reduced when the two microphones are located in a single physical unit, and the small distance between the two microphones can preclude the most efficient processing of a binaural signal (Maxon, Deutsch and Mazor, 1972). The necessity for a binaural receiver unit must be weighted individually, in terms of the child's candidacy for binaural amplification, the relative time he spends receiving group or individual instruction, and the organization of classroom and out-of-classroom activities. When in doubt, it makes sense to ensure that the group system offers binaural possibilities.

Simplicity and Stability of Operation

The likelihood of a classroom amplification system being used effectively, or being used at all, is much increased when its operation is simple and clearly defined and trouble-free. Classroom teachers are easily intimidated, for which one can hardly fault them, when they are confronted with an imposing array of dials, switches, adjustments, and check procedures. To manufacturers and salesmen, and even sometimes audiologists, the proper operation of a system may appear to be an uncomplicated simple procedure. These individuals are often amazed at the apparent stupidity of the classroom teacher, who evidently can't figure out or use properly what to them is really a very simple device. They should keep in mind that even teachers of the deaf receive very little training in classroom amplification systems, that the little training they do receive is frequently irrelevant and shortly outmoded, and that their days are fully occupied in the very trying task of teaching a class of hearing-impaired children. These concerns are even more applicable to the regular teacher in whose classroom a hearing-impaired child may be placed. The point is that the manufacturer of classroom systems must take responsibility for simple and effective operational design, and not ask teachers to compensate for poor engineering. Other aspects being equal, the classroom systems which are the simplest to operate, the easiest to trouble-shoot, which demonstrate the best performance stability, and provide for rapid and accurate repair and replacement, are to be preferred.

In some RF systems, the carrier wave frequency can be changed by a flick of a switch; in others, a module must be replaced, which, because it requires more effort, sometimes gets ignored in the press of other business. The battery operation in many units has been greatly improved in recent years. Improvements include a pilot light on the child's receiver to signal when the battery is going dead, pilot lights on the charger to indicate when the microphone-transmitter and student receiver is charging or fully charged, provision for a complete recharge in just 1 hour rather than overnight, and a realistic battery tester which places the proper electrical load on the battery when it is being checked. One system includes a visual indicator on the microphone-transmitter to show the proper volume level on the auxiliary input (TV, audio, tape recorder, phonograph, etc.) feeding into it. A number of the newer RF auditory trainers incorporate in the battery charger the appropriate circuitry for toubleshooting the cords, transducers, and the receivers in a simple and accurate manner. One innovative development includes a "muting" circuit, which automatically reduces the signal received through the child's environmental microphones as the teacher is talking, and, when she stops, automatically reactivates them. Theoretically, this should improve the S/N ratio both when the teacher and the children are talking.

Classroom systems requiring an intermediate stage or device between the teacher microphone and the student receiver are less advisable than those which do not have this requirement. Examples of this are units which necessitate an external FM table-model tuner to detect and retransmit the signal from the teacher's microphone, or those which require both FM and magnetic field variations for their operation. In this latter type of system, the teacher transmits an RF signal to a receiver worn by the child: this signal is then converted to electromagnetic field variations, which are picked up by the telephone coil of the child's personal hearing aid and finally then converted into sound. Several studies have warned of the increased possibility of acoustic response irregularities and poorer speech intelligibility scores when a classroom amplification system uses both an FM and an induction loop amplification (magnetic field variations) mode of operation (Matkin and Olsen, 1973; Sung et al., 1973). As a general principle a classroom amplification system is preferred when it requires the fewest signal conversions, when its operation is most simple and clear-cut, and when troubleshooting and repair can be carried out with the least amount of difficulty.

TYPES OF CLASSROOM AMPLIFICATION SYSTEMS

There will be three general types of systems discussed in this section: the hard-wire system, the induction loop amplification (ILA) system, and the radio frequency (RF) carrier-wave systems. It is these latter units which shall occupy us most fully, since they offer the most versatility and have seen the greatest recent proliferation in their use and number. Of the different types of RF systems which have been developed, we shall be concerned here only with the completely portable, wireless, frequency-modulated (FM) system. In the course of the RF device development, there have been those which required a loop antenna around the room, and which necessitated a table-model receiver and transmitter connected to the teacher's microphone via a wire cord. These complex units operated on the amplitude-modulated (AM) rather than the FM band, and included an adapter to couple the transmitted signal through the telephone coil of the child's personal hearing aid. A description of the various units can be found in Matkin and Olsen (1973). All of these served a very useful purpose at one time, and many are still being used. In keeping with the perspective of this chapter, however, we shall be minimizing the historical development of classroom amplification systems, and focusing on current and future need and what appears to me to be educationally most defensible.

Hard-Wire Systems

A typical hard-wire system arrangement is shown in Figure 13-2. This was the first type of electronic classroom amplification system made and

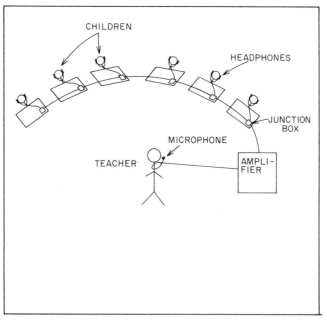

FIG. 13-2. A typical hard-wire auditory trainer arrangement.

the one which dominated the market for many years. In the simplest case, there is one microphone, an amplifier, and a number of earphones. The units were called "hard-wire" systems because both the teachers and the students were tethered to the amplifier by means of a wire cord, thus limiting their mobility to the length of the cord. During the years before miniaturization of electronic circuitry became perfected, the greater size of these systems permitted the incorporation of a number of desirable acoustic features. Working and used properly, they could provide a high level acoustic signal of excellent quality. However, except for adjustments in the relative intensity of a diotic signal to the two ears, these units typically did not permit individualized adjustments in electroacoustic dimensions. This factor is not intrinsic to a hard-wire system, since it is possible to design a unit which would provide desired electroacoustic features on an individualized basis. However, the advent of other types of classroom systems, which appear to have more educational desirability, has essentially obviated further commercial developments in this area.

Utilization

In Figure 13-2, notice the short distance between the teacher and the microphone, a precondition for assuring a high S/N ratio between the teacher's voice and the background sounds. Notice, too, however, that in order for the children to hear themselves or the other children, their speech signal has to travel to the teacher's microphone before it is picked up and delivered back to them. As Figure 13-1 indicates, the intensity of the speech signal will diminish with distance. If the ambient noise is moderately high, a not unusual condition, then auditory self-monitoring and child-to-child communication will be negatively affected by the resulting poor S/N ratio. It is precisely this factor — where to locate the microphone — which presents the biggest single drawback to the use of hard-wire systems for classroom amplification purposes. This drawback is probably greater than the loss of mobility engendered by the wire cord.

There have been a number of attempts to circumvent the limitations imposed by the single microphone. Some manufacturers provide a microphone for the teacher and another one centered among the children, for self-monitoring and child-to-child communication purposes. This arrangement is not much better. In this arrangement, the children are now too far from the microphone for optimum self-monitoring and child-to-child communication. One group system provides an automatic volume control circuit in connection with a single, centered microphone, which automatically increases the level of soft speech and decreases the level of more intense speech. This appears to be a logical solution, until one reflects on the fact that the device cannot distinguish between speech and the varying background sounds. This would work well in a quiet environment, but would not improve the S/N ratio in noisy circumstances.

Hirsh (1968) discussed some other pitfalls and some of the attempts which have been made to circumvent the microphone's placement problems. He described the use of multiple microphones, one for each child or one between each pair of children. Experiences with multiple microphones have not been too positive. With all the microphones "live," all sounds impinging on each microphone are delivered to each child in the room. Such extraneous noises as pencil scratching, foot shuffling, paper rattling, and irrelevant vocalizations mask the wanted speech and make the acoustic situation very undesirable. Damashek and Boothroyd (1973) described a miniature boom microphone fixed to the earphone transducer and situated a few inches to the side of the student's mouth. The microphone leads are fed to the room amplifier and thence to each transducer. With this arrangement they showed a highly significant improvement in child-to-child communication—measured via speech intelligibility tests—and good subjective reactions in regards to the self-monitoring aspects. The only extraneous sounds which constitute a major problem with this arrangement are unwanted and inadvertent vocalizations. These, perhaps, could be remedied if each of the miniature boom microphones was voice-actuated with a reasonably high actuating threshold.

Several research studies have evaluated the presumed benefits of group hard-wire amplification systems with hearing-impaired children. Hudgins (1953) and Clarke (1957) both found that children who used the group systems improved significantly in some academic areas and in speech production and perception compared to children who did not use the group system. However, since an auditory training component was a major factor in both these studies, it is difficult to attribute the improvement to the use of a classroom amplification system per se, as opposed to the systematic training which accompanied its use.

The hard-wire classroom amplification system reflects an educational era which stressed small, structured, and self-contained classes of hearing-impaired students away from the educational "mainstream." An educational philosophy which emphasized teacher input happened to coincide with the technical possibilities at the time. As awareness grew regarding the interdependence of speech output and auditory input, as educational theory began to stress a more individualized and "open" classroom environment, the limitations of hard-wire systems became more apparent. In certain situations, they can be used effectively, particularly if the teacher is a master at microphone technique (the proper microphone placement) but the life span of hard-wire systems is probably limited. Nothing they can do cannot also be accomplished with portable units, which offer the advantages that the hard-wire system cannot match.

Induction Loop Amplification (ILA)

Description

The lack of physical mobility of both children and teachers fostered the development, and rapid acceptance, of ILA devices. Later, claims regarding the superiority of the ILA system in terms of the consistency of the auditory signal in group and individual situation would also be made, but this presumed advantage was a post-hoc thought, and in any event, not supported by empirical research.

An ILA system consists of a microphone, an amplifier, and instead of earphones or a speaker, a coil of wire placed around the room in any one of a number of geometrical configurations. The amplified electrical analog of sound waves is fed to the coil of wire, producing electromagnetic variations in the room. These variations represent a conversion of the sound waves into another form of energy. The electromagnetic field then crosses a tiny induction coil in the child's hearing aid and induces an electrical current in the coil. This current is then amplified and reconverted to sound waves by the student's hearing aid receiver.

The coil was originally designed for electromagnetic pickup of telephone conversations. The original ILA system simply used the existing telephone coils in hearing aids, which made no provision for the reception of an auditory signal from any other source. That is, the child could hear the teacher, but not himself or the other children directly. Later modifications of hearing aids permitted the reception of a signal from either the microphone or the induction coil. Aids with this modification have a three way input switch: microphone only, telecoil only, or combined microphone-telecoil input. A block diagram of a typical ILA installation is shown in Figure 13-3. Only one configuration of a loop is shown. In practice, various kinds of configurations are possible, from a "grid" to a "clover leaf" design.

Utilization

With an ILA arrangement, the children theoretically have the advantages of a hard-wire system (group reception of the teacher's signal at a favorable S/N ratio) plus the advantages of using their personal hearing aids for improved mobility, self-monitoring, and child-to-child communication. In practice, the situation has been found to be quite different. The many and variable pitfalls which have been found, while not uncorrectable, have discouraged the continued acceptance of this system. Only a brief summary will be provided of the major problems of ILA systems; for a more detailed examination, the reader is referred to the extensive literature which rapidly developed on this topic (Bellefleur and McMenamin, 1965; Borrild, 1967; Calvert et al., 1965; Klijn, 1961; Ling, 1966; Matkin and Olsen, 1970a and b, 1973; Ross, 1969; Sung and Hodgson, 1971; Sung, Sung, and Hodgson, 1974).

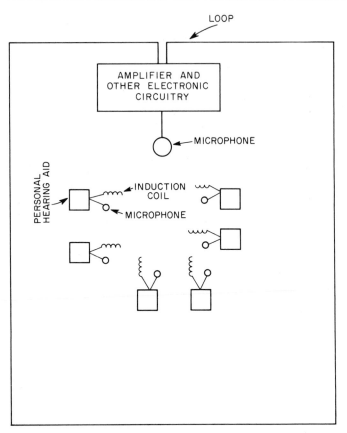

F_IG_. 13-3. An induction loop amplification arrangement, showing microphone and induction coil pick-up.

These investigators established that the electroacoustic characteristics of a hearing aid are frequently modified when it is used with a telephone coil in the place of a microphone. The output may be reduced, the low frequencies may be extended or otherwise modified, and the high frequency range may be sharply curtailed. The strength of the electromagnetic field emitted from the coil can, and usually does, show great variations in the room, with differential interactions between separate ILA systems and different hearing aids. The physical orientation of the telephone coil in the hearing aid will markedly effect the acoustic characteristics of the signal the child receives. In buildings where more than one ILA system is installed, signals may "spill over" between rooms, masking desired signals and generally confusing the children.

During the period when only ILA systems permitted both the freedom of movement in the classroom and the convenience of using the same instrument in and out of group situations, the profession wrestled with the above problems so as to achieve the presumed advantages. With the advent of RF classroom amplification systems, however, which solved many of these problems and minimized others, the motivation for continued involvement with ILA instruments has essentially disappeared. It is now very rare to find a manufacturer of classroom amplification equipment displaying ILA systems at professional conventions. They served an important purpose, and some obeisance to their presence should be made for historical purposes, but their eventual demise is not to be regretted.

Radio-Frequency (RF) Frequency-Modulated (FM) Systems

Description

The newest generation of FM classroom amplification systems consists of a microphone-transmitter worn by the teachers and an FM receiver-hearing aid worn by the child. Except for battery rechargers, that's all. The microphone is normally suspended around the teacher's neck, thus ensuring a favorable microphone-talker distance with a resulting good S/N ratio (see Figure 13-1). The transmitters, which ordinarily broadcast in the 72–76 MHz band, are permitted sufficient power by FCC regulations virtually to guarantee equal signal strength within the confines of even very large classrooms. Sufficiently distinct transmitting frequencies are available to obviate problems of interference from other channels, except perhaps in the very largest special schools which contain more than 32 classrooms, which is the number of carrier-wave frequencies potentially available in the 72–76 MHz band. The children's receivers are tuned to the required frequency, either with plug-in modules or with a two or three position channel selection switch. One or two environmental microphones are incorporated within the receiver units, permitting it to serve also as a body-worn monaural or binaural hearing aid. These microphones provide the requirement of auditory self-monitoring and child-to-child communication. Most of the systems are powered by rechargeable energy cells. Essentially, the system can be conceptualized as no more than an FM radio, with the teacher broadcasting a signal which the child detects via his own "radio."

A microphone-transmitter and a receiver hearing aid are shown in Figure 13-4. Note that each unit has an input jack for battery charging as well as an auxiliary input for signals from a tape recorder, phonograph or other source. Figure 13-5 shows an FM system in use (*a*) in a conventional classroom situation and (*b*) as an individual child studies a tape-recorded lesson. Figure 13-6 shows an FM system encased in its battery charger-storage compartment.

Utilization

The educational purposes and electroacoustic dimensions offered by the older classroom systems can also be found in the more recent RF systems.

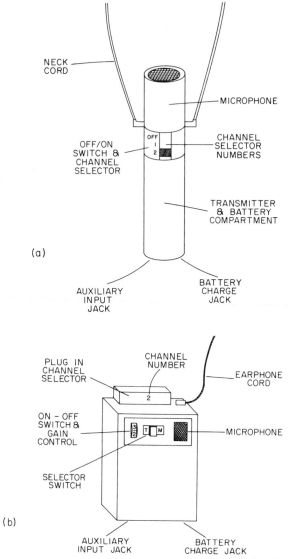

NECK CORD

MICROPHONE

OFF/ON SWITCH & CHANNEL SELECTOR

OFF
1
2

CHANNEL SELECTOR NUMBERS

TRANSMITTER & BATTERY COMPARTMENT

(a)

AUXILIARY INPUT JACK

BATTERY CHARGE JACK

PLUG IN CHANNEL SELECTOR

CHANNEL NUMBER

EARPHONE CORD

2

ON – OFF SWITCH & GAIN CONTROL

MICROPHONE

SELECTOR SWITCH

(b)

AUXILIARY INPUT JACK

BATTERY CHARGE JACK

FIG. 13-4. (a) FM microphone-transmitter. (b) Receiver-hearing aid.

The sticking point, until quite recently, was the presumably superior acoustic characteristics found in some of the hard-wire systems. When used appropriately, it is true that they could deliver to the child an excellent quality amplified version of the teacher's speech. As seen above, however, this advantage was offset by the difficulty of achieving the goals of good self-monitoring and child-to-child communication. The advantage was further eroded by the practice in many classes of substituting hearing aid transducers for the headphones. This practice wrought a number of undesirable side effects on the published electroacoustic specifications

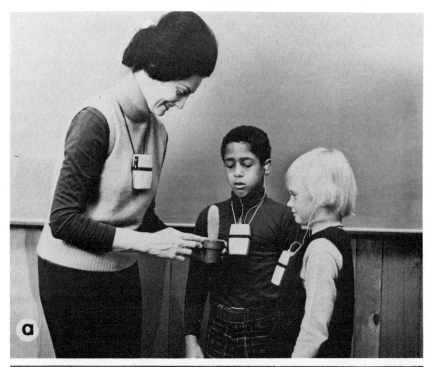

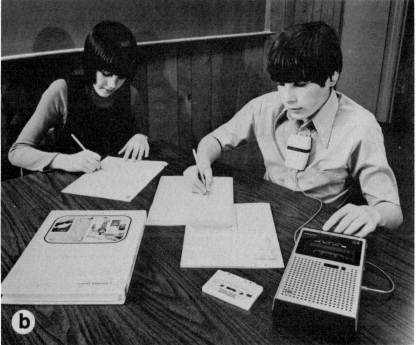

FIG. 13-5. (*a*) Classroom situation showing teacher transmitter and student receiver. (*b*) Receiver used with auxiliary patchcord (photo by permission of Electronics Future, Inc.)

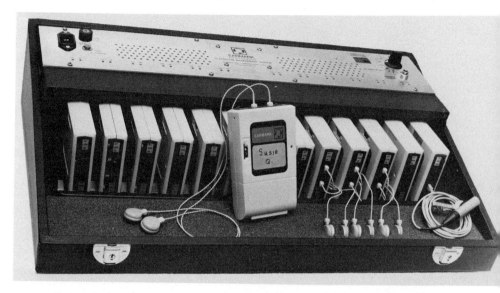

Fig. 13-6. Complete package, showing wireless microphone and receivers, and charger with cord and transducer testing facility and SPL calibration binaurally (photo by permission of Earmark, Inc.).

which many teachers were apparently not aware of, such as reducing the bandwidth of the amplified signal and increasing its maximum power output to dangerously high levels (Ross, 1969).

The FM auditory training systems can be used individually or with groups. They are engineered to accept an input into the transmitter of auxiliary sound sources (tape recorders, etc.). They can be used in and out of the classroom and require no permanent classroom installation of any kind. Different transmission frequencies permit several activities to be carried out with different groups of children in the same classroom. Any teacher who can successfully cope with the average home stereo unit should be able to operate one with relatively little difficulty. Correct utilization, however, requires a conscious and ongoing awareness of the basic principles discussed in this chapter. Children are no longer being educated very much as a group in the same classroom by the same teacher for the entire school day. Every changing educational circumstance demands an explicit analysis of the effect of this change upon the reception of the highest quality amplified signal (Ross, 1973).

Self-Contained Classes

The use of an FM system for purposes of group communication in a self-contained classroom is very straightforward and needs very little elaboration. All that is required is for the children to tune their units to the teacher's broadcast frequency, and to ensure that their personal environmental microphones are also operative. It is when modifications are made in this basic educational paradigm that the understanding of basic principles are required. For example, the teacher in the self-contained class may prefer to organize much of her day around "activity centers" located in different portions of her classroom and to individually program different children into different activities at different times. She will not be able to use her microphone-transmitter at these times, since she is no longer broadcasting to the group as a whole. If she forgets and leaves her microphone "open," then everything she says to each child will be presented with equal facility to every child in the room. Perhaps some children are engaged in intense and highly motivating child-to-child communication and the teacher's voice, while she is talking to another child in a separate location in the room, obliterates their attempts at verbal communication. And suppose that this happens repeatedly during the school day (how often do teachers *not* talk?). One possible effect is the de-emphasis of the auditory signal for children, who have been finding it an irrelevant and annoying distraction. It should be pointed out that a similar situation does not occur with normal hearing children in the same kind of educational situation. They tend to hear loudest those voices which are closest. With an RF system, the hearing-impaired child hears the signal at equal strength no matter where he is in the room and no matter what he is doing.

In this kind of situation, it is necessary to use the environmental microphones on the receiver unit for the reception of sounds; in other words, to employ the receiver as a hearing aid. If enough time during the school day is devoted to individualized activities, then we must devote some serious attention to the characteristics of the receiver unit when functioning as a hearing aid. Often, we find ourselves concentrating on the RF aspects of a classroom system, when in actuality it is used as a hearing aid for more time during the day then it is for group transmission. This is the major reason why, in the general principles outlined above, the binaural factor was included, since this will result in generally superior verbal reception for most children.

"Mainstream" Settings

The educational emphasis nowadays is to "normalize" a hearing-impaired child through integration in the mainstream educational setting. The theoretical advantages are many, but so is the potential for mischief. It is a step which must be done carefully, sequentially, and with built-in mechanisms for alternatives and frequent re-evaluations (Ross, 1976a). Generally speaking, the child with more residual hearing will tend to be the one who is "mainstreamed" (Ross, 1976b). This child's progress, educationally and socially, will depend on the use he makes of his residual hearing. In a mainstream setting, the auditory tool most likely to permit maximum utilization of residual hearing is the FM wireless auditory training system. Ross and Giolas (1971), and Ross, Giolas, and Carver (1973) evaluated the effect upon intelligibility scores of using a wireless microphone in a regular school setting. Both times it was found that the use of the wireless microphone, compared to the hearing-impaired child's usual listening situation in the regular classroom, resulted in a highly significant increase in intelligibility scores. The improvement was attributed to the improved S/N ratio due to the decreased microphone-mouth distance.

If a child is fully integrated in a "mainstream" setting, or is placed in a resource room in such a setting, there are going to be a number of times during the school day when he is engaged in different activities with different teachers. For the most part, whenever a teacher is instructing or addressing a group or the class as a whole, it is appropriate to use the FM microphone-transmitter. This means the child must take responsibility for bringing the unit from class to class. The teacher must take responsibility for determining when it can and cannot be used effectively. All teachers working with the hearing-impaired child must receive an orientation dealing with the need for the FM units, its physical operation, and the basic principles underlying its effective employment.

Whenever the hearing-impaired child in the regular class is not receiving generalized instruction from the teacher, it is necessary for the teacher to shut off the transmission from her microphone-transmitter. It is convenient if the unit permits this to be accomplished both at the receiver and in the microphone-transmitter. On many occasions teachers have forgotten to shut off their transmitter, walked to a different part of the room, or a different room, and engaged in what they thought was private conversation, only to find that the hearing-impaired child was privy to their personal thoughts and comments. During periods when group instruction is not taking place, the unit must be used as a personal hearing aid. If there is more than one hearing impaired child in a school, and they are likely to be receiving an FM signal at the same time, then the same number of complete FM units are required as there are children.

In most "mainstream" settings, there are going to be periods during the day when an individual hearing-impaired child leaves the resource room to engage in some outside academic or non-academic activities. At these times, the child must be able to turn off the RF transmission at the receiver unit, else he will be bombarded by the signals emanating from the resource room or other room using the same carrier frequency. These signals, having nothing to do with the activities in which he is engaged, are confusing, irrelevant, distracting, and can generate a negative listening attitude.

In short, the correct utilization of an FM auditory training system in a "mainstream" setting is, to be blunt, often a pain the neck. The teacher must be aware at all times during the day when the unit is to be worn for group transmission, or the FM transmitter turned off for individualized instruction. She must deal with the needs for different transmitting and receiving frequencies for different children at the same time, or the same child at different times. She must manage the reluctance of children to part with their cosmetically desirable ear-level hearing aids during some or all of the school day and wear a relatively bulky FM receiver-hearing aid. She must switch between the child's hearing aids and the auditory trainer several times each day. She must ensure that the units are charging before leaving school every day. We are, it seems, making yet more demands upon the time of already harried and overloaded teachers, and I can understand the reservations many of them have regarding FM classroom systems. What must be emphasized, however, as an overriding consideration, is that the payoff is worth the effort. If the child can hear better, he will learn more. It's as simple as that.

THE "OPTIMUM" UNIT

It is a very simple, yet frustrating, task for the audiologist in rehabilitation to "prescribe" all the features desirable in a classroom system. Simple, because we can define our needs fairly accurately; frustrating, because so often our pleas seem to be falling on deaf ears. Nevertheless, speaking as one who has expressed more than his share of skepticism and discouragement, the signs of significant progress are clearly discernible and appear to be accelerating. Manufacturers have been demonstrating an increasing sensitivity to consumer needs, with their ever-increasing number evidently stimulating a healthy competitive situation. Many of the different brands have some unique desirable features; none have every one, and some major developments are apparently still gestating. To carry the analogy further, the needs have been conceived; they just haven't been delivered.

Our most crucial need is the final breakdown of the distinction between personal hearing aids and classroom amplification systems. Each hearing-impaired child should possess a personal amplification instrument (call it a hearing aid or whatever) appropriate for all of the personal and academic situations he finds himself in. He should be able to put it on in the morning and wear it to school. At school, he should be able to switch to any one of a number of FM frequencies for group and classroom communication, and then easily switch off the FM mode for individual and social experiences. After school, he should be able to wear it for all of his home activities, recharging or exchanging the batteries at night. Such an "optimal" unit should permit binaural reception of acoustic stimuli at ear level, though FM reception would of necessity be diotic, since it is transmitted by a single microphone. It should include the capability of many potentially desirable electroacoustic adjustments to each ear separately. The representatives of several manufacturers have personally indicated to this writer the current technical feasibility of this "optimum" unit, in which the microphones and hearing aid transducers would be located at ear level, and wired to the associated circuitry and power supply contained in a body pack located on the chest. Bolt, Beranek, and Newman have already manufactured a prototype "master hearing aid" which is being evaluated by Dr. Harry Levitt and his colleagues at the City University of New York, which has been constructed in exactly this manner. The unit provides for an impressive number of electroacoustic adjustments, and except for the lack of FM capability, which should not be too difficult to include, it appears to meet all the requirements of the optimal unit.

Such a device should include all the desirable features now found in a number of systems. Some of the more intriguing ones are the use of pilot lights to signify whether the unit is charging or completely recharged, pilot lights to warn of impending battery failure, and light dimmers to indicate proper intensity level when auxiliary inputs are used (tape recorders, etc.). Some battery chargers will permit a full charge, in emergency situations, in approximately an hour. Some chargers incorporate troubleshooting provisions to check the functioning of the transducers, cords, batteries, and receivers. One FM unit includes a "muting" circuit, referred to earlier, which automatically reduces environmental sound competition during teacher transmission. The incorporation of all these desirable features, plus no doubt others presently available, would greatly enhance the performance of an optimal unit.

The development and dissemination of such a device can finally lay to rest the "consistent versus inconsistent" amplification debate. Children can hopefully receive the consistent amplification emphasized by the hearing aid advocates combined with the high quality possibilities stressed by the auditory trainer partisans. The job of parents and professionals will be made much easier, since they will now have only one system to troubleshoot and maintain, rather than two separate and distinct instruments. With everybody's attention focused on the single amplification device used by the child, malfunctions should be detected sooner and repairs expedited. Extra time should then be available to ensure that the electroacoustic pattern was most appropriate for a particular child. Additionally, the time-consuming and annoying chore of replacing aids with auditory trainers in the morning, troubleshooting both devices, and then exchanging the auditory trainers for a personal hearing aid in the afternoon can be made much easier if a single device could meet the needs of both classroom and personal amplification.

The major obstacle impeding the dissolution of the differences between personal hearing aids and classroom amplification systems has little to do with technical feasibility. It has chiefly to do with customs and regulatory practices based on historical precedents. Simply stated, hearing aids are purchased and owned privately; even when some agency assists in the hearing aid's purchase, they are used as private property. Classroom amplification systems, on the other hand, belong to the school system and remain in the premises after school. Many agencies which are mandated to assist in the purchase of personal hearing aids would balk, get confused, require a large number of meetings and new guidelines from their superiors, etc., if they were informed that their "hearing aids" were also "classroom amplifiers." A similar confusion would no doubt exist in the minds of many school officials, if they were to learn that their "classroom amplifiers" were also personal hearing aids. No doubt this kind of bureaucratic impediment can ultimately be resolved. Unfortunately, time is not on the side of the hearing-impaired child whose development of maximum auditory potential is a time-limited function.

OVERVIEW

The formal education of hearing-impaired children takes place in school. Typically, they enter school with deficiencies in speech and language. We then expect them to overcome these deficiencies while staying abreast of the academic material being presented to them. Yet this material presumes a higher level of language competence than hearing-impaired children ordinarily demonstrate. The literature is replete with instances of our failure. That we shall ever succeed in educating the majority of hearing-impaired children commensurate with their intellectual ability is problematic. Perhaps someday we will be able to. That we can do better than we are, however, seems certain. One prerequisite, at least, for the accomplishment of this goal is to conceptualize the education of hearing-impaired children in a somewhat more unified manner than we have been.

The "education" of hearing-impaired children should begin at age of detection, hopefully before age one. The parents must be enlisted as the prime movers, and assisted by professionals so that they can effectively carry out their filial responsibilities. The separation of audiologic clinics from the educational setting erects immense barriers of continuity and communication; these barriers must be obliterated either physically or administratively. The entrance of the child in the formal educational setting does not obviate the need for continued clinical and parental input and participation. The classroom amplification requirements are a minor, though indispensable component of a unified educational approach. Our ultimate goal, it must be emphasized, is not limited to the provision of effective amplification, but participation in the growth of a human being, in all his many varied, unique, and wondrous dimensions.

hearing aid facilities and delivery systems

Theodore J. Glattke, Ph.D.

INTRODUCTION

An audiologic facility involved in a program of total rehabilitation for the hearing impaired must incorporate several features that might not be required in the course of a more limited audiologic practice. These physical aspects of the facility can be grouped according to three general topics: basic construction, sound proofing, and specialized equipment. In addition, the form of the facility will be influenced by the type of delivery system. Traditional delivery systems and possible alternatives are considered in this chapter.

PHYSICAL FACILITIES

Figure 14–1 provides an example of a floor plan for a minimum facility that would accommodate the audiologic services essential to a rehabilitation program as well as supporting activities. The floor plan may be divided into five areas: (1) waiting-reception; (2) threshold and suprathreshold hearing evaluations; (3) individual or group therapy; (4) counseling and other consultation in a private office; and (5) analysis of hearing aid electroacoustic performance. The facility includes 1125 square feet in order to accommodate these activities, and there are several special features which should be noted.

The hallways and doorways in rooms that are likely to be used by patients are all of a greater width than might normally be found in a small office suite. This is because a significant number of patients seen in a full-service facility may not be ambulatory. Non-ambulatory individuals will

244

require sufficient space to manipulate wheelchairs and other assistance devices. Doorways built to 40 inch widths, rather than the more typical 36 or 30 inch widths will make the transportation of non-ambulatory patients more convenient. If the clinic is located within a hospital facility, it is also possible that some of the patients will be bedridden, and will use a gurney for transportation. Because of this, the hallway having access to the patient examining room should be at least 6 to 7 feet in width. Consideration of the non-ambulatory patient also extends to the dimensions of the examining room and its door. In order to enable the use of a gurney, the room should be at least 7 feet square along its inside dimensions, and the doorways should be 36 to 40 inches wide.

While the facility shown in Figure 14-1 is free-standing, it is likely that an actual clinical facility would occupy a portion of a larger building. If that is the case, the clinic must be accessible to the non-ambulatory patient. This may be accomplished with ramps or elevators of adequate size, and preferably both, so that elevators could be used routinely and ramps in the case of fire or other emergency.

If the clinic does occupy space in a larger building, several other considerations should be kept in mind. The foremost is the weight of the audiologic test suite. A combined single wall-double wall suite such as that shown in Figure 14-1 will weigh more than 11,000 pounds. Modern commercial buildings will accommodate such loads, but older frame structures

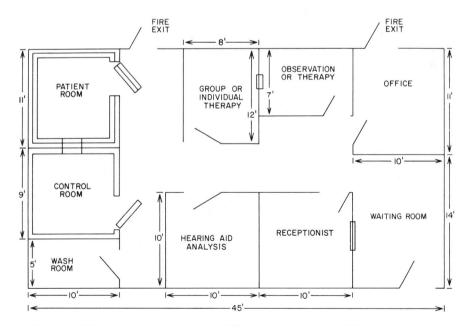

FIG. 14-1. Floor plan for a minimum facility to accommodate audiologic services essential to a rehabilitation program.

may not, even on the "ground" floor if there is excavation under the building. The test suites have limited ventilation, and heat generated within them or stored in them (e.g. from direct sunlight) dissipates very slowly. For this reason, it is prudent to place the suites away from any heat-generating machinery within the building and away from forced air heating conduit. If the test suite is to be placed near an outside building wall, it would be best to avoid locations on the western or southern side of buildings in the Northern Hemisphere, due to solar heat. Such considerations will make the facility more comfortable for long periods of use, and they will also favor the performance of electronic instruments housed within the test booths. The stability and life span of most instruments will be adversely affected by ambient temperatures which are too high.

The electrical power requirements of an audiology facility are not stringent. The use of transistor or integrated circuits in audiometric equipment has reduced the amount of required power to levels which should be compatible with most modern wiring systems. Three-wire receptacles with true grounds should be used whenever possible. Grounded systems of that type are now usually required by the building codes that are applicable to patient care areas. If a true grounded system is not available, special care should be taken to ensure that all pieces of electronic equipment that are to be coupled together or used simultaneously have the *same electrical reference point*. If they do not have the same reference point, a shock hazard can exist. While a mild shock may be a source on inconvenience for the clinic staff, it may be especially dangerous to the debilitated patient, to those with implanted pacemaker devices, or to individuals who cannot report the sensation associated with a shock.

Consideration of the safety of individuals should also extend to *any* electrical conductor within the test facility, including the metal sound suite, metal tables and chairs, and other metal fixtures which might be present. Regardless of the grounding techniques that are to be used, it is wise to have a complete system certified by an individual who is trained in biomedical engineering measurement prior to any patient use. Electronic devices may develop faulty ground systems as a result of the aging of components in their power supplies, and the devices should be rechecked periodically to ensure that their grounding characteristics have not changed.

Soundproofing

Obviously, the major soundproofing effort in an audiologic facility will deal with the test suite itself. The applicable standard for background noise in test facilities (American National Standards Institute (ANSI) S 3.1–1960) has not yet been modified to accommodate the difference between the previous standards for hearing threshold values (American Standards

Association Z24.5 1951) and the current threshold standard (ANSI S 3.6–1969). Since the current threshold values are substantially lower than the previous values, it follows that less noise should be permitted in the test facility. As a general rule of thumb, one may take the old standard value for background noise at a given frequency and subtract the difference between the old and current threshold standards in order to arrive at a suitable background noise level. This has been done for octave band measurements in Table 14–1.

The background noise within a test facility is, of course, the result of the ambient noise outside of the facility, the attenuation provided by the test suite, and the noise generated within the facility. Because the ambient noise in buildings where clinics are housed may vary considerably, it is impossible to specify the minimum attenuation requirements that might apply for a specific facility. However, the single-double wall combination illustrated in Figure 14–1 is typical of a suite which should be satisfactory under the most adverse conditions. Indeed, the single-double configuration will be mandatory for most full-service facilities. The configuration will be required primarily for threshold measurements, but one must also remember that hearing aid and other sound field assessments may require the use of live voice stimuli and high signal sound pressure levels. The single wall control booth will ensure that an open microphone can be used without ambient interference. The double-walled examination room will reduce the possibility of sound-field acoustic feedback to the control room, as well as attenuating the outside noise.

Regardless of the choice of room configuration and attenuation characteristics, it should be remembered that the ambient noise outside of the test facility must be measured before a meaningful choice can be made. Further, one should be mindful of the possibility that the ambient noise may not be constant. Buildings located in urban areas may experience differing levels of noise due to automobile traffic conditions. Clinics located within buildings that have multiple uses may experience different noise levels because of the air conditioning system, the presence of large numbers of people, and other factors. A clinic located adjacent to elevator machinery may experience noise levels which fluctuate with the volume of pedestrian traffic.

The other soundproofing requirements of a clinic facility are somewhat more subtle. Speech privacy is one concern. When used in this sense, speech privacy refers to some individual's awareness of a conversation, and not necessarily to perfect intelligibility of an overheard conversation. Poor speech privacy can have a distracting and inhibiting effect on individuals, and while these effects are difficult to measure with precision, they should be avoided whenever possible. If the long term level of conversational speech is taken to be about 65 dB sound pressure level (SPL), and if

TABLE 14-1. **Suggested allowable background noise levels for audiometric test facilities**

	Test Frequency						
	125 Hz	250 Hz	500 Hz	1000 Hz	2000 Hz	4000 Hz	8000 Hz
ANSI S 3.1, 1960 Standard Level in dB (SPL)*	40 dB	40 dB	40 dB	40 dB	47 dB	57 dB	67 dB
Difference (dB) between ANSI-1969 and ASA-1951 reference threshold levels†	−9 dB	−15 dB	−14 dB	−10 dB	−8.5 dB	−6 dB	−11.5 dB
Suggested new levels in dB (SPL)*	31 dB	25 dB	26 dB	30 dB	38.5 dB	51 dB	55.5 dB

* All measurements are for octave bandwidths with the indicated test frequency at the approximate center of the band. ANSI, American National Standards Institute; SPL, sound pressure level.
† ASA, American Standards Association.

shouting corresponds to about 80 dB SPL, then the common walls of a clinic facility must offer 60 dB or more of attenuation for broad band signals in order to ensure speech privacy. Conventional frame construction techniques offer only 30 to 45 dB attenuation. Therefore, one should consider *room placement* as a means of assisting speech privacy. This can take the form of separating therapy rooms by a space which is normally quiet and enclosed, thereby obtaining the attenuation effects of two walls (60 to 90 dB total). In Figure 14-1, this is accomplished by placing the office-consultation room and therapy room on opposite sides of an observation facility. Placement of this type would, under most circumstances, permit conversation at high sound pressure levels to occur in the therapy room without undue loss of privacy.

In most cases, *doors* are the weakest link in the soundproofing characteristics of conventional construction. This is because a hollow door, itself, provides little attenuation, and also because the fit of the door in the jamb and threshold is not sufficiently close to provide for a good acoustic seal. Transmission losses of only 15 to 20 dB are common for typical office and residential construction. Therefore, even if great care is taken to provide for adequate isolation of common walls, the doorways can defeat this effort. Where speech privacy is critical, weatherstripping, thresholds that extend below the door on closure, and the more expensive solid doors should be considered.

Modern commercial construction often contains an additional fault that precludes speech privacy. While the walls of most facilities are a standard 8 feet in height, the ceilings may be 10 feet or more above the floor. The apparent ceiling in the room is "false" and is suspended from the actual ceiling (or floor of the next story) by 2 or more feet. False ceilings are convenient because they allow for the passage of heating and cooling conduit, telephone cables, electrical wiring, and antennas for paging systems, but they provide for little sound isolation. In the worst case, one could imagine a large space divided into cubicles with no ceilings at all. In that instance, the walls of the cubicles would provide for some small amount of attenuation depending on their height, distance from the source, and construction material. A loose-fitting ceiling made of sound-absorbing materials may add as much as 10 dB to the isolation provided by walls, but a rigid, sealed enclosure would be required to reach the 30 to 45 dB isolation which is possible with single wall construction. An additional fault is often encountered with air ducts which run for long distances through hallways, and which couple many rooms to a source of air conditioning. From a sound isolation viewpoint, a radial system with many short ducts feeding off from the machinery would be preferred.

In addition to soundproofing, audiologic facilities must be protected from electromagnetic radiation and other forms of radiated energy, such as strong radio, television, or diathermy signals. Protection from electromagnetic radiation is necessary to enable the use of the induction telephone pick-up coils on hearing aids, and to permit accurate measurements of the hearing aid's performance when the telephone pick-up is in use. In addition, the clinic may use auditory training equipment which works on an induction principle, and such equipment would be adversely affected by strong radiation. Radio-frequency or diathermy radiation may be detected by the electronic components of audiometers and other equipment, and may add additional unwanted noise to the hearing evaluation situation or to the hearing aid analysis equipment.

One who is fortunate to be planning an entirely new facility, or substantial renovation of an existing building, should most certainly enlist the services of an architectural firm experienced in acoustics in order to avoid the pitfalls described here, and others which may be peculiar to a particular location.

Specialized Equipment

When providing amplification in the context of a comprehensive rehabilitation program, the clinic facility must first be a *diagnostic* facility. This is not to say that every patient who may be a candidate for amplification must undergo the most exotic of contemporary diagnostic routines, but the facility and its personnel must be competent to obtain a complete discription of the patient's sensory and communicative disability. The key item required for diagnostic facilities is, of course, an audiometer. This instrument must conform to the minimum requirements for a wide range audiometer and a speech audiometer as described in sections 2.1.1 and 2.2 in the applicable standard (ANSI S 3.6–1969). In addition, some means of obtaining audiologic measurements in sound field must be avilable. Even though sound field measurements are not yet described in terms of standard values, clinics employ them for pediatric audiometry. Visual reinforcement audiometry is an example of the use of sound field measures for threshold estimation. Sound field measures may also be used for threshold and suprathreshold evaluation with speech signals in the process of identifying candidates for amplification and evaluating their performance with amplification. All of the signals normally routed to earphones should be available for sound field testing, and if tones are used in sound field situations, provision should be made for warbled (frequency-modulated) tones to avoid standing waves in the test suite.

There are a number of optional items which may be of value. Acoustic impedance measurements (tympanometry) would be an important addition to a full-service facility. Additionally, studies of acoustic reflex behavior, "automatic" Bekesy-type audiometers, and some means of obtaining "objective" threshold measurements would be of utility in a large number of clinic facilities. A portable pure-tone audiometer with air, bone, and masking capacity should be considered if difficult-to-test patients are anticipated. The portable instrument will allow the clinician to work in the room with the patient for the purpose of conditioning the patient to the test signals. The masking feature on the portable instrument is essential if the existence of audiometric air-bone gaps or significant unilateral hearing loss is to be confirmed.

Additional specialized equipment that may be useful depends upon the extent of the clinic's involvement with the hearing aid after it has been provided to the patient. The following comments are based on the assumption that the clinic will provide complete services. The essential equipment for postfitting follow-up consists of the sound field measurement equipment and some means of evaluating the basic electroacoustic characteristics of the hearing aid itself. In the most elegant systems, measurements of gain, frequency response, distortion, and maximum power output are made semiautomatically with results plotted on standardized graphs. The more humble systems require considerable manual effort and will measure the basic parameters of hearing aids only at certain fixed frequencies. The instrumentation and procedure for measuring electroacoustic characteristics of hearing aids are described above in Chapter Five. It might be well to note here that the *measurement* portions of a hearing aid evaluation system, together with appropriate couplers, can also be used to obtain basic calibration measurements for the audiometric equipment, as well as the hearing aids.

Regardless of whether or not a clinic facility stocks hearing aids for demonstration purposes, the facility should have the capacity to make minimal adjustments and repairs for the aids used by its patients. Thus, a selection of appropriate tools and hearing aid parts might be included. Adjustment of earmolds will require, in addition, small motor-driven tools suitable for working with plastic materials. Finally, an adequate battery tester should be included. An "adequate" tester is not a typical volt-ohmmeter or electronic voltmeter, because they draw very little current from the source which they are measuring. Rather, the meter must place an electrical load on the battery that is similar to the load provided by a normal hearing aid. A meter providing a load of 2000 to about 5000 ohms should be satisfactory, and these can be obtained from hearing aid or camera accessory suppliers.

Any additional equipment which might be included will depend on the facility skills and interest in more detailed repair services for hearing aids. Modern assembly techniques which involve integrated circuits have resulted in a situation where replacement of an entire amplifier is simpler and less costly than replacement of specific components in the older transistor instruments. As the repair procedures become simpler, clinics or other facilities independent from the manufacturers may begin to engage in detailed repair.

Some Comments on Cost

It is difficult to make general statements regarding costs of facilities that will be valid throughout the United States because of widely varying factors related to labor, materials, shipping, and distribution. However, the following general guidelines might apply for a moderate-sized urban area. Construction of an 1100 square foot facility at $60 per square foot would amount to $66,000 in 1976. This figure does not include the land and adjacent parking and service areas which could add $20,000 to $30,000 to the basic construction costs. Standard office furnishings would add an additional 15% to the building construction costs. The prospect of a large capital investment in the region of $100,000 might lead one to conclude that leasing of existing space would be preferred over actual construction. Typical commercial leases pay back about 10% of the value of the property per year, in this case about $10,000 annually, or about $833 monthly.

The sound suite depicted in Figure 14-1 is of rather generous proportions, and would cost between $13,000 and $15,000 in 1976. The audiometric equipment meeting the minimum ANSI standards would cost $4000 to $6000, depending upon accessories. Acoustic impedance and reflex measurement equipment would add $2000 to $4000. Finally, the hearing aid measurement equipment can range in cost from about $1500 for manual devices to more than $6000 for the most complete automatic equipment. Using the minimum equipment figures just described, the total cost would be approximately $20,500, and the maximum figure would sum to about $31,000. If equipment of this caliber were assumed to have a useful life of 10 years, the average monthly cost would range between $170 and $300. Obviously, the establishment of a full-service facility is not inexpensive, but the development of a facility which has less instrumentation and space than that described here would also mean that only limited services could be provided. Additional fixed costs related to a clinic will include insurance on the facility and its contents. This insurance may be particularly important if the clinic maintains a stock of hearing aids for demonstration purposes. Clinics should not neglect to consider professional liability insurance for their staff members. Information about this insurance is available from the American Speech and Hearing Association.

DELIVERY SYSTEMS

The procedures, personnel, and avenues involved in the actual delivery of a hearing aid to a patient represent an emotionally charged and controversial topic of consideration. The underlying questions surrounding the various delivery systems are much too complex and extensive to be considered adequately in this chapter. Rather than attempt to resolve the questions, this chapter will simply describe those systems that are in use. The discussion will not include the hearing aid services provided by the United States Government through the Veterans Administration, but will be restricted to a description of activity in the "private sector." Figure 14-2 outlines several approaches that are in use, and each will be described below.

1. Physician-audiologist-retail dealer. When this system functions, the patient may consult his or her family physician or an otolaryngologist regarding a hearing, vestibular, or communication problem. Subsequent to a medical examination, or as a part of it, the audiologist may be consulted for an assessment of the patient's sensory and communicative impairment, and the disability resulting from that impairment. Based upon the medical findings, the physician will arrive at a diagnosis and make a recommendation regarding medical or surgical treatment. If medical or surgical treatment is not indicated, the patient returns to the audiologist for a hearing aid recommendation. The patient then goes to a retail hearing aid salesperson who provides the instrument, the earmold, and all subsequent adjustments related to the instrument. The audiologist

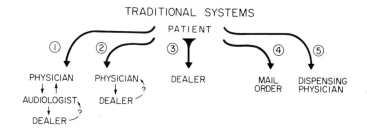

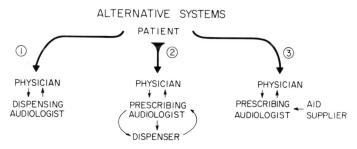

FIG. 14-2. Hearing aid delivery systems.

might see the patient following provision of the hearing aid for therapy and/or orientation sessions as well as for continued evaluation of the patient's performance with amplification. In other instances, this follow-up care will be assumed by the salesperson who provided the hearing aid.

As with all cases of individuals with hearing impairment, three types of decisions have been made in this sequence of events: a diagnosis, a recommendation for treatment, and an implementation of that treatment. In addition, three individuals are involved with the care of the patient.

2. Physician-dealer. In this instance, the patient consults a family physician or specialist who collects the medical and audiometric information, obtains a diagnosis, and refers the patient to the dealer for selection of a hearing aid (or aids) and subsequent care. The patient may be followed by the physician, but often the patient will utilize the dealer for all services related to hearing aid selection, counseling, repair and modification of the aid, and the purchase of additional hearing aids. In this instance, the physician has made the diagnosis and ruled out additional medical or surgical intervention, and the salesperson has assumed the responsibility for the services that accrue following the physician's decision.

3. Dealer. A substantial number of hearing aids are sold to individuals who have contact only with a retail hearing aid salesperson. In this case, the patient does not consult with either a physician or an audiologist prior to obtaining a hearing aid. In the broadest interpretation of this means of hearing aid delivery, the salesperson and patient have arrived at a diagnosis, recommendation, and implementation of treatment. The subsequent source of advice for the patient is also the dealer.

4. Mail Order. It is possible to purchase a hearing aid through mail order from the catalogs of retail merchandising companies. The patient who chooses this route has somehow assessed the handicap, medical status, and rehabilitation route, and acts entirely on behalf of himself. This self-treatment may also extend to fabrication of an impression for an earmold, which is ultimately provided by the company.

5. Dispensing physician. When this route is used, the patient consults with a physician who assumes complete responsibility for measurement, diagnosis, provision of the instrument, and subsequent patient care related to the hearing aid. In those states where hearing aids are provided through Medicaid laws, single individuals may be precluded from serving all of these functions for a patient in order to avoid the appearance of conflict-of-interest regarding the sale of the hearing aid.

Alternative Systems

Several alternatives to these first five delivery systems are now in use. In general, they reflect an increase in the involvement of the audiologist in provision of the hearing aid and an increase in the involvement of the audiologist in the overall rehabilitation program for the patient. The alternative systems include the following:

1. Physician-dispensing audiologist. In this instance, the patient consults with a physician who may or may not use the services of an audiologist in obtaining the information necessary to arrive at a diagnosis and decision regarding medical or surgical intervention. The patient then consults with an audiologist who selects a hearing aid and provides it along with attendant services and subsequent follow-up care. Medicaid restrictions which might apply to a dispensing physician in certain states also apply to dispensing audiologists.

2. Physician-prescribing audiologist-dispenser: When this alternative is used, the physician will subsequently refer the patient to an audiologist for consultation regarding rehabilitative measures. The audiologist conducts evaluations as needed and issues a *prescription* for a hearing aid that specifies its output characteristics, along with the form and type of earmold. This prescription is filled by a dispenser who serves the role of stocking the instruments and arranging for the finished earmold and implementation of the guarantee or insurance for the instrument. The patient returns to the audiologist for initial fitting of the aid and for subsequent evaluations, counseling and rehabilitative measures. Adjustments to the earmold and ancillary problems are handled by the audiologist. Warranty service is provided through the dispenser.

3. Physician-prescribing audiologist-supplier: This plan differs from the previous plan in that the hearing aid supplier is not a local dispenser. Rather, the supplier is essentially a "jobber," not unlike a wholesaler, who obtains hearing aids directly from the manufacturer. The supplier stocks the aids and mails them to patients only upon receipt of a prescription from a physician or audiologist. The supplier is not involved in the selection or fabrication of the earpiece or any other accessory and does not have contact with the patient except through written correspondence. The audiologist performs all other functions related to the hearing aid and to the rehabilitation of the patient.

Some Implications of the Alternative Delivery Systems

The alternative delivery systems might be viewed from several facets, including economic, service-related, and professional viewpoints. From an economic viewpoint, a hearing aid dispensing or supply facility differs considerably from the conventional retail sales office. Since the dispenser, unless an audiologist, does not engage in testing or other services related to patient evaluation, no testing facility is required. In addition, since the dispenser functions solely on a prescription basis, no local expenses related to product promotion should be involved. Such expenses include advertising, "gifts," travel, and even the selection of suitable office space which might require greater capital investment or higher rental fees than a simple dispensing facility. Savings of this nature can contribute to a significant lowering of the retail cost of the aid itself. While it is impossible to state the extent of these savings accurately in every situation, a reduction in net cost of 50% or more from the conventional retail price structure might be anticipated.

This is not to say that the total cost of a rehabilitation program which included the provision of a hearing aid would be reduced, for the services provided by the audiologist in recommending the aid and in postfitting care would be billed to the patient on a fee-for-service basis. If an individual patient required little care associated with his rehabilitation program, the total cost would be lower than the cost under traditional delivery systems. If a substantial amount of rehabilitative care were necessary, the total cost might exceed that found in conventional delivery systems, with the obvious benefits accruing from the professional care afforded the patient.

When viewed from the standpoint of the population at large, the cost reduction may be considerable. This is because the alternative delivery systems have in common a prescription issued by an individual who does not profit from the sale of the hearing aid. Under such circumstances, one might comfortably speculate that hearing aids would not be prescribed unless their utility could be demonstrated. The consequence of this is that those aids which were actually provided would be so within the context of total rehabilitation of the patient. Thus, the patient would be more likely to become a fully contributing member of society. In addition, the alternative delivery systems provide substantial insurance against inappropriate sales in the case of medical or surgical problems, and in the case of those individuals who will not benefit from the use of amplification.

From a service-related viewpoint, the alternative systems place the responsibilities of patient rehabilitation squarely with the audiologist. This means that the patient is not passed to and fro between dealer and audiologist for the purpose of adjustments or changes, re-evaluation, and patient dissatisfaction. Elimination of the to and fro pattern will certainly make the acquisition of the aid more convenient than under conventional systems in which an audiologist may be involved. If the patient's convenience is improved, then it is safe to speculate that the patient will be more likely to seek out required services rather than discontinue the use of a hearing aid which is not providing satisfaction.

From a professional viewpoint, the three steps involved in the acquisition of assistance for hearing disability should again be considered. They are: (1) development of a medical diagnosis with implementation of medical or surgical treatment; (2) formulation of a recommendation for treatment; and (3) implementation of the treatment with appropriate follow-up to determine its effectiveness. All three of these steps occur regardless of the route selected by an individual patient in obtaining a hearing aid. Physicians, by virtue of their training and experience, as well as their legal status, are the only individuals from whom a medical diagnosis should be obtained. An audiologist, hearing aid dealer, or the patients themselves do not appear to be the appropriate individuals with whom this responsibility should be placed. Physicians in the United States are, by and large, not actively involved in the actual delivery of hearing rehabilitative services apart from medical and surgical treatment. The alternative plans place the responsibility for delivery of those services directly with the audiologist. The audiologist possesses special skills related to the measurement of sensory dysfunction and the handicap resulting from that dysfunction. Further, the audiologist has the knowledge necessary to plan and execute a program designed to ameliorate the handicap. The hearing aid, while important, is only one part of the program. Under conventional delivery systems, the acquisition of the instrument is likely to signal the end of any effort at patient rehabilitation, whereas the alternative systems provide the environment for an audiologist to use the special skills that have been acquired through formal training and clinical experience. If we assume this to be so, it would appear that the audiologist is in a unique position to provide competent services related to the non-medical and non-surgical rehabilitation of a patient who requires those services.

Some Suggestions for Guidelines

In recent years there has been much formal testimony under the auspices of the United States Food and Drug Administration regarding the nature of hearing aids, and the role of physicians, audiologists, and retail hearing aid dealers in the provision of services to the hearing impaired. The Federal Trade Commission has evoked additional testimony regarding hearing aid distribution practices. If that testimony is reviewed along with the Code of Ethics of the American Speech and Hearing Association, one must conclude that audiologists comprise a service-oriented profession. Involvement with the dispensing of a product must result in some change in the way in which the profession functions, as has been the case for other health-related professions which engage in some form of dispensing. Can this change be made without destruction of the audiologists' real or perceived role in the care of the hearing impaired? The answer is not likely to be available on an a priori basis, but will evolve with experiences gained from the alternate delivery systems described in this chapter. The following comments are made with the intention of stimulating thought and discussion regarding the optimal way of preserving the traditional professional status of the audiologist who may choose to become more actively involved in the provision of hearing aid-related services.

The key danger which must be avoided if an audiologist is to maintain the public trust is an apparent *conflict of interest*. In order to avoid this danger, the audiologist must establish the dispensing procedure in a manner so as to preclude the augmentation of income through the actual dispensing activity. This is not to say the practice of audiology should not expand, for such expansion would be a natural consequence of the provision of more complete rehabilitative services. However, the dispensing of a given hearing aid should have absolutely no influence on the audiologist's net income.

Perhaps the easiest way in which an audiologist can increase his involvement with the hearing aid patient without entering into a situation that might be construed as conflict of interest would be to use the services of a dispenser as described in the alternative delivery systems. If the dispenser functions primarily to procure instruments on a prescription basis, many of the problems identified with the traditional retail system would be eliminated, and the audiologist's role would clearly be limited to the services which he is prepared to provide. Furthermore, the utilization of a dispenser corresponds well with the spirit and intent of hearing aid dealer licensing laws which are becoming more commonplace. The hearing aid supplier system offers many of the same advantages as the dispenser system in terms of clear definition of the roles of the audiologist and ultimate provider of the hearing aid.

If an audiologist chooses to serve the role of both the provider of service and provider of the hearing aid, he should be mindful of the guidelines suggested by the American Speech and Hearing Association, even if he does not choose to be a member of that organization. The guidelines contain several important elements, including the following: (1) the dispensing activity must be independent of the services provided by the audiologist and the ultimate fees charged by the audiologist for services; (2) the patient must have a basis on which to give his informed consent to accepting both the services and hearing aid that would be provided by the audiologist; and (3) the patient's costs for the hearing aid must be based solely upon recovery of cost incurred by the audiologist in the process of acquiring the instrument and actually dispensing it to the patient. The overall philosophy resulting in these guidelines is that the hearing aid be delivered to the patient within the context of total rehabilitative care. Within the context of total rehabilitative care, the audiologist is bound to a responsibility for continuing evaluation of the effectiveness of that care.

By virtue of an academic tradition, membership in professional societies, licensing by state consumer protection agencies, and other routes of communication with peers, the audiologist is in a unique position to provide continuing evaluation through a peer-review system. A peer-review system that functions optimally can detect abuses in an efficient and timely manner and can anticipate future difficulties. Correction of abuses or avoidance of difficulties will be very important ingredients in any dispensing system.

If the public trust and confidence in audiologists is to be preserved, steps taken toward a departure from traditional dispensing systems must be made only after thoughtful consideration and great care. It is probably safest to say that significant changes will occur over the next few years, but that these changes will be successful from the patients' viewpoint only if their welfare is kept uppermost in the minds of individuals involved in the dispensing procedures.

RECOMMENDED READINGS*

BERANEK, L., *Acoustics*. New York: McGraw-Hill Book Co., Inc. (1954).

KRYTER, K., *The Effects of Noise on Man*. New York: Academic Press (1970).

PETERSON, A., AND GROSS, E., JR., *Handbook of Noise Measurement*. Concord: General Radio Co. (1972).

* References cited in this chapter are included in the bibliography at the end of the book.

chapter *15*

some implications for research

Theodore J. Glattke, Ph.D.

INTRODUCTION

There are several approaches to the general problem of prosthetic assistance to the hearing impaired. These include:

1. Wearable electroacoustic amplification systems
2. Wearable electromechanical systems for bone conduction
3. Non-wearable aids intended for group use
4. Devices for stimulation of alternate sensory systems
5. Implantable devices for electrical stimulation of the nervous system
6. Prosthetic surgical modification of the outer and middle ear structures.

The progress in the design and implementation of all of these approaches have been quite dramatic in the past 45 years, and the unanswered questions related to each pose many interesting and important research topics. In general terms, the research questions fall into two categories: (1) those related to optimal hardware or surgical techniques; and (2) those related to the patient's interaction with the device or procedure. Whereas this chapter will emphasize hardware and procedural questions, some aspects of patient interaction will also be considered, particularly with respect to the newer developments in unconventional prosthetics.

WEARABLE AND GROUP AMPLIFICATION SYSTEMS

The efficiency, portability, and flexibility of conventional hearing aids have extended their usefulness significantly in the past decade. These features of the aids have been made possible by the miniaturization of the transducers and electronic components that comprise the devices and by the speed with which the manufacturers have adopted new materials. Among the advantages of modern hearing aids, their flexibility has been crucial in expanding their usefulness. The key to the flexibility lies in the modification of the acoustic signal using acoustic devices or modification of the instrument's internal electrical signals using electronic devices. The acoustic devices include direction-specific microphones, microphones and electroacoustic transducers with extended frequency response, and the vented earmold coupling systems.

One persistent problem in the evaluation of acoustic devices of this type is the lack of a suitable laboratory environment in which to measure their effects. Direction-sensitive or frequency response measurements that are made within an anechoic environment simply are not applicable to the normal acoustic environment in which hearing aids are used. The real environment includes not only the hard-walled enclosures in which individuals spend much of their time, but also the effects of the individual's own body within the acoustic environment. The body effects can be evaluated in terms of the diffraction or sound shadow characteristics of the head and in terms of the acoustic characteristics of the ear canal, pinna, and related structures. Two recent developments hold great promise for the alleviation of the previous lack of control for such body-induced effects. These are the development of an acoustic coupler system which reproduces the acoustic properties of the ear canal and middle ear systems as a whole (Zwislocki, 1971), and the use of these couplers in a mannekin which is a near replica of the human head in terms of its acoustic properties (Knowles and Burkhard, 1975). The introduction of these coupler-mannekin combinations should provide for new and relevant specifications of the acoustic properties of hearing aids in the future, and offers a significant step in the development of new research protocols under controlled acoustic environments.

Electronic modification of the hearing aid's internal electrical signals has employed the use of filters and "automatic gain control" or other forms of non-linear amplification. When filters or amplifiers are combined appropriately, frequency- and gain-selective devices can be produced, and hearing aids incorporating frequency- and gain-selective characteristics have been particularly useful for individuals with unusual audiometric configurations or loudness tolerance problems. Amplifiers and filters that have been used in the past are called analog devices because they operate on the electrical analogy of the acoustic signals. Analog approaches to signal modification offer some degree of flexibility through the use of adjustable resistors or capacitors, but the use of *digital* processing may offer significant advances in flexibility in the future.

Digital processing schemes are very commonplace today in the form of hand-held electronic calculators. In the case of those calculators, information is led to the processor by pressing a sequence of keys. The processor then acts upon the information and displays the results of that action in a form that is readable by the user. A digital processing scheme that could be incorporated into a hearing aid is shown in Figure 15-1. The incoming information is detected by a microphone and converted to an electrical analog of the signal, as is the case in a standard hearing aid. Subsequently, the electrical version of the signal is sampled for a brief instant and assigned some digital value by an analog-to-digital converter. This conversion may be completed within 5 to 10 microseconds. The numerical representation of the signal that results from the analog-to-digital conversion can then be led to a very small general purpose *micro*-computer. This computer can modify the digital representation of the signal according to rules stored in the computer memory.

The rules for processing the digital signal could be invariant. For example, multiplication of every incoming voltage by a factor of 32 would provide for a gain of about 36 dB for all incoming signals. Alternatively, the device could provide for variable gain and multiply small incoming signals by a factor of 32, but larger signals by only 16. The device could also provide for automatic gain control only when energy in some restricted frequency region exceeded some critical sound pressure level. All of these

CONVENTIONAL AMPLIFICATION

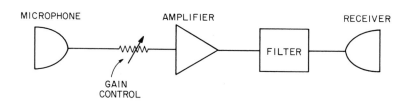

DIGITAL PROCESSING

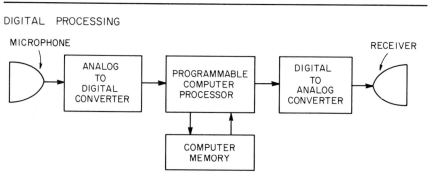

FIG. 15-1. Schematics of a conventional analog hearing aid and of an amplification system that would use digital processing.

features are possible with conventional analog equipment, but only with the addition of relatively cumbersome electronic devices.

An additional favorable aspect of a digital device of the type illustrated in Figure 15-1 is that its flexibility would be limited only by the programmed instructions actually loaded into the computer memory. The set of instructions could be changed at will to provide for different frequency response and gain characteristics.

The digital representation of speech signals also has important potential for solving special problems associated with hearing aid use. One of these involves the use of amplification in noisy situations. Present devices use either an indiscriminate automatic gain control or direction-specific microphone (or both) to provide assistance in this regard. If incoming signals were processed digitally, however, it would be possible to store recent signals and to compare the most recent sample with previously stored information to determine if the last incoming data were part of a novel "signal" or not significantly different from the ongoing "noise." If the recent data met the criteria for a "signal," they could be processed differently from the noise. There are several mathematical routines that can be put into effect in order to enhance desired signals which are embedded in noise. Such routines include auto- and cross-correlation. When cross-correlation is used, an incoming signal is compared with some standard signal, and the output of the correlator fluctuates in a manner which is proportional to the value of the computed correlation from moment to moment. An autocorrelator compares an incoming signal with itself after some small time delay has been imposed. If the incoming signal is periodic, the output of the correlator will vary periodically according to the signal's characteristics. If it is not periodic, the output will remain at zero. An example of the signal enhancement provided by an autocorrelation routine is shown in Figure 15-2. The *upper tracing* shows the waveform of a signal consisting of 500 Hz plus wide-band noise. When that signal was led through a digital autocorrelator, the waveform shown in the bottom trace appeared at the output. While the correlator output was an imperfect sinusoidal waveform, the general enhancement of the 500 Hz component can be seen clearly.

Group amplification systems may also derive significant benefit from digital processors. At present, group systems are either "hard-wired," audio induction, or radio-frequency types. The "hard-wired" system is essentially a master amplifier to which are attached the receivers worn by members of the group. Each receiver circuit may be controlled independently of the others, but the system has two serious disadvantages. The first is that the hardware coupling the earphones to the amplifier curbs the mobility of the user, and the second results from the fact that the master amplifier has a single microphone. This means that the members of the

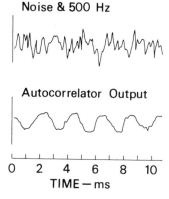

FIG. 15–2. An example of an autocorrelation analysis of a noisy signal. The *upper tracing* consists of a 500 Hz sinusoid mixed with wide band noise. The autocorrelation analysis of the noisy signal is shown in the *bottom tracing*. Note the periodic changes in the autocorrelation function corresponding to the period of the 500 Hz sinusoid. *ms* = milliseconds.

group can receive speech only when someone is using the master system microphone, and communication between members of the group who are not near the microphone is not possible. The induction and radio frequency systems alleviate the hardware problem and they function somewhat like a standard radio broadcast system with individual receivers. They may be influenced by unwanted signals, "crosstalk" between transmitters in adjacent classrooms, and unequal transmission within a classroom.

The *digital* transmission of speech signals through a radio frequency broadcast device offers several advantages over the conventional systems. The advantages include the possibility of selective addressing of receivers worn by members of the group and selective modification of the gain and frequency response of individual receivers while signals are actually being transmitted. If each individual's unit were activated only by a specific digital code, two way communication could be established between a number of wearable receiver-transmitters without crosstalk and other interference problems that are associated with conventional systems.

The technology for such signal processing is already in use, as the majority of long distance telephone communication is carried between cities by digital codes. Only shrinking of the components to wearable dimensions remains to be accomplished, and the techniques for that step are also available from the semiconductor industry. To date, there has been no great pressure on the hearing aid manufacturers to adopt digital processing techniques, but it is likely that such forms of processing will influence future trends.

SURGICAL MODIFICATION OF THE EAR

Modern approaches to the surgical treatment of hearing loss began with Lempert (1938) who refined the fenestration procedure. The true fenestration procedure involves opening the horizontal semicircular canal of a patient from whom stapes mobility cannot be created safely. When a patient has a mobile stapes footplate, any of several tympanoplasty procedures may be used to restore the middle ear mechanism and, hence, improve hearing (Wullenstein, 1956). The structural effects of some of these procedures, as well as the fenestration procedure, are shown in Figure 15-3. When all middle ear structures are present, but the tympanic membrane is perforated, the simplest form of tympanoplasty may be used. This involves closure of the perforation with a graft. If the malleus and incus are absent, the graft may be placed between the inner end of the ear canal and a mobile stapes. If all ossicles are absent, the graft may be placed between the canal and the cochlear promontory, thereby sealing off a small space containing the round window and leaving the footplate open to the outside and its attendant acoustic energy.

Surgical procedures may also be used to reconstruct the middle ear mechanism with man-made materials such as stainless steel or teflon. Usually, reconstruction of this type is limited to ossicular replacements. Reconstruction using man-made materials has one serious limitation: namely, the use of dissimilar materials within the middle ear must eventually lead to failure of the least noble material. Therefore, a stainless steel rod attached to an ossicle must eventually lead to erosion of the ossicle. Because of this limitation, the use of *homograft transplantation materials* has received much attention in the past decade.

Homograft, literally, refers to the grafting of man's body parts, and the source of such parts may be either the recipient or another donor. In the case of ear surgery, parts that may be transplanted from one individual to another include the tympanic membrane and ossicles, and a portion of the bony external auditory canal. Transplanted ossicles do not require a new blood supply to be useful to the recipient, and they are not detected as "foreign" by the recipient's immune system. Therefore, the tissue rejection problems common to more heroic transplantation procedures do not occur. The transplanted tympanic membrane serves as a foundation for new skin growth, and is eventually replaced by the recipient's own skin, which forms a new (if imperfect) tympanic membrane. Descriptions of the various approaches to homograft transplantation may be found in Goodhill (1975).

To be considered minimally successful, a homograft transplantation involving the tympanic membrane and ossicles must provide the patient who has undergone a radical mastoidectomy with a closed middle ear space. This will enable normal bathing and water recreation activities. A better result occurs when an individual who required an extremely high gain hearing aid prior to the procedure is able to use a mild to moderate gain instrument afterwards. The best result occurs when transplanted middle ear parts function to close an audiometric air-bone gap and amplification is no longer required. Homograft procedures have yet to undergo

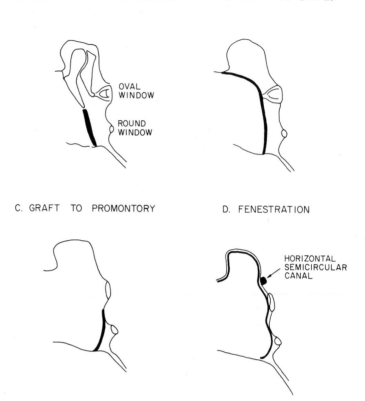

A. REPAIR OF A PERFORATION

OVAL WINDOW

ROUND WINDOW

B. GRAFT TO STAPES

C. GRAFT TO PROMONTORY

D. FENESTRATION

HORIZONTAL SEMICIRCULAR CANAL

Fig. 15-3. Examples of surgical reconstruction for the treatment of hearing loss.

long term evaluations with emphasis on their stability and the incidence of recurrent middle ear disease. Nonetheless, they may offer a distinct advantage over the more conventional artificial prosthesis techniques in the amelioration of hearing loss.

Another surgical approach which is undergoing scrutiny involves the modification of a normal air conduction apparatus to provide assistance to patients with sensorineural hearing loss (Goode and Cooper, 1975). Several structures of the air conduction apparatus present themselves as possible candidates for surgical modification. The first of these is the ear canal itself. Since the canal functions as a resonator with a preferential response in the 2500 to 4000 Hz region, the canal might be modified surgically with the goal of changing that resonance. An individual with a precipitously sloping hearing loss might benefit from a slight lowering of the canal's resonant frequency, and the lowering could be accomplished by lengthening the canal. The initial report of this work has shown the feasibility of an approach of this type (Goode and Cooper, 1975). Additional modification of the middle ear mechanism also presents an intriguing research question.

It may be that changes in the effective area of the tympanic membrane or changes in the ossicular lever system will warrant increased scrutiny in the near future.

IMPLANTATION TECHNIQUES

The implantation of electromechanical devices has undergone study by several individuals in recent years (Fredrickson et al., 1973; Goode and Glattke, 1973). The essence of these techniques involves the use of a conventional external hearing aid microphone and amplifier and an *implanted transducer*, rather than a conventional earphone or bone conduction driver. As illustrated in Figure 15-4, the transducer is a moving element which is coupled directly to a movable portion of the middle ear apparatus. This could be the malleus, in the case of a normal middle ear apparatus, or the cochlear promontory or stapes footplate, in the case of absent middle ear parts. The transducer may consist of a lightweight magnet surrounded by a coil or a piezoelectric device which changes its dimensions when an electrical current is applied to it. The transducer's

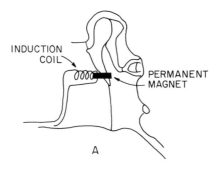

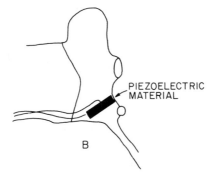

FIG. 15-4. Examples of implantable hearing aid transducers.

role is to produce *motion*, but not sound energy, even though some acoustic energy must be the consequence of such motion. This motion, whether it be introduced to the ossicles or promontory, results in motion of the cochlear fluid to produce auditory sensation.

Implanted transducers offer two advantages over conventional air conduction hearing aids. The first is that the external ear canal need not be occluded by the device. Therefore, individuals who cannot tolerate earmolds are potential candidates for this type of implantation. Second, since very little acoustic energy is produced with the implanted device, there is little opportunity for feedback to occur. The implication of the reduced feedback is that very high gain and wide frequency response may be incorporated into an implantable system, and certain patterns of frequency-selective responses that are now difficult to achieve due to mechanical or acoustic feedback problems might be used.

Human subject investigations (Goode and Glattke, 1973) have shown that devices operating on this principle can transmit intelligible speech, but they are not efficient. The implantable transducers require either a considerable voltage (piezoelectric devices) or a large amount of current (coil-magnet induction), and conventional battery supplies cannot be used. If the efficiency problems can be solved, this approach will warrant further study.

ELECTRICAL STIMULATION

Attempts at direct stimulation of the nervous system of a hearing-impaired individual have received a great deal of public attention in recent years, and they are certainly the most controversial of the approaches to providing auditory sensation. The essential features of all such approaches include a microphone and electronic components which convert the microphone's output into a stimulus that is transmitted to the central nervous system or cochlea by indwelling electrodes. The active electronic elements are worn on the outside of the body. Only the electrodes and some means of coupling them to the active electronics are actually implanted. Beyond this general scheme, there is wide diversity among the approaches various investigators have used.

The disagreement begins with the choice of the site for the electrodes. Five approaches have been described, and some of these are illustrated in Figure 15-5. The first (A) involves placement of a single wire electrode on the round window (Vernon, 1974). The second (B) approach uses small unsupported electrodes placed within the scala tympani (House, 1974). In another approach (C), several electrodes are fitted to a silastic "cast" that is inserted into the scala tympani and fills it, thereby providing support for the electrodes (Merzenich et al., 1973). The fourth approach (D) involves the placement of electrodes directly into auditory nerve tissue by first

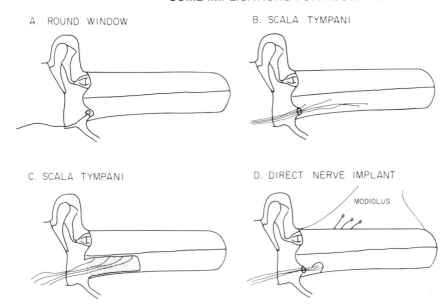

FIG. 15-5. Examples of the placement of electrodes for prosthetic electrical stimulation of the auditory nerve in man.

passing them through the round window and then through a perforation made intentionally in the wall of the modiolus (Simmons, 1966). Finally, there has been some preliminary study of the effects of electrodes placed directly on the auditory cortex (Dobelle et al., 1973).

There is no doubt that electrical current passed into the central nervous system or the auditory nerve by these techniques will produce sensation. However, there are several critical problems that must receive attention if the electrical stimulation techniques are to become successful. These problems include the choice of materials used for the electrodes (White and Mercer, 1974). The implanted materials must not be toxic to the nervous system and must dissolve slowly as a result of the application of the electrical current. Further, its insulation must be complete and impervious to body fluids if the implanted portion is to have a long useful life. Additional problems are discussed below and include the feasibility of using several electrical channels simultaneously (Merzenich, Schindler, and White, 1974); shrinking of the electronic components to implantable dimensions so that they, too, can be implanted (Gheewala, Melen, and White, 1975); and the development of a suitable "code" for the artificial stimuli that are actually sent to the nervous system (Kiang and Moxon, 1972).

It is difficult to rank such problems in their order of importance, because failure in any one of these areas would render the device useless. However, when one considers the experiences that have been reported with human subjects, it becomes apparent that the development of a suitable artificial code may be the most complex and elusive of all of the problems. In the present state of the implant systems, human subjects are able to perceive electrical stimulation over a wide range of frequencies, but they are unable to differentiate among those frequencies when they are above about 500 Hz (Michelson et al., 1973; Simmons, 1966). In the frequency range below 500 Hz, the change in frequency necessary to detect a change is quite large. The best results are that changes of 10 to 15% are necessary, and the poorest suggest that a 100% change is necessary (Michelson et al., 1973; Simmons, 1966). The 100% finding, of course, means that a full octave change in frequency must be introduced before that change can be detected by a user. This should be considered in the light of the 0.2% frequency change which may be detected by normal-hearing individuals. The loudness perception associated with artificial stimulation is also abnormal. Most observations on the loudness change with changes in electrical stimulation suggest that the dynamic range, from threshold to maximum tolerable levels, is not more than 20 dB. Findings from human subjects have disasterous implications for speech perception. The few quantitative studies that have actually involved speech as stimuli have suggested that little intelligence can be transmitted to the nervous system using a single pair of stimulating electrodes (Owens, 1974). Without speechreading, individuals can be expected to operate at a chance level in speech perception tasks, though there is some evidence that the prosodic cues afforded by electrical stimulation may combine with speechreading to improve an individual's overall performance.

Animal studies using single electrodes or electrode pairs have suggested the physiological correlates for the poor perceptual skills of human subjects implanted in the same fashion (Glattke, 1974; Merzenich et al., 1973). In brief, those studies have suggested that single electrodes will provide for information about the temporal cadence of the incoming speech signal, but single electrodes cannot supply information that would be like the spatial array of stimulation provided by the normal cochlea. Animal studies have also shown evidence of a limited dynamic range, in that the stimulus intensity range from threshold to maximum number of neural discharges or maximum amplitude of evoked response is approximately 20 dB. The perfect artificial electrical stimulation device would duplicate the analysis performed by the cochlea and present the results of that analysis to the auditory nerve in a form normally used by the cochlea. It is for this reason that multiple-channel stimulation is now under consideration (Merzenich et al., 1974; Gheewala, Melen, and White, 1975). While preliminary results of multiple channel feasibility studies are promising, the problem, of how to selectively activate the individual channels in a manner similar to cochlear activation of neurons remains elusive. It is clear that a great amount of investigation in both normal and pathological hearing processes will have to be undertaken before artificial stimulation of the nervous system earns the title "artificial ear" that has been given it by the popular press.

The research into artificial stimulation of the ear has raised some additional questions which bear not only upon that problem, but also upon the general problem of rehabilitation of the hearing-impaired individual. The utility of any type of hearing aid that is designed to offer auditory sensation is dependent upon the presence of viable auditory nerve fibers. Current knowledge suggests that certain classes of hearing loss may be the result of selective destruction of hair cells. Drug-induced loss is an example. There is no evidence to suggest that the auditory nerve will not degenerate eventually in patients with hair cell loss. The histologic evidence regarding this question is simply not available at the present time. One must also be concerned about the damaging effects of implantation, and whether electrode implantation into already damaged ears will accelerate destruction of the auditory nerve (Schindler and Merzenich, 1974).

Related to the general problem of the status of the auditory system in a hearing loss patient, Shuknecht (1974) has offered evidence that the common presbycusis may be the result of any one of four types of damage that can occur individually or in concert with one another. The damage types include (1) atrophy of the basal organ of Corti; (2) atrophy of the stria vasculaires; (3) loss of central nervous system function; and (4) mechanical anomalies within the cochlea that disrupt the normal motion of the basilar membrane and organ of Corti. At first consideration, such information may seem to have little relevance to patient rehabilitation. In fact, these clinical entities can be recognized through careful audiometric and diagnostic procedures, and their recognition may be very helpful in patient counseling and the selection of candidates for amplification or other rehabilitative measures. One should not lose sight of the need for constant refinement of diagnostic skills, so that the rehabilitation effort can proceed on solid grounds.

STIMULATION OF ALTERNATE SENSORY SYSTEMS

The use of visual or tactile stimulation in the rehabilitation of the deaf and hearing loss population continues to be an important and critical area of research. In general terms, stimulators for visual or tactile senses consist of a sound-receiving apparatus and an analysis device which subsequently provides for a display of the temporal or spectral features of the incoming stimulus. The display could take the form of an oscilloscope screen, a series of lights, or an array of vibro-tactile stimulators placed at some suitable and convenient location on the body (Pickett, 1968, 1963). Audition is most certainly a temporal sense primarily, and devices which attempt visual or tactile displays have not been successful in recoding auditory signals in a form which is useful and highly discriminable. One major problem common to the visual and tactile systems is the question of which features of speech must be recoded in order to produce intelligible messages. Another serious question stems from the fact that the visual and tactile sensory systems are not usually involved with the discrimination of spoken language, though they do play an important role in supporting auditory perception. Thus, future research in this area must not only include device selection, but also basic questions of visual and tactile function, language recognition and competence, and other broadly based avenues of inquiry (Pickett, 1975).

Questions related to patient interaction with the prosthetic method used in an individual case span the entire range of rehabilitation measures. One of the most critical, and yet elusive, of these questions relates to patient motivation. At a recent conference on artificial stimulation of the auditory nerve House (1974) provided filmed and live testimonials by patients underscoring the high degree of motivation common to them. After witnessing their testimonials, one cannot help but consider that, no matter how carefully a patient has been counseled, the patient's expectations of the utility of an approach will affect the success of the approach. One wonders how a conventional hearing aid, or a vibro-tactile device, can be fairly evaluated against the more exotic implantable devices when individuals receiving the various forms of treatment evidence significantly different levels of motivation toward the treatments. The complexity of the problem of patient motivation is sufficiently great to make the technical, surgical, and engineering aspects of prosthesis development seem relatively simple, and it is a problem which deserves and requires considerable attention in the future.

bibliography

ALPINER, J., Aural rehabilitation and the aged client. *Maico Audiological Library Series*, 4, 9–12 (1967).

American Standard Criteria for Background Noise in Audiometer Rooms, S3.1. New York: American National Standards Institute (1960).

American National Standard Method for Coupler Calibration of Earphones, S3.7-1973. New York: American National Standards Institute (1973).

American National Standard Method of Expressing Hearing Aid Performance, S3.8-1967 (R-1971). New York: American National Standards Institute (1967).

American National Standard Methods for Measurement of Electroacoustical Characteristics of Hearing Aids, S3.3-1960 (R-1971). New York: American National Standards Institute (1960).

American National Standard Specifications for Audiometers, S3.6. New York: American National Standards Institute (1969).

ANGEL, J., AND FITE, W., The monaural localization of sound. *Psychol. Rev.*, 8, 225 (1901).

ANONYMOUS, *Prices of Hearing Aids*. Hearings before the Subcommittee on Antitrust and Monopoly of the Committee on the Judiciary, United States Senate. Washington, D. C.: U. S. Government Printing Office (1962).

ASHA Committee on Rehabilitative Audiology, The audiologist: Responsibilities in the habilitation of the auditorily handicapped. *Asha*, 16, 14–18 (1974).

AUFRICHT, H., A follow-up study of the CROS hearing aid. *J. Speech Hear. Disord.*, 37, 113–117 (1972).

BALLENGER, H., The "aural or acoustic" method of treating deafness: Further investigation. *Am. Ann. Rhinol. Laryngol.*, 45, 632–637 (1936).

BARNET, A., Biology of sensory deprivation. *Acta Otolaryngol.*, Supplement 206, 210–214 (1965).

BAUER, B., Electroacoustic transducers. In GERBER, S. (Ed.), *Introductory Hearing Science*, Chapter 3. Philadelphia: W. B. Saunders Co. (1974).

BELENDIUK, K., AND BUTLER, R., Monaural localization of low-pass noise bands in the horizontal plane. *J. Acoust. Soc. Am.*, 58, 701–705 (1975).

BELLEFLEUR, P., AND MCMENAMIN, S., Problems of induction loop amplification. *Volta Rev.*, 67, 559–563 (1965).

BELLEFLEUR, P., AND VAN DYKE, R., The effects of high gain amplification on children in a residential school for the deaf. *J. Speech Hear. Res.*, 11, 343–347 (1968).

BENNETT, D., AND BYERS, V., Increased intelligibility in the hypacusic by slow-play frequency transposition. *J. Auditory Res.*, 7, 107–118 (1967).

BERANEK, L., *Acoustics*. New York: McGraw-Hill Book Company, Inc. (1954).

BERGER, K., *The Hearing Aid: Its Operation and Development*. Detroit: The National Hearing Aid Society (1970).

BERGER, K., *The Hearing Aid: Its Operation and Development*, Second Edition. Livonia, Mich.: The National Hearing Aid Society (1974).

BERGMAN, M., Binaural hearing. *Arch. Otolaryngol.*, 66, 572–578 (1957).

BERGMAN, M., A master hearing aid. *Asha*, 1, 140–141 (1959).

BIRT, B., AND ALBERTI, P., Evaluation of hearing aid assessment and quality control of hearing aids. *Can. J. Otolaryngol.*, 2, 63–71 (1973).

BODE, D., AND OYER, H., Auditory training and speech discrimination. *J. Speech Hear. Res.*, 13, 839–855 (1970).

BOOTHROYD, A., Distribution of hearing levels in the student population of Clarke School for the Deaf. SARP #3, Clarke School for the Deaf, Northampton (1970).

BORRILD, K., Electroacoustic aids applied in the training of deaf and hard of hearing children. *Proceedings of the 1967 International Congress on Oral Education of the Deaf*, 564–576 (1967).

BOYD, J., AND JAMROZ, A., A comparison of group hearing aid systems. *Am. Ann. Deaf*, 108, 245–250 (1963).

BRANDER, R., Personal communication with members of the ANSI writing group (1974).

BRESSON, K., Open ear-mould treatment versus closed. In EWERTSEN, H. (Ed.), Electroacoustic characteristics relevant to hearing aids. *Scand. Audiol.*, Supplement 1, 40–44 (1971).

BRISKEY, R., AND WRUK, K., Acoustic influence of insert vents. *Hear. Instruments*, 25, 12–13 (1974).

BRISKEY, R., GREENBAUM, W., AND SINCLAIR, J., Pitfalls in hearing aid response curves. *J. Audio Engineering Soc.*, 14, 317–323 (1966).

BRITE, R., *Transistor Fundamentals*, Vol. 1, *Basic Semiconductor and Circuit Principles*. Kansas City: The Bobbs-Merrill Co., Inc. (1972).

BROWN, A., AND HOPKINS, H., Interaction of the auditory and visual sensory modalities. *J. Acoust. Soc. Am.*, 41, 1–6 (1967).

BURKHARD, M., AND SACHS, R., KEMAR, the Knowles electronics manikin for acoustic research. Report Number 20032-1 of Project 20032. Elk Grove Village, Ill.: Industrial Research Products (1973).

BURNEY, P., A survey of hearing aid evaluation procedures. *Asha*, 14, 439–444 (1972).

BYMAN, J., Testing of auditory and audiovisual speech perception related to everyday communication. *Scand. Audiol.*, Supplement 4, 58–66 (1974).

BYRNE, D., Some implications of body baffle for hearing aid selection. *Sound*, 6, 86–91 (1972).

273

CALVERT, D., REDDEL, R., DONALDSON, R., AND PEW, L., A comparison of auditory amplifiers for the deaf. *Except. Child.*, 32, 247–253 (1965).

CARHART, R., Selection of hearing aids. *Arch. Otolaryngol.*, 44, 1–18 (1946a).

CARHART, R., Tests for selection of hearing aids. *Laryngoscope*, 56, 780–794 (1946b).

CARHART, R., Volume control adjustment in hearing aid selection. *Laryngoscope*, 56, 510–521 (1946c).

CARHART, R., The usefulness of the binaural hearing aid. *J. Speech Hear. Disord.*, 23, 41–51 (1958).

CARHART, R., Problems in the measurement of speech discrimination. *Arch. Otolaryngol.*, 82, 253–260 (1965).

CARHART, R., POLLACK, K., AND LOTTERMAN, S., Comparative efficiency of aided binaural hearing. Paper presented at the 39th annual meeting of the American Speech and Hearing Association (1963).

CARHART, R., AND TILLMAN, T., Individual consistency of hearing for speech across diverse listening conditions. *J. Speech Hear. Res.*, 15, 105–113 (1972).

CARHART, R., TILLMAN, T., AND JOHNSON, K., Release of masking for speech through interaural time delay. *J. Acoust. Soc. Am.*, 42, 124–138 (1967).

CARLISLE, R., AND MUNDEL, A., Practical hearing aid measurements. *J. Acoust. Soc. Am.*, 16, 45–51 (1944).

CARLSON, E., Smoothing the hearing aid frequency response. Paper presented at the 48th Audio Engineering Society Convention (1974).

CARLSON, E., AND KILLION, M., Subminiature directional microphones. *J. Audio Engineering Soc.*, 22, 92–96 (1974).

CARMEL, N., Open forum: Dispensing. *Audiol. Hear. Educ.*, 1, 50, 52–53 (1975).

CARSON, E., Rehabilitation of the deafened. In Coates, G. (Ed.), *Otolaryngology*. Hagerstown, Md.: W.F. Prior (1960).

CASTLE, W. (Ed.), A conference on hearing aid evaluation procedures. *A.S.H.A., Reports*, Number 2 (1967).

CHERRY, C., Two ears—but one world. In Rosenblith, W. (Ed.), *Sensory Communication*, 99–117. Boston: Massachusetts Institute of Technology Press (1959).

CHERRY, E., AND SAYERS, B., Human "cross-correlator"—A technique for measuring certain parameters of speech perception. *J. Acoust. Soc. Am.*, 28, 889–895 (1956).

CILIAX, D., Lipreading performance as affected by continuous auditory distractions. Unpublished Doctoral Dissertation, Michigan State University (1973).

CLARKE, B., Use of a group hearing aid by profoundly deaf children. In EWING, A. (Ed.), *Educational Guidance and the Deaf Child*, 128–159. Manchester: Manchester University Press (1957).

CONKEY, H., AND SCHNEIDERMAN, C., The effect of a contralateral routing of sound on auditory localization and mobility of a blind person. *Except. Child.*, 34, 705–706 (1968).

COOPER, W., FRANKS, J., McFALL, R., AND GOLDSTEIN, D., Variable venting valve for earmolds. *Audiology*, 14, 259–267 (1975).

CRANDALL, K., A study of the production of chers and related sign language aspects by deaf children between the ages of three and seven years. Doctoral Dissertation, Northwestern University (1974).

Custom Earmold Manual. Pittsburgh, Pa.: Microsonic (1974).

DAMASHEK, M., AND BOOTHROYD, A., Student to student communication in a group hearing aid. Paper presented at the American Speech and Hearing Association Convention, Detroit (1973).

DANAHER (NÉE MARTIN), E., OSBERGER, N., AND PICKETT, J., Discrimination of formant frequency transitions in synthetic vowels. *J. Speech Hear. Res.*, 16, 439–451 (1973).

DANAHER, E., AND PICKETT, J., Some masking effects produced by low frequency vowel formants in persons with sensorineural hearing loss. *J. Speech Hear Res.*, 18, 261–271 (1975).

DAVID, E., JR., GUTTMAN, N., AND VAN BERGEIJK, W., Letter to the editor. *J. Acoust. Soc. Am.*, 30, 801–803 (1958).

DAVIS, H., *Hearing and Deafness: A Guide for Laymen*. New York: Rinehart Books (1947).

DAVIS, H., ET AL., The selection of hearing aids. *Laryngoscope*, 56, 85–115, 135–163 (1946).

DAVIS, H., ET AL., *Hearing Aids: An Experimental Study of Design Objectives*. Cambridge, Mass.: Harvard University Press (1947).

DAVIS, H., AND SILVERMAN, S., *Hearing and Deafness*. New York: Holt, Rinehart and Winston (1960, third edition: 1970).

DAVIS, R., AND GREEN, S., The influence of controlled venting on discrimination ability. *Hear. Aid J.*, 27, 6 (1974).

DE BOER, B., Tolerance of components for hearing aids. *J. Audiol. Tech.*, 9, 142–150 (1970).

DI CARLO, L., Auditory training for the adult. *Volta Rev.*, 50, 490–496 (1948).

DIRKS, D., AND CARHART, R., A survey of reaction from users of binaural and monaural hearing aids. *J. Speech Hear. Disord.*, 27, 311–322 (1962).

DIRKS, D., AND WILSON, R., The effect of spatially separated sound sources on speech intelligibility. *J. Speech Hear. Res.*, 12, 5–38 (1969).

DOBELLE, W., STENSAAS, S., MLADEVJOVSKY, M., AND SMITH, J., A prosthesis for the deaf based on cortical stimulation. *Ann. Otol. Rhinol. Laryngol.*, 82, 445–463 (1973).

DODDS, E., AND HARFORD, E., Modified earpieces and CROS for high frequency hearing losses. *J. Speech Hear. Res.*, 11, 204–218 (1968a).

DODDS, E., AND HARFORD, E., Application of a lipreading test in a hearing aid evaluation. *J. Speech Hear. Disord.*, 33, 167–173 (1968b).

DODDS, E., AND HARFORD, E., Follow-up report on modified earpieces and CROS for high frequency losses. *J. Speech Hear. Res.*, 13, 41–43 (1970).

DOWNS, M., The establishment of hearing aid use: A program for parents. *Maico Audiological Library Series*, 4, 13–15 (1967).

DOWNS, M., The deafness management quotient. *Hearing and Speech News*, 42, 8–28 (1974).

ELLIOTT, L., Prediction of speech discrimination scores from other test information. *J. Auditory Res.*, 3, 35–45 (1963).

ERBER, N., Interaction of audition and vision in the recognition of oral speech stimuli. *J. Speech Hear. Res.*, 12, 423–434 (1969).

ERBER, N., Auditory, visual, and auditory-visual recognition of consonants by children with normal and impaired hearing. *J. Speech Hear. Res.*, 15,

413–422 (1972).

ERBER, N., Body-baffle and real-ear effects in the selection of hearing aids for deaf children. *J. Speech Hear. Disord.*, 38, 224–231 (1973).

EWERTSEN, H., Hearing aid distribution in Denmark. *Scand. Audiol.*, 1, 77–79 (1972).

EWERTSEN, H., Hearing rehabilitation in Denmark. *Hear. Instruments*, 25, 20–21 (1974).

FANT, G., *Acoustic Theory of Speech Production.* The Hague: Mouton (1960).

FINITZO-HIEBER, T., The influence of reverberation and noise on the speech intelligibility of normal and hard of hearing children in classroom size listening environments. Doctoral Dissertation, Northwestern University (1975).

FISHER, H., AND FREEDMAN, S., The role of the pinna in auditory localization. *J. Auditory Res.*, 8, 15–26 (1968).

FLETCHER, H., *Speech and Hearing.* New York: D. Van Nostrand, Co. (1929).

FLETCHER, H., *Speech and Hearing in Communication.* Princeton, N.J.: D. Van Nostrand, Co. (1953).

FLOTTORP, G., Intermodulation in hearing aids. *Scand. Audiol.*, Supplement 1 (1971).

FORESTER, C., Residual hearing and its bearing on oral training. *Am. Ann. Deaf*, 73, 796–804 (1928).

FOWLER, E., Bilateral hearing aids for monaural total deafness: A suggestion for better hearing. *Arch. Otolaryngol.*, 72, 57–58 (1960).

FRANK, T., AND GOODEN, R., The effect of hearing aid microphone types on speech discrimination scores in a background of multitalker noise. *Maico Audiological Library Series*, 2, 5 (1973).

FRANSSON, A., Geriatric rehabilitation. In LIDEN, G. (Ed.), *Geriatric Audiology.* Stockholm: Almqvist and Wiksell (1968).

FREDRICKSON, J., TOMLINSON, D., DAVIS, E., AND ODKVIST, L., Evaluation of an electromagnetic implantable hearing aid. *Can. J. Otolaryngol.*, 2, 53–62 (1973).

FRENCH, N., AND STEINBERG, J., Factors governing the intelligibility of speech sounds. *J. Acoust. Soc. Am.*, 19, 90–119 (1947).

FRY, D., Acoustic cues in the speech of the hearing and the deaf. *Proc. R. Soc. Med.*, 66, 959–969 (1973).

GAETH, J., Verbal and nonverbal learning in children including those with hearing losses. Cooperative Research Project, Number 1001, Wayne State University (1963).

GAETH, J., Learning with visual and audiovisual presentation. In McCONNELL, F., AND WARD, J. (Eds.), *Deafness in Childhood.* Nashville, Tenn.: Vanderbilt University Press (1967).

GAETH, J., AND LOUNSBURY, E., Hearing aids for children in elementary schools. *J. Speech Hear. Disord.*, 31, 283–289 (1966).

GALLOWAY, A., A review of hearing aid fittings on young adults with severe to profound hearing impairment. Paper presented to the Academy of Rehabilitative Audiology, July (1974).

GALLOWAY, A., AND GAUGER, J., Personal communication (1975).

GANG, R., The effects of age on the diagnostic utility of the rollover phenomenon. *J. Speech Hear. Disord.*, 41, 63–69 (1976).

GARDNER, M., Historical background of the Haas and/or precedence effect. *J. Acoust. Soc. Am.*, 43,

1243–1248 (1968).

GENGEL, R., Acceptable speech-to-noise ratios for aided speech discrimination by the hearing-impaired. *J. Audiol. Res.*, 11, 219–222 (1971).

GENGEL, R., AND FOUST, K., Some implications of listening level for speech reception by sensorineural hearing impaired children. *Language, Speech and Hearing Services in Schools*, 6, 14–20 (1975).

GERBER, S., *Introductory Hearing Science.* Philadelphia: W. B. Saunders, Co. (1974).

GHEEWALA, T., MELEN, R., AND WHITE, R., A CMOS implantable multielectrode auditory stimulator for the deaf. *IEEE J. Solid State Circuits*, SC-10, 472–479 (1975).

GIOLAS, T., AND EPSTEIN, A., Comparative intelligibility of word lists and continuous discourse. *J. Speech Hear. Res.* 6, 349–358 (1963).

GLATTKE, T., Electrical stimulation of the auditory nerve in animals. In MERZENICH, M., SCHINDLER, R., AND SOOY, F. (Eds.), *Proceedings of the First International Conference on Electrical Stimulation of the Acoustic Nerve as a Treatment for Profound Sensorineural Deafness in Man*, 63–78. San Francisco: Velo-bind, Inc. (1974).

GOLDBERG, H., Telephone amplifying pick-up devices. *Hear. Instruments*, 26, 19–20 (1975).

GOLDSTEIN, M., *The Acoustic Method for the Training of the Deaf and Hard-of-Hearing Child.* St. Louis, Mo.: Laryngoscope Press (1939).

GOODE, R., AND COOPER, K., Prosthetic modification of ear canal resonance. *Asha*, 17, 671 (1975).

GOODE, R., AND GLATTKE, T., Audition via electromagnetic induction. *Arch. Otolaryngol.*, 98, 23–26 (1973).

GOODFELLOW, L., The re-education of defective hearing. *J. Psychol.*, 14, 53–58 (1942).

GOODHILL, V., Surgical management of hearing loss. In TOWER, D. (Ed.), *The Nervous System*, Vol. 3, *Human Communication and its Disorders*, 273–290. New York: Raven Press (1975).

GRAMMATICO, L., The development of listening skills. *Volta Rev.*, 77, 303–308 (1975).

GREEN, D., Non-occluding earmolds with CROS and IROS hearing aids. *Arch. Otolaryngol.*, 89, 512–522 (1969).

GREEN, D., AND HENNING, G., Audition. *Ann. Rev. Psychol.*, 20, 105–128 (1969).

GREEN, D., AND ROSS, M., The effects of a conventional versus a non-occluding "CROS-type" earmold upon the frequency response of a hearing aid. *J. Speech Hear. Res.*, 11, 638–647 (1968).

GRIFFING, T., Variable venting of earmolds. *Hear. Dealer*, 22, 23 (1971).

HAIC Standards for Hearing Aids. New York: Hearing Aid Industry Conference (1974) .

HALLE, M., HUGHES, G., AND RADLEY, J., Acoustic properties of stop consonants. *J. Acoust. Soc. Am.*, 29, 107–116 (1957).

HANSON, W., The baffle effect of the human body on the response of a hearing aid. *J. Acoust. Soc. Am.*, 16, 60–62 (1944).

HARFORD, E., Bilateral CROS: Two-sided listening with one hearing aid. *Arch. Otolaryngol.*, 84, 426–432 (1966).

HARFORD, E., AND BARRY, J., A rehabilitative approach to the problem of unilateral hearing impairment: The contralateral routing of signals (CROS). *J. Speech Hear. Dis.*, 30, 121–138 (1965).

HARFORD, E., AND DODDS, E., The clinical application of CROS: A hearing aid for unilateral deafness. *Arch. Otolaryngol.*, 83, 455–464 (1966).

HARFORD, E., AND DODDS, E., Versions of the CROS hearing aid. *Arch. Otolaryngol.*, 100, 50–57 (1974).

HARFORD, E., AND MARKLE, D., The atypical effect of a hearing aid on one patient with congenital deafness. *Laryngoscope*, 65, 970–972 (1955).

HARFORD, E., AND MUSKET, C., Binaural hearing with one hearing aid. *J. Speech Hear. Disord.*, 29, 133–146 (1964a).

HARFORD, E., AND MUSKET, C., Some considerations in the organization and administration of a clinical hearing aid selection program. *Asha*, 66, 35–40 (1964b).

HARRIS, J., Monaural and binaural speech intelligibility and the stereophonic effect based upon temporal cues. *Laryngoscope*, 75, 428–446 (1965).

HARRIS, J., HAINES, H., KELSEY, P., AND CLACK, T., The relation between speech intelligibility and the electroacoustic characteristics of low fidelity circuitry. *J. Auditory Res.*, 5, 357–381 (1961).

HARRIS, K., Cues for the discrimination of American English fricatives in spoken syllables. *Lang. Speech*, 1, 1–7 (1958).

HASKINS, H., AND HARDY, W., Clinical studies in stereophonic hearing. *Laryngoscope*, 70, 1427–1432 (1960).

HEBRANK, J., AND WRIGHT, D., Are two ears necessary for localization of sound sources on the median plane? *J. Acoust. Soc. Am.*, 56, 935–938 (1974).

HEYNE, K., Construction and function of sound transducers. In *Hearing Instrument Technology*, Chapter 5.6. Compiled by Hans-Jürgen von Kilisch-Horn, Median Verlag, Heidelberg, West Germany (1975).

HIEBER, T., MATKIN, N., CHEROW-SKALKA, E., AND RICE, C., A preliminary investigation of a sound effects recognition test (SERT). Paper presented at the American Speech and Hearing Association Convention (1975).

HIRSH, I., Binaural summation and interaural inhibition as a function of the level of the masking noise. *Am. J. Physiol.*, 56, 205–213 (1948).

HIRSH, I., The relation between localization and intelligibility. *J. Acoust. Soc. Am.*, 22, 196–200 (1950).

HIRSH, I., *The Measurement of Hearing*. New York: McGraw Hill Book Co., Inc. (1952).

HIRSH, I., Use of amplification in educating deaf children. *Am. Ann. Deaf*, 113, 92–100 (1968).

HIRSH, I., REYNOLDS, E., AND JOSEPH, M., Intelligibility of different speech materials. *J. Acoust. Soc. Am.*, 26, 530–538 (1954).

HOCHBERG, I., Most comfortable listening for the loudness and intelligibility of speech. *Audiology*, 14, 27–33 (1975).

HODGSON, W., AND MURDOCK, C., Effect of the earmold on speech intelligibility in hearing aid use. *J. Speech Hear. Res.*, 13, 290–297 (1970).

HODGSON, W., AND SUNG, R., Comparative performance of hearing aid microphone and induction coil for a sentence intelligibility test. *J. Auditory Res.*, 12, 261–264 (1972).

HORTON, K., Every child should be given a chance to benefit from acoustic input. *Volta Rev.*, 75, 348–350 (1973).

HOUSE, W., Multichannel electrical stimulation in man. In MERZENICH, M., SCHINDLER, R., AND SOOY, F. (Eds.), *Proceedings of the First International Conference on Electrical Stimulation of the Acoustic Nerve as a Treatment for Profound Sensorineural Deafness in Man*, 127–132. San Francisco: Velo-bind, Inc. (1974).

HUDGINS, C., The responses of profoundly deaf children to auditory training. *J. Speech Hear. Disord.*, 18, 273–288 (1953).

HUDGINS, C., Auditory training: Its possibilities and limitations. *Volta Rev.*, 56, 339–349 (1954).

HUGHES, G., AND HALLE, M., Spectral properties of fricative consonants. *J. Acoust. Soc. Am.*, 28, 303–310 (1956).

JEFFERS, J., Formants and auditory training of deaf children. *Volta Rev.*, 68, 418–423, 449 (1966).

JERGER, J., CARHART, R., AND DIRKS, D., Binaural hearing aids and speech intelligibility. *J. Speech Hear. Res.*, 4, 137–148 (1961).

JERGER, J., AND HAYES, D., Hearing aid evaluation: Clinical experience with a new philosophy. *Arch. Otolaryngol.*, 102, 214–221 (1976).

JERGER, J., AND JERGER, S., Diagnostic significance of PB word functions. *Arch. Otolaryngol.*, 93, 573–580 (1971).

JERGER, J., AND LEWIS, N., Binaural hearing aids: Are they dangerous for children? *Arch. Otolaryngol.*, 101, 480–483 (1975).

JERGER, J., SPEAKS, C., AND MALMQUIST, C., Hearing aid performance and hearing aid selection. *J. Speech Hear. Res.*, 9, 136–149 (1966).

JERGER, J., AND THELIN, J., Effects of electroacoustic characteristics of hearing aids on speech understanding. *Bull. Prosthet. Res.*, 11, 159–197 (1968).

JETTY, A., AND RINTELMANN, W., Acoustic coupler effects on speech audiometric scores using a CROS hearing aid. *J. Speech Hear. Res.*, 13, 101–114 (1970).

JIRSA, R., AND HODGSON, W., Effects of harmonic distortion in hearing aids on speech intelligibility for normals and hypacusics. *J. Auditory Res.*, 10, 213–217 (1970).

JIRSA, R., HODGSON, W., AND GOETZINGER, C., Reliability of PB half-lists. *J. Am. Audiol. Soc.*, 2, 47–49 (1975).

JOHANSSON, B., The use of the transposer for the management of the deaf child. *Int. Audiol.*, 5, 362–372 (1966).

JOHANSSON, B., The hearing aid as a technical-audiological problem. *Scand. Audiol.*, Supplement 3, 55–76 (1973).

JOHNSON, E., Testing results of acoustic training. *Am. Ann. Deaf*, 84, 223–229 (1939).

JOHNSON, E., The ability of pupils in a school for the deaf to understand various methods of communication, II. *Am. Ann. Deaf*, 93, 280–314 (1948).

JONGKEES, L., AND VAN DER VEER, R., On directional sound localization in unilateral deafness and its explanation. *Acta Otolaryngol.*, 49, 119–131 (1958).

KAISER, J., AND DAVID, E., JR., Reproducing the cocktail party effect. *J. Acoust. Soc. Am.*, 32, 918 (1960).

KARLOVICH, R., Sensory interaction: Perception of loudness during visual stimulation. *J. Acoust. Soc. Am.*, 44, 570–575 (1968).

KASTEN, R., Electroacoustic measurements of hearing aids. Paper presented at the annual convention of the American Speech and Hearing Association, Denver (1968).

KASTEN, R., Body and over-the-ear hearing aids. In KATZ, J. (Ed.), *Handbook of Clinical Audiology*. Baltimore: Williams and Wilkins Company (1972).

KASTEN, R., AND LOTTERMAN, S., Azimuth effects with ear-level hearing aids. *Bull. Prosthet. Res.*, 10, 50-61 (1967).

KASTEN, N., AND LOTTERMAN, S., The influence of hearing aid gain control rotation on acoustic gain. *J. Auditory Res.*, 9, 35-39 (1969).

KASTEN, R., LOTTERMAN, S., AND BURNETT, E., The influence of non-linear distortion on hearing aid processed signals. Paper presented at the annual convention of the American Speech and Hearing Association, Chicago (1967).

KASTEN, R., LOTTERMAN, S., AND HINCHMAN, S., Head shadow and head baffle effects in ear level aids. *Acustica*, 17, 154-160 (1967-68).

KASTEN, R., LOTTERMAN, S., AND REVOILE, S., Variability of gain versus frequency characteristics in hearing aids. *J. Speech Hear. Res.*, 10, 377-383 (1967).

KASTEN, R., AND TILLMAN, T., Effects of azimuth on monaural and binaural speech discrimination under conditions simulating aided listening. Paper presented at the annual convention of the American Speech and Hearing Association, San Francisco, Calif., Nov. (1964).

KEIL, J., The effects of peripheral visual stimuli on lipreading performance. Unpublished Doctoral Dissertation, Michigan State University (1968).

KIANG, N., AND MOXON, E., Physiological considerations in artificial stimulation of the inner ear. *Ann. Otol. Rhinol. Laryngol.*, 81, 714-731 (1972).

KILLION, M., AND CARLSON, E., A wide-band miniature microphone. Paper presented at the 37th Audio Engineering Society (1969).

KILLION, M., AND CARLSON, E., A subminiature electret-condenser microphone of new design. *J. Audio Engineering Soc.*, 22, 237-243 (1974).

KLEFFNER, F., Hearing losses, hearing aids, and children with language disorders. *J. Speech Hear. Dis.*, 38, 232-239 (1973).

KLIJN, J., The electronic link between teacher and child. *Proceedings of the 2nd International Course in Paedo-Audiology, Groningen University*, 96-102. The Netherlands (1961).

KNOWLES, H., AND BURKHARD, M., Hearing aids on KEMAR. *Electron. Instruments*, 32, 19-24 (1975).

KODMAN, F., Techniques for counseling the hearing aid client. *Maico Audiological Library Series*, 4, 23-25 (1967).

KOENIG, W., Subjective effects in binaural hearing. *J. Acoust. Soc. Am.*, 22, 61-62 (1950).

KONKLE, D., AND BESS, F., Custom-made vs. stock earmolds in hearing aid evaluations. *Arch. Otolaryngol.*, 99, 140-144 (1974).

KRYTER, K., *The Effects of Noise on Man*. New York: Academic Press (1970).

LACH, R., LING, D., LING, A., AND SHIP, N., Early speech development in deaf infants. *Am. Ann. Deaf*, 115, 522-526 (1970).

LANGFORD, B., Why binaural? *Audecibel*, 151-158 (1970).

LANKFORD, J., AND BEHNKE, C., Bacteriology of and cleaning merthods for stock earmolds. *J. Speech Hear. Res.*, 16, 325-329 (1973).

LARIVIERE, C., WINITZ, H., AND HERRIMAN, E., The distribution of perceptual cues in English prevocalic fricatives. *J. Speech Hear. Res.*, 18, 613-622 (1975).

LEMPERT, J., Improvement of hearing in cases of otosclerosis. *Arch. Otolaryngol.*, 28, 42-97 (1938).

LENNEBERG, E., *Biological Foundations for Language*. New York: John Wiley and Sons (1967).

LENTZ, W., Speech discrimination in the presence of background noise using a hearing aid with a directionally-sensitive microphone. *Maico Audiological Library Series*, 10, Report 9 (1972a).

LENTZ, W., Assessment of performance using hearing aids with directional and nondirectional microphones in a highly reverberant room. Paper presented to the annual convention of the American Speech and Hearing Association, San Francisco (1972b).

LEONARD, R., The effects of continuous auditory distractions on lipreading performance. Unpublished Master's Thesis, Michigan State University (1962).

LIBERMAN, A., COOPER, G., SHANKWEILER, D., AND STUDDERT-KENNEDY, M., Perception of the speech code. *Psychol. Rev.*, 74, 431-461 (1967).

LIBERMAN, A., DELATTRE, P., GERSTMAN, L., AND COOPER, F., Tempo of frequency change as a cue for distinguishing classes of speech sounds. *J. Exp. Psychol.*, 52, 127-137 (1956).

LICKLIDER, J., The influence of interaural phase relations upon the masking of speech by white noise. *J. Acoust. Soc. Am.*, 20, 150-159 (1948).

LIDEN, G., AND KANKKUNEN, A., Visual reinforcement audiometry in the management of young deaf children. *International Audiol.*, 8, 99-106 (1969).

LING, D., Implications of hearing aid amplification below 300 cps. *Volta Rev.*, 66, 723-729 (1964).

LING, D., Loop induction for auditory training of deaf children. *Maico Audiological Library Series*, 5, Report 2 (1966).

LING, D., Installation and operation of loop induction systems in real-life situations. *Audecibel*, Spring, 61-70 (1967).

LING, D., Comment on "Sensorineural loss and upward spread of masking." *J. Speech Hear. Res.*, 14, 222-223 (1971).

LING, D., It is through meaningful communication that speech and language skills are acquired and perfected. *Volta Rev.*, 75, 354-356 (1973).

LING, D., Amplification for speech. In CALVERT, D., AND SILVERMAN S. (Eds.), *Speech and Deafness*, Chapter 3. Washington, D.C.: A.G. Bell Association for the Deaf (1975).

LING, D., AND DOEHRING, D., Learning limits for deaf children for coded speech. *J. Speech Hear. Res.*, 12, 83-94 (1969).

LING, D., AND DRUZ, W., Transposition of high frequency sounds by partial vocoding of the speech spectrum: Its use by deaf children. *J. Auditory Res.*, 7, 133-144 (1967).

LISKER, L., AND ABRAMSON, A., Some effects of context on voice onset time in English stops. *Lang. Speech*, 10, 1-28 (1967).

LLOYD, N., Behavioral audiometry viewed as an operant procedure. *J. Speech Hear. Disord.*, 31, 128-135 (1966).

LOTTERMAN, S., AND KASTEN, R., Non-linear distortion in modern hearing aids. *J. Speech Hear. Res.*, 10, 586-592 (1967a).

LOTTERMAN, S., AND KASTEN, R., The influence of gain control rotation on nonlinear distortion in hearing aids. *J. Speech Hear. Res.*, 10, 593-599

(1967b).

LOTTERMAN, S., AND KASTEN, R., Examination of the CROS type hearing aid. *J. Speech Hear. Res.*, 14, 416–420 (1971).

LOTTERMAN, S., KASTEN, R., AND MAJERUS, D., Battery life and non-linear distortion in hearing aids. *J. Speech Hear. Dis.*, 32, 274–278 (1967).

LOTTERMAN, S., KASTEN, R., AND REVOILE, S., Acoustic gain and threshold improvement in hearing aid selection. *J. Speech Hear. Res.*, 10, 856–858 (1967).

LUDVIGSEN, C., Construction and evaluation of an audio-visual test (the Helen test). *Scand. Audiol.*, Supplement 4, 67–75 (1974).

LUNDBORG, T., LINZANDER, S., ROSENHAMER, H., LINDSTROM, B., SVARD, I., AND FRANSSON, A., Experiences with hearing aids in adults. *Scand. Audiol.*, Supplement 3, 9–46 (1973).

LYBARGER, S., *The Ear Mold as a Part of the Receiver Acoustic System*. Canonsburg, Pa: Radioear Corp. (1958).

LYBARGER, S., Earmold acoustics. *Audecibel*, 16, 9–20 (1967).

LYBARGER, S., Earmolds. In KATZ, J. (Ed.), *Handbook of Clinical Audiology*. Baltimore: Williams and Wilkins Company (1972).

LYBARGER, S., Advantages and limitations of the 'Y' cord. *Hear. Aid J.*, 26, 6, 34 (1973).

LYBARGER, S., Electroacoustic measurements. In DONNELLY, K. (Ed.), *Interpreting Hearing Aid Technology*. Springfield: Charles C Thomas (1974).

LYBARGER, S., AND BARRON, F., Head-baffle effect for different hearing aid microphone locations. (Abstract) *J. Acoust. Soc. Am.*, 38, 922 (1965).

LYNNE, G., AND CARHART, R., Influence of attack and release in compression amplification on understanding of speech by hypoacusics. *J. Speech Hear. Disord.*, 28, 124–140 (1963).

MACRAE, J., TTS and recovery from TTS after use of powerful hearing aids. *J. Acoust. Soc. Am.*, 43, 1445–1446 (1968).

MACRAE, J., AND FARRANT, R., The effect of hearing aid use on the residual hearing of children with sensorineural deafness. *Ann. Otol., Rhinol., and Laryngol.*, 74, 409–419 (1965).

MAIER, H., *The Psychoanalytic Theory of Erik H. Erikson. Three Theories of Child Development*, Chapter 2. New York: Harper and Row, Publishers (1969).

MALLES, I., Hearing aid effect in unilateral conductive deafness. *Arch. Otolaryngol.*, 77, 406–408 (1963).

MARTIN, E., AND PICKETT, J., Sensorineural hearing loss and upward spread of masking. *J. Speech Hear. Res.*, 13, 426–437 (1970).

MARTIN, E., PICKETT, J., AND COLTEN, S., Discrimination of vowel formant transitions by listeners with severe sensorineural loss. In FANT, G. (Ed.), *Speech Communication Ability and Profound Deafness*, Paper 9. Washington, D.C.: A.G. Bell Association for the Deaf (1972).

MATKIN, N., Hearing aids for children. Paper presented at the symposium: Amplification for Sensorineural Hearing Loss. Audiology Center of Redlands, July (1971).

MATKIN, N., Some essential features of a pediatric audiologic evaluation. Evaluation of Hearing Handicapped Children, Chapter 7. Denmark: Fifth Danavox Symposium (1973).

MATKIN, N., AND OLSEN, W., Response of hearing aids with induction loop amplification systems. *Am. Ann. Deaf*, 115, 73–78 (1970a).

MATKIN, N., AND OLSEN, W., Induction loop amplification systems: Classroom performance, *Asha*, 12, 239–244 (1970b).

MATKIN, N., AND OLSEN, W., An investigation of radio frequency auditory training units. *Am. Ann. Deaf*, 118, 25–30 (1973).

MATKIN, N., AND THOMAS, J., CROS hearing aids for children. *Maico Audiological Library Series*, 10, Report 8 (1971a).

MATKIN, N., AND THOMAS, J., CROS hearing aids for children. Paper presented at the annual convention of the American Speech and Hearing Association, Chicago, Ill., Nov. (1971b).

MATKIN, N., AND THOMAS, J., The utilization of programmed instruction with parents of hearing impaired children. Paper presented at the annual convention of the American Speech and Hearing Association (1973).

MAXON, T., DEUTSCH, L., AND MAZOR, M., The effect of microphone spacing on auditory localization and speech intelligibility. Paper presented at the American Speech and Hearing Association Convention, San Francisco (1972).

MCCLELLEN, M., Aided speech discrimination in noise with vented and unvented earmolds. *J. Auditory Res.*, 7, 93–99 (1967).

MCCROSKEY, R., Progress report on a home training program for deaf infants. *Int. Audiol.*, 6, 171–177 (1967).

McDONALD, F., AND STUDEBAKER, G., Earmold alteration effect as measured in the human auditory meatus. *J. Acoust. Soc. Am.*, 48, 1366–1372 (1970).

MERZENICH, M., MICHELSON, R., PETTIT, C., SCHINDLER, R., AND REID, M., Neural encoding of sound sensation evoked by electrical stimulation of the acoustic nerve. *Ann. Otol. Rhinol. Laryngol.*, 82, 486–503 (1973).

MERZENICH, M., SCHINDLER, D., AND WHITE, M., Feasibility of multichannel scala tympani stimulation. *Laryngoscope*, 84, 1887–1893 (1974).

MICHELSON, R., MERZENICH, M., PETTIT, C., AND SCHINDLER, R., A cochlear prosthesis, further clinical observations and preliminary results of physiological studies. *Laryngoscope*, 83, 1166–1172 (1973).

MILLER, A., A case of severe unilateral loss helped by a hearing aid. *J. Speech Hear. Disord.*, 30, 186–187 (1965a).

MILLER, C., Lipreading performance as a function of continuous visual distraction. Unpublished Master's Thesis, Michigan State University (1965b).

MILLER, G., AND NICELY, P., An analysis of perceptual confusions among some English consonants. *J. Acoust. Soc. Am.*, 27, 338–352 (1955).

MILLER, J., An analytical evaluation of speech discrimination scores prior to and following an auditory training program. Unpublished Master's Thesis, University of Maryland (1952).

MILLS, W., Auditory localization. In TOBIAS, J. (Ed.), *Foundations of Modern Auditory Theory*, Vol. 2, Chapter 8. New York: Academic Press (1972).

MINIFIE, F., Speech acoustics. In MINIFIE, F., HIXON, T., AND WILLIAMS, F., Normal Aspects of Speech, Hearing, and Language, Chapter 7. Englewood Cliffs, N.J.: Prentice-Hall, Inc. (1973).

MONCUR, J., AND DIRKS, D., Binaural and monaural

speech intelligibility in reverberation. *J. Speech Hear. Res.*, 10, 186–195 (1967).

MONTGOMERY, G., Analysis of pure-tone audiometric responses in relation to speech development in the profoundly deaf. *J. Acoust. Soc. Am.*, 41, 53–59 (1967).

NABELEK, A., AND PICKETT, J., Reception of consonants in a classroom as affected by monaural and binaural listening, noise, reverberation and hearing aids. *J. Acoust. Soc. Am.*, 65, 628–639 (1974a).

NABELEK, A., AND PICKETT, J., Monaural and binaural speech perception through hearing aids under noise and reverberation with normal and hearing impaired listeners. *J. Speech Hear. Res.*, 17, 724–739 (1974b).

NAVARRO, M., AND VOGELSON, D., An objective assessment of a CROS hearing aid. *Arch. Otolaryngol.*, 100, 58–59 (1974).

NEWBY, H., *Audiology: Principles and Practice*. New York: Appleton-Century-Crofts., Inc. (1958).

NEWBY, H., *Audiology* (rev. ed.). New York: Appleton-Century-Crofts., Inc. (1964).

NICHOLS, R., JR., ET AL., Electroacoustic characteristics of hearing aids. Section I of OSRD Report Number 4666 (1945).

NICHOLS, R., JR., MARQUIS, R., WIKLUND, W., FILLER, A., HUDGINS, C., AND PETERSON, G., The influence of body-baffle effects on the performance of hearing aids. *J. Acoust. Soc. Am.*, 19, 943–951 (1947).

NIELSEN, T., Information about: The directional microphone. Oticongress, 2 (1972).

NIEMOELLER, A., SILVERMAN, S., AND DAVIS, H., Hearing aids. In DAVIS, H., AND SILVERMAN, S. (Eds.), *Hearing and Deafness*, Third Edition, Chapter 10, Chicago: Holt, Rinehart and Winston (1970).

NINDS, *Human Communication and Its Disorders: An Overview*. U. S. Department of Health, Education, and Welfare, Public Health Service, National Institutes of Health, NINDS Monograph No. 10, 13 (1969).

NIX, G., *Mainstream Education for Hearing Impaired Children and Youth*. New York: Grune and Stratton, Inc. (1976).

NORDLUND, B., AND FRITZELL, B., The influence of azimuth on speech signals. *Acta Otolaryngol.*, 632–642 (1963).

NORTHCUTT, W., *The Hearing Impaired Child in a Regular Classroom*. Washington, D. C.: A.G. Bell Association for the Deaf (1973).

NORTHERN, J., CILIAX, D., ROTH, R., AND JOHNSON, R., JR., Military patient attitudes toward aural rehabilitation. *Asha*, 11, 391–395 (1969).

NORTHERN, J., AND DOWNS, M., *Hearing in Children*. Baltimore: Williams and Wilkins Company (1974).

NORTHERN, J., AND HATTLER, K., Earmold influence on aided speech identification tasks. *J. Speech Hear. Res.*, 13, 162–172 (1970).

OBNESORGE, H., Introduction to functional principles of a hearing aid. In *Hearing Instrument Technology*, Chapter 5.1. Compiled by Hans-Jürgen von Killisch-Horn, Median Verlag, Heidelberg, West Germany (1975).

OEKEN, S., Can the Hearing of patients suffering from high-tone perceptive deafness be improved by frequency transposition? *Int. Audiol.*, 2, 263–266 (1963).

OLSEN, W., The influence of harmonic and intermodulation distortion on speech intelligibility. *Scand. Audiol.*, Supplement 1, 109–123 (1971).

OLSEN, W., AND CARHART, R., Development of test procedure for evaluation of binaural hearing aids. *Bull. Prosthet. Res.*, 10, 22–49 (1967).

OLSEN, W., AND CARHART, R., Head diffraction effects on ear-level hearing aids. *Audiology*, 14, 244–258 (1975).

OLSEN, W., AND TILLMAN, T., Hearing aids and sensorineural loss. *Ann. Otol.*, 77, 717–727 (1968).

OLSEN, W., AND WILBUR, S., Physical performance characteristics of different hearing aids and speech discrimination scores achieved with them by hearing impaired persons. Paper presented at the annual convention of the American Speech and Hearing Association (1967).

OLSEN, W., AND WILBUR, S., Hearing aid distortion and speech intelligibility. Paper presented at the annual convention of the American Speech and Hearing Association (1968).

O'NEILL, J., Contributions of the visual components of oral symbols to speech comprehension. *J. Speech Hear. Disord.*, 19, 429–439 (1954).

O'NEILL, J., Recognition of intelligibility test materials in context and isolation. *J. Speech Hear. Disord.*, 22, 87–90 (1957).

ORWALL, B., The problems of the aged in adapting themselves to the use of a hearing aid. In LIDEN, G. (Ed.), *Geriatric Audiology*. Stockholm: Almqvist and Wiksell (1968).

OWENS, E., Rehabilitation of implanted patients. In MERZENICH, M., SCHINDLER, R., AND SOOY, F. (Eds.), *Proceedings of the First International Conference on Electrical Stimulation of the Acoustic Nerve as a Treatment for Profound Sensorineural Deafness in Man*, 151–160. San Francisco: Velobind, Inc. (1974).

OYER, H., AND DOUDNA, M., Structural analysis of word responses made by hard-of-hearing subjects on a discrimination test. *Arch. Otolaryngol.*, 70, 357–364 (1959).

OYER, H., AND DOUDNA, M., Word familiarity as a factor in testing discrimination of hard-of-hearing subjects. *Arch. Otolaryngol.*, 72, 351–355 (1960).

OYER, H., AND FRANKMANN, J., *The Aural Rehabilitation Process, A Conceptual Framework Analysis*. New York: Holt, Rinehart, and Winston (1975).

PALMER, J., The effect of speaker differences on the intelligibility of phonetically balanced word lists. *J. Speech Hear. Dis.*, 20, 192–195 (1955).

PASCOE, D., Frequency responses of hearing aids and their effects on the speech perception of hearing impaired subjects. *Ann. Otol., Rhinol., Laryngol.*, Supplement 23, 84, No. 5, Part 2 (1975).

Paying Through the Ear. Washington: Retired Professional Action Group (1973).

PETERSON, A., AND GROSS, E., JR., *Handbook of Noise Measurement*. Concord: General Radio (1972).

PETERSON, G., AND BARNEY, H., Control methods used in a study of the vowels. *J. Acoust. Soc. Am.*, 24, 175–184 (1952).

PICKETT, J., Tactual communication of speech sounds to the deaf. Comparison with lipreading. *J. Speech Hear. Dis.*, 28, 315–330 (1963).

PICKETT, J., Proceedings of the conference on speech analyzing aids for the deaf. *Am. Ann. Deaf*, 113, 116–330 (1968).

PICKETT, J., Speech processing aids for communication handicaps: Some research problems. In

Tower, D., (Ed.), *The Nervous System*, Vol. 3, *Human Communication and its Disorders*, 299–304. New York: Raven Press (1975).

Pike, C., *Transistor Fundamentals*, Vol. 2, *Basic Transistor Circuits*. Kansas City: The Bobbs-Merrill Company, Inc. (1974).

Plenge, G., On the differences between localization and lateralization. *J. Acoust. Soc. Am.*, 56, 944–951 (1974).

Pollack, D., *Educational Audiology for the Limited Hearing Infant*. Springfield, Ill.: Charles C Thomas (1970).

Pollack, D., Denver's acoupedic program. *Peabody J. Educ.*, 5, 180–185 (1974).

Pollack, M., Electroacoustic characteristics. In Pollack, M. (Ed.), *Amplification for the Hearing-Impaired*. New York: Grune and Stratton (1975).

Porter, T., Hearing aids in a residential school. *Am. Ann. Deaf*, 118, 31–33 (1973).

Prall, J., Lipreading and hearing aids combine for better comprehension. *Volta Rev.*, 59, 64–65 (1957).

Preves, D., Some considerations in using KEMAR to measure hearing aid performance. Paper presented before Conference on Manikin Measurement Techniques, Washington (1976).

Raas, M., Your custom earmold. *The Hearing Dealer*, 16 (1972).

Recommended Methods for Measurements of the Electroacoustical Characteristics of Hearing Aids. Publication 118. Geneva: International Electrotechnical Commission (1959).

Reddell, R., and Calvert, D., Selecting a hearing aid by interpreting audiologic data. *J. Auditory Res.*, 6, 445–452 (1966).

Resnick, D., and Becker, M., Hearing aid evaluation—A new approach. *Asha*, 5, 695–699 (1963).

Rintelmann, W., Harford, E., and Burchfield, S., A special case of auditory localization: CROS for blind persons with unilateral loss. *Arch. Otolaryngol.*, 91, 284–288 (1970).

Ritsma, R., Speech intelligibility with eye and ear. *Scand. Audiol.*, Supplement 4, 231–242 (1974).

Roberts, C., Can hearing aids damage hearing? *Acta Otolaryngol.*, 69, 123–125 (1970).

Robinson, D., and Gaeth, J., A procedure for testing/training prelinguistic hearing impaired children. *Volta Rev.*, 77, 249–254 (1975).

Rosenberg, P., Case history: The first test. In Katz, J. (Ed.), *Handbook of Clinical Audiology*, 60–66. Baltimore: Williams and Wilkins Company (1972).

Rosenthal, A., The effects of power supply on the electroacoustic characteristics of modern hearing aids. Unpublished Master's Thesis, University of Kansas Medical Center (1975).

Ross, M., Loop auditory training systems for preschool hearing impaired children. *Volta Rev.*, 71, 289–295 (1969).

Ross, M., Classroom acoustics and speech intelligibility. In Katz, J. (Ed.), *Handbook of Clinical Audiology*, 756–771. Baltimore: Williams and Wilkins Company (1972a).

Ross, M., Principles of Aural Rehabilitation. New York: Bobbs-Merrill Company (1972b).

Ross, M., Considerations underlying the selection and utilization of classroom amplification systems. *J. Acad. Rehab. Audiol.*, 6, 33–42 (1973).

Ross M., Hearing aid selection for the preverbal hearing impaired child. In Pollack, M. (Ed.), *Amplification for the Hearing-Impaired*. New York: Grune and Stratton, Inc. (1975).

Ross, M., Assessment of the hearing-impaired prior to mainstreaming. In Nix, G. (Ed.), *Mainstream Education for Hearing Impaired Children and Youth*. New York: Grune and Stratton, Inc. (1976).

Ross, M., Model educational cascade for hearing impaired children. In Nix, G. (Ed.), Mainstream *Education for Hearing Impaired Children and Youth*. New York: Grune and Stratton, Inc. (1976).

Ross, M., Barrett, L., and Trier, T., Ear-level hearing aids for motivated patients with minimal hearing losses. *Laryngoscope*, 76, 1555–1561 (1966).

Ross, M., Duffy, R., Cooker, H., and Sergeant, R., Contribution of the lower audible frequencies to the recognition of emotions. *Am. Ann. Deaf.*, 118, 37–42 (1973).

Ross, M., and Giolas, T., Effect of three classroom listening conditions on speech intelligibility. *Am. Ann. Deaf*, 116, 580–584 (1971).

Ross, M., Giolas, T., and Carver, P., Effect of three classroom listening conditions on speech intelligibility: A replication in part. *Language, Speech Hear. Serv. Schools*, 4, 72–76 (1973).

Ross, M., Hunt, M., Kessler, M., and Henniges, M., The use of a rating scale to compare binaural and monaural amplification with hearing impaired children. *Volta Rev.*, 76, 93–99 (1974).

Ross, M., Kessler, M., Phillips, M., and Lerman, J., Visual, auditory, and combined mode presentations of the WIPI test to hearing impaired children. *Volta Rev.*, 74, 90–96 (1972).

Ross, M., and Lerman, J., Hearing aid usage and its effect upon residual hearing. *Arch. Otolaryngol.*, 86, 639–644 (1967).

Ross, M., and Lerman, J., A picture identification test for hearing-impaired children. *J. Speech Hear. Res.*, 13, 44–53 (1970).

Rubenstein, H., and Pickett, J., Word intelligibility and word position in sentences. *J. Acoust. Soc. Am.*, 29, 1263 (1957).

Rudmose, H., Clark, K., Carlson, F., Eisenstein, J., and Walker, R., Voice measurements with an audio spectrometer. *J. Acoust. Soc. Am.*, 20, 503–512 (1948).

Sanders, D., *Aural Rehabilitation*. Englewood Cliffs, N.J.: Prentice-Hall, Inc. (1971).

Sanders, D., and Goodrich, S., The relative contribution of visual and auditory components of speech to speech intelligibility as a function of three conditions of frequency distortion. *J. Speech Hear. Res.*, 14, 154–159 (1971).

Sayers, B., and Cherry, E., Mechanism of binaural fusion in the hearing of speech. *J. Acoust. Soc. Am.*, 29, 973–987 (1957).

Schaudinischky, L., New hearing-aid for the monaurally deaf restoring binaural hearing. *Acta Otolaryngol.*, 60, 461–466 (1965).

Schindler, R., and Merzenich, M., Chronic intracochlear electrode implantation: cochlear pathology and acoustic nerve survival. *Ann. Otol., Rhinol., Laryngol.*, 83, 202–215 (1974).

Schmitz, H., Loudness discomfort level modification. *J. Speech Hear. Res.*, 12, 807–817 (1969).

Schubert, E., Some preliminary experiments on

binaural time delay and intelligibility. *J. Acoust. Soc. Am.*, 28, 895–901 (1956).

SEDGE, R., An investigation of the difference between auditory and auditory-visual articulation curves. Unpublished Master's Thesis, Michigan State University (1965).

SESSLER, G., AND WEST, J., Electret transducers: A review. *J. Acoust. Soc. Am.*, 53, 1589–1600 (1973).

SHAPIRO, I., Hearing aid fitting by prescription. *Audiology*, 15, 163–173 (1976).

SHORE, I., BILGER, R., AND HIRSH, I., Hearing aid evaluation: Reliability of repeated measurements. *J. Speech Hear. Disord.*, 25, 152–170 (1960).

SHUKNECHT, H., *Pathology of the Ear.* Cambridge: Harvard University Press (1974).

SIEGENTHALER, E., A study of the relationship between measured hearing loss and intelligibility of selected words. *J. Speech Hear. Disord.*, 14, 111–118 (1949).

SILVERMAN, S., Tolerance for pure tones and speech in normal and defective hearing. *Ann. Otol., Rhinol., Laryngol.*, 56, 658–677 (1947).

SILVERMAN, S., TAYLOR, S., AND DAVIS, H., Hearing aids. In DAVIS, H., AND SILVERMAN, S. (Eds.), *Hearing and Deafness*, Chapter 10. Chicago, Holt, Rinehart and Winston, Inc. (1960).

SIMMONS, F., Electrical stimulation of the auditory nerve in man. *Arch. Otolaryngol.*, 84, 2–54 (1966).

SIVIAN, L., AND WHITE, S., On minimum audible sound fields. *J. Acoust. Soc. Am.*, 4, 288–321 (1933).

SMITH, C., Residual hearing and speech production in deaf children. Communication Sciences Laboratory Report No. 4, CUNY Graduate Center, New York (1973).

SMITH, G., The telephone adapter and other telephone aids for the hard of hearing. *Volta Rev.*, 76, 474–484 (1974).

SMITH, K., Variability of battery life in children's hearing aids. *Audecibel*, 21, 148–152 (1972).

SMITH, K., BALDWIN, R., AND HETSEL, G., A study of discharge characteristics of modern hearing aids as a function of their power supply. Paper presented at the annual convention of the American Speech and Hearing Association, San Francisco (1971).

SORTINI, A., Hearing aids for pre-school children. *Volta Rev.*, 58, 103–106 (1956).

SPEAKS, C., AND JERGER, J., Method for measurement of speech identification. *J. Speech Hear. Res.*, 8, 185–194 (1965).

SPEAKS, C., KARMEN, J., AND BENITEZ, L., Effect of a competing message on synthetic sentence identification, *J. Speech Hear. Res.*, 10, 390–396 (1967).

Special Report: Senate subcommittee looks at hearing aids. *Washington Sounds*, 7, 1–6 (1973).

Standard for Hearing Aids, FDA-MDS-071-0002. Washington, D. C.: Food and Drug Administration (1974; 1975).

STEWART, J., The hearing aid – Investment in the child's future lifetime potential. *Volta Rev.*, 75, 350–352 (1973).

STREVENS, P., Spectra of fricative noise in human speech. *Lang. Speech*, 3, 32–49 (1960).

STUDEBAKER, G., AND ZACHMAN, T., Investigation of the acoustics of earmold vents. *J. Acoust. Soc. Am.*, 47, 1107–1115 (1970).

SULLIVAN, E., Feedback controlled. *Hearing Instruments*, 24, 27, 35 (1973a).

SULLIVAN, E., Fine tuning – A study on earmold modifications. *Mercury Laboratory Monograph* (1973b).

SULLIVAN, E., Tips about children's earmold fittings. *Hear. Aid J.*, 8, 33 (1974).

SUMBY, W., AND POLLACK, I., Visual contribution to speech intelligibility in noise. *J. Acoust. Soc. Am.*, 26, 212–215 (1954).

SUNG, G., SUNG, R., AND ANGELELLI, R., Hearing aid frequency response and speech intelligibility. *J. Auditory Res.*, 11, 318–321 (1971).

SUNG, G., SUNG, R., AND ANGELELLI, R., Directional microphone in hearing aids. *Arch. Otolaryngol.*, 101, 316–319 (1975).

SUNG, G., SUNG, R., HODGSON, W., AND ANGELELLI, R., Intelligibility of speech transduced via classroom-installed FM and conventional audio induction loop amplification systems. Paper presented at the American Speech and Hearing Association Convention, Detroit (1973).

SUNG, R., AND HODGSON, W., Performance of individual hearing aids utilizing microphone and induction coil input. *J. Speech Hear. Res.*, 14, 365–371 (1971).

SUNG, R., SUNG, G., AND HODGSON, W., A comparative study of physical characteristics of hearing aids on microphone and telecoil inputs. *Audiology*, 13, 78–89 (1974).

SUZUKI, T., AND OGIBA, Y., Conditioned reflex audiometry. *Arch. Otolaryngol.*, 74, 192–198 (1961).

TEMBY, A., Sound diffraction in the vicinity of the human ear. *Acustica*, 15, 219–222 (1965).

THOMPSON, G., AND LASSMAN, F., Relationship of auditory distortion test results to speech discrimination through flat versus selective amplifying systems. *J. Speech Hear. Res.*, 12, 594–606 (1969).

TILLMAN, T., AND CARHART, R., An expanded test for speech discrimination utilizing CNC monosyllabic words: Northwestern University Test No. 6. USAF School of Aerospace Medicine SAM-TR-66-55 (1966).

TILLMAN, T., CARHART, R., AND OLSEN, W., Hearing aid efficiency in a competing speech situation. *J. Speech Hear. Res.*, 13, 789–811 (1970).

TILLMAN, T., KASTEN, R., AND HORNER, J., Effect of head shadow on reception of speech. Paper presented at the annual convention of the American Speech and Hearing Association, Chicago, Ill., November (1963).

TRUAX, R., Amplifier to prosthesis. In DONNELLY, K. (Ed.), *Interpreting Hearing Aid Technology*, 3–39. Springfield, Ill.: Charles C Thomas (1974).

VAN EYSBERGEN, H., AND GROEN, J., The 2-ML coupler in the high frequency performance of hearing aids. *Acustica*, 9, 381–388 (1959).

VAN WINKLE, D., Earmold effects on the pure tone thresholds of normal and hearing impaired listeners. Unpublished Master's Thesis, University of Kansas Medical Center (1975).

VARGO, S., TAYLOR, S., TANNAHILL, J., AND PLUMMER, S., The intelligibility of speech by hearing aids on inductance loop and microphone modes of signal reception. *J. Speech Hear. Res.*, 13, 87–91 (1970).

Variables in Fitting. *Maico Training Manual*, 302–305. Minneapolis: Maico Hearing Instruments (1974).

VENTRY, I., WOODS, R., AND HILL, N., Most comfortable loudness for pure tones, noise, and speech. *J. Acoust. Soc. Am.*, 49, 1805–1813 (1971).

VERNON, J., Round window stimulation in man. In MERZENICH, M., SCHINDLER, R., AND SOOY, F. (Eds.), *Proceedings of the First International Conference on Electrical Stimulation of the Acoustic Nerve as a Treatment for Profound Sensorineural Deafness in Man*, 63–78. San Francisco: Velo-bind, Inc. (1974).

VERNON, M., Mind over mouth: A rationale for total communication. *Volta Rev.*, 74, 529–540 (1972).

Veterans Administration Hearing Aid Performance Measurement Data and Hearing Aid Selection Procedures, Contract Year 1975. Washington: Veterans Administration (1975).

VIET, I., A short introduction to the circuitry and function of hearing aid amplifiers. In *Hearing Instrument Technology*, Chapter 5.7. Compiled by Hans-Jürgen von Killisch-Horn, Median Verlag, Heidelberg, West Germany (1975a).

VIET, I., Short introduction to electrical science. In *Hearing Instrument Technology*, Chapter 4.1. Compiled by Hans-Jurgen von Killisch-Horn, Median Verlag, Heidelberg, West Germany (1975b).

WALDEN, B., PROSEK, R., AND WORTHINGTON, D., Auditory and audiovisual feature transmission in hearing impaired adults. *J. Speech Hear. Res.*, 18, 272–280 (1975).

WALLACH, H., On sound localization. *J. Acoust. Soc. Am.*, 10, 270–274 (1939).

WALLACH, H., The role of head movements and vestibular and visual cues in sound localization. *J. Exp. Psychol.*, 27, 339–368 (1940).

WANSDRONK, D., On the influence of the diffraction of sound waves around the human head on the characteristics of hearing aids. *J. Acoust. Soc. Am.*, 31, 1609–1612 (1959).

WARREN, M., AND KASTEN, R., Efficacy of hearing aid repairs by manufacturers and by alternative repair facilities. *J. Acad. Rehab. Audiol., 9, 38–47 (1976).*

WATSON, L., AND TOLAN, T., *Hearing Tests and Hearing Instruments*. Baltimore: Williams and Wilkins Company (1949).

WATSON, T., *The Use of Residual Hearing in the Education of Deaf Children*. Reprint Number 770. Washington, D. C.: The Volta Bureau (1961).

WATSON, T., The use of hearing aids by hearing impaired children in ordinary schools. *Volta Rev.*, 741–744, 787 (1964).

WEATHERTON, M., AND GOETZINGER, C., The effects of various modified earmolds on hearing sensitivity. *J. Auditory Res.*, 11, 25–32 (1971).

WHITE, R., AND MERCER, H., Microelectrodes for biorecording and biostimulation fabricated by integrated circuit techniques. In MILLER, H., AND HARRISON, D. (Eds.), *Biomedical Electrode Technology*, 159–168. New York: Academic Press (1974).

WIENER, F., On the diffraction of a progressive sound wave by the human head. *J. Acoust. Soc. Am.*, 19, 143–146 (1947).

WINITZ, H., *From Syllable to Conversation*. Baltimore: University Park Press (1975).

WINITZ, H., LA RIVIERE, C., AND HERRIMAN, E., Variations in VOT for English stops. *J. Phonetics*, 3, 41–52 (1975).

WITTER, H., Quality judgments of hearing aid transduced speech. *J. Speech Hear. Res.*, 14, 312–322 (1971).

WRIGHT, H., Binaural hearing and the hearing-impaired. *Arch. Otolaryngol.*, 70, 485–494 (1959).

WRIGHT, J., Auricular education of deaf children. *Medical Rev.*, 92, 241–242 (1917).

WULLENSTEIN, H., Theory and practice of tympanoplasty. *Laryngoscope*, 66, 1076–1093 (1956).

WULLENSTEIN, H., AND WIGAND, M., A hearing aid for single ear deafness and its requirements. *Acta Otolaryngol.*, 54, 136–142 (1962).

YONOVITZ, A., AND CAMPBELL, I., Speech discrimination in noise: A test of binaural advantage in normal and hearing impaired children. Paper presented at the American Speech and Hearing Association Convention, Las Vegas (1974).

ZINK, G., Hearing aids children wear: A longitudinal study of performance. *Volta Rev.*, 74, 41–51 (1972).

ZWISLOCKI, J., *An Ear-Like Coupler for Earphone Calibration*. Syracuse: Laboratory of Sensory Communication, Syracuse University (1971).

Abramson, A., 101
Alberti, P., 138
Alpiner, J., 204
Angel, J., 116, 117
Angelelli, R., 104, 124, 155
Armbruster, V., 168
Aufricht, H., 177
Baldwin, R., 62
Ballenger, H., 210
Barnet, A., 147
Barney, H., 96, 97, 99, 100
Barrett, L., 129
Barron, F., 122
Barry, J., 174, 175, 183
Bauer, B., 40
Becker, M., 137
Behnke, C., 45
Belendiuk, K., 116
Bellefleur, P., 168, 216, 233
Bender, R., 168
Benitez, L., 114
Bennett, D., 216
Beranek, L., 259
Berger, K., 5, 7, 8, 10, 12, 14, 43, 56
Bergman, M., 138, 173
Bess, F., 135
Bilger, R., 136
Birt, B., 138
Blair, J., 168
Bode, D., 215
Boothroyd, A., 168, 224, 232
Borrild, K., 233
Boyd, J., 211
Brander, R., 89
Bresson, K., 181, 182
Bricker, D., 168
Bricker, W., 168
Briskey, R., 58, 67, 68, 70
Brite, R., 40
Brown, A., 218
Burchfield, S., 175
Burkhard, M., 89, 261
Burnett, E., 89
Burney, P., 140
Butler, R., 116
Byers, V., 216
Byman, J., 220
Byrne, D., 122
Calvert, D., 114, 133, 233
Campbell, I., 228
Carhart, R., 92, 108–110, 113, 118–122, 134, 142, 168, 171, 211, 224
Carlisle, R., 122
Carlson, E., 40
Carmel, N., 212
Carson, E., 170
Carver, P., 240
Castle, W., 143, 168

Cherry, C., 116
Cherry, E., 116, 118, 120
Ciliax, D., 219
Clarke, B., 232
Colten, S., 100
Conkey, H., 175
Cooker, H., 224, 227
Cooper, K., 266
Cooper, W., 56
Crandall, K., 146
Damashek, M., 232
Danaher, E., 100, 227
David, E., Jr., 118, 120
Davis, H., 7, 15, 17, 91, 112, 114, 131, 133, 136–138, 145
Davis, R., 58
de Boer, B., 40, 168
Deutsch, L., 228
Di Carlo, L., 212
Dirks, D., 118, 120, 121
Dobelle, W., 269
Dodds, E., 131, 176, 179, 181, 182, 185, 219
Doehring, D., 216
Doudna, M., 210
Downs, M., 168, 201, 214
Druz, W., 216
Duffy, R., 224, 227
Elliott, L., 96, 97, 168
Epstein, A., 125
Erber, N., 122, 168, 217–219
Ewertsen, H., 199, 203
Fant, G., 101
Farrant, R., 216
Finitzo-Hieber, T., 162
Fisher, B., 168
Fisher, H., 116
Fite, W., 116, 117
Fletcher, H., 90, 91, 221
Flottorp, G., 113
Forester, C., 210
Foust, K., 224, 226
Fowler, E., 174
Frank, T., 124, 143
Frankmann, J., 207
Fransson, A., 205
Fredrickson, J., 267
Freedman, S., 116
French, N., 95, 96, 114
Fritzell, B., 119, 120, 172
Fry, D., 224
Gaeth, J., 166, 189, 215, 218
Galloway, A., 204
Gang, R., 93
Gardner, M., 120
Gauger, J., 204
Gengel, R., 224, 226
Gerber, S., 93, 103
Gheewala, T., 269, 270

Giolas, T., 125, 240
Glattke, T., 267, 268, 270
Goetzinger, C., 56, 137, 179
Goldberg, H., 31
Goldstein, M., 209, 221
Goode, R., 266–268
Gooden, R., 124, 143
Goodfellow, L. 210
Goodhill, V., 265
Goodrich, S., 217
Grammatico, L., 146, 212
Green, D., 120, 179, 182
Green, R., 168
Green, S., 58
Greenbaum, W., 58, 67, 70
Griffing, T., 55
Groen, J., 58
Guttman, N., 118
Halle, M., 101
Hanson, W., 122
Hardy, W., 173
Harford, E., 131, 136, 173–176, 178, 178–183, 185, 216, 217, 219
Harris, J., 89, 93, 113, 120
Harris, K., 101
Haskins, H., 173
Hayes, D., 137
Hebrank, J., 116, 117
Henning, G., 120
Herriman, E., 101, 102
Hetsel, G., 62
Heyne, K., 40
Hieber, T., 151
Hinchman, S., 119, 171
Hirsch, I., 95, 96, 116, 118, 120, 136, 232
Hochberg, I., 108
Hodgson, W., 56, 57, 113, 125, 142, 180, 181, 233
Hopkins, H., 218
Horner, J., 119, 142, 171
Horton, K., 212
House, W., 268, 272
Hudgins, C., 98, 212, 232
Hughes, G., 101
Jamroz, A., 211
Jeffers, J., 96
Jerger, J., 93, 113, 114, 118, 137, 216
Jerger, S., 93
Jetty, A., 58, 180
Jirsa, R., 113, 137
Johansson, B., 111, 216
Johansson, R., 168
Johnson, E., 210
Johnson, K., 118
Jongkees, L., 116
Joseph, M., 95, 96
Kaiser, J., 120
Kankkunen, A., 149
Karlovich, R., 218
Karmen, J., 114
Kasten, R., 62, 74, 89, 107–109, 113, 119, 122, 138, 142, 171–173, 183, 195, 200

Keil, J., 219
Kiang, N., 269
Killion, M., 40
Kleffner, F., 213
Klijn, J., 233
Knowles, H., 261
Kodman, F., 191
Koenig, W., 116, 118, 168
Konkle, D., 135
Kryter, K., 259
Kuyper, P., 168
Lach, R., 212
Langford, B., 121
Lankford, J., 45
LaRiviere, C., 101, 102
Lassman, F., 134
Leckie, D., 168
Lempert, J., 264
Lenneberg, E., 147
Lentz, W., 123, 124, 143
Leonard, R., 219
Lerman, J., 151, 160, 168, 216
Lewis, D., 168
Lewis, N., 216
Liberman, A., 102, 103, 111
Licklider, J., 118
Liden, G., 149
Ling, D., 61, 99, 103, 104, 155, 168, 212, 216, 233
Lisker, L., 101
Lloyd, N., 149
Lotterman, S., 62, 89, 107–109, 113, 119, 122, 138, 142, 171, 183, 195
Lounsbury, E., 166, 189
Ludvigsen, C., 220
Lundborg, T., 215
Luterman, D., 168
Lybarger, S., 43, 49, 51, 53, 56, 57, 74, 121, 122, 178
Lynne, G., 110
Macrae, J., 164, 216
Maier, H., 147
Majerus, D., 195
Malles, I., 173
Malmquist, C., 113
Markle, D., 216, 217
Martin, E., 100, 104
Matkin, N., 126, 145, 149, 150, 154, 156, 167, 168, 177, 182, 229, 230, 233
Maxon, T., 228
Mazor, M., 228
McClellen, M., 57
McCroskey, R., 212
McDonald, E., 168
McDonald, F., 58, 179
McMenamin, S., 233
Melen, R., 269, 270
Mercer, H., 269
Merzenich, M., 268–271
Michelson, R., 270
Miller, A., 175
Miller, C., 219

Miller, G., 98, 210
Miller, J., 212
Mills, W., 117
Minifie, F., 98, 99, 101–103
Moncur, J., 118
Montgomery, G., 224
Moxon, E., 269
Mundel, A., 122
Murdock, C., 57, 180, 181
Musket, C., 136, 173
Nabelek, A., 118, 142, 159, 228
Navarro, M., 184
Newby, H., 136, 170
Nicely, P., 98, 210
Nichols, R., 73, 122
Nielsen, T., 40
Niemoeller, A., 40
Nix, G., 223
Nordlund, B., 119, 120, 172
Northcutt, W., 223
Northern, J., 201, 203, 212
Obnesorge, H., 41
Oeken, S., 216
Ogiba, Y., 149
Olsen, W., 93, 113, 119, 120, 122, 123, 126, 141, 142, 158, 224, 229, 230, 233
O'Neill, J., 210, 217
Orwall, B., 205
Osberger, N., 100
Owens, E., 270
Oyer, H., 207, 210, 215
Palmer, J., 210
Pascoe, D., 114
Peterson, A., 259
Peterson, G., 96, 97, 99, 100
Pickett, J., 100, 104, 118, 142, 155, 159, 210, 227, 228, 271, 272
Pike, C., 41
Plenge, G., 116
Pollack, D., 202, 212
Pollack, I., 217
Pollack, K., 119, 142
Pollack, M., 89
Porter, T., 166, 189, 199
Prall, J., 217
Preves, D., 89
Prosek, R., 218
Raas, M., 45
Radley, J., 101
Reddell, R., 114, 133
Resnick, D., 137
Revoile, S., 89, 107, 138
Reynolds, E., 95, 96
Rintelmann, W., 58, 175, 180
Ritsma, R., 218
Roberts, C., 216
Robinson, D., 215
Rosenberg, P., 191
Rosenthal, A., 62
Ross, M., 129, 151, 158, 160, 168, 179, 216, 218, 222–224, 227, 228, 233, 238–240
Rubenstein, H., 210

Rudmose, H., 94
Sachs, R., 89
Sanders, D., 169, 217, 222
Sayers, B., 116, 118, 120
Schaudinischky, L., 175, 186
Schindler, D., 269
Schindler, R., 271
Schmitz, H., 112
Schneiderman, C., 175
Schubert, E., 118
Sedge, R., 217
Sergeant, R., 224, 227
Sessler, G., 41
Shapiro, I., 138
Shore, I., 136, 137
Shuknecht, H., 271
Siegenthaler, E., 211
Silverman, S., 17, 91, 145, 212
Simmons, F., 269, 270
Sinclair, J., 58, 67, 70
Sivian, L., 122, 172
Smith, C., 224
Smith, G., 31
Smith, K., 62, 195
Sortini, A., 147, 169
Speaks, C., 113, 114, 137
Staab, W., 169
Steinberg, J., 95, 96, 114
Stewart, J., 212
Strevens, P., 101
Studebaker, G., 57, 58, 179
Sullivan, E., 56, 57, 59
Sumby, W., 217
Sung, G., 56, 104, 124, 142, 155, 233
Sung, R., 56, 104, 124, 125, 142, 155, 229, 233
Suzuki, T., 149
Taylor, S., 17
Temby, A., 122
Thelin, J., 114
Thomas, J., 156, 167, 168, 177, 182
Thompson, G., 134
Tillman, T., 93, 118–120, 141, 142, 159, 171–173, 224
Tolan, T., 7, 8, 11, 12, 221
Trier, T., 129
Truax, R., 41
Van Bergeijk, W., 118
van der Veer, R., 116
Van Dyke, R., 168, 216
Van Eysbergen, H., 58
Van Winkle, D., 57, 58
Vargo, S., 125
Vegely, A., 168
Ventry, I., 108
Vernon, J., 268
Vernon, M., 213
Viet, I., 41
Vogelson, D., 184
Walden, B., 218
Wallach, H., 117, 120
Wansdronk, D., 122
Warren, M., 200

Watson, L., 7, 8, 11, 12, 221
Watson, T., 93, 141
Weatherton, M., 56, 179
Whetnall, E., 169
White, M., 269
White, R., 269, 270
White, S., 122, 142, 172
Wiener, F., 122
Wigand, M., 174
Wiig, E., 168
Wilbur, S., 113, 123
Wilson, R., 120

Winitz, H., 101, 102, 104
Witter, H., 89
Worthington, D., 218
Wright, D., 116, 117
Wright, H., 121
Wright, J., 210
Wullenstein, H., 174, 265
Yonovitz, A., 228
Zachman, T., 57, 58
Zink, G., 166, 189, 199
Zwislocki, J., 261

Accesories for hearing aids, 60–61
Amplifiers, 110, 192
ANSI standards, 68, 73–89
Auditory training, 211–212, 215–216
  classroom systems, 221–243, 263–264
    binaural, 227–228, 239
    child-to-child communication, 225–226, 231–232, 235, 239
    electroacoustics, 227, 238
    hardwire, 230–232, 263
    induction loop, 229, 233–235
    microphones, 232
    operation, 228–229
    optimum unit, 241–243
    RF systems, 229, 230, 235–241, 264
    self-monitoring, 224–225, 231, 235
    signal-to-noise ratio, 223–224, 226, 231–232, 235, 240
Audiologic habilitation, 1–2, 207
  amplification and, 208, 212–213, 215
  concepts, 207–208
  history, 209–210
  research, 217, 220
  speechreading, 215, 217–220
Aural rehabilitation (see Audiologic habilitation)
Automatic Gain Control (AGC), 35, 39, 110–112, 131, 140, 160, 217, 261
  measurement (see also Electroacoustic measurements), 85–86
Batteries, 20–22, 61–66, 192, 194–195
  discharge patterns, 63, 64, 66
  electroacoustic modifications, 62
  life, 64, 65, 189
  tester, 61, 62, 195, 251
  types, 62
BICROS (see also CROS amplification), 156, 174, 178, 186
Binaural hearing, 13, 115–121, 142, 158–159, 173, 211, 227–228
Body aids, 113, 127, 132, 153–155, 156–158, 193
Body baffle, 121–123
BOHA (see also CROS amplification), 173–174
Bone conduction aids, 7, 154
Capacitor, 23–24, 38
Children's hearing aids, 145–169, 177, 201–202, 208, 212–213, 216
  parent management, 165–167, 207
  rationales, 146–147
  readings, 168–169
  selection procedures, 147–163
Couplers, 68, 76–77, 261
  2cc, 58, 67, 107
  Zwislocki, 58, 77, 261
CRISCROS (see also CROS amplification), 185

CROS amplification, 59, 131, 160, 170–187
  BICROS, 156, 174, 178, 186
  BOHA, 173–174
  clinical evaluation, 183–185
  CRISCROS, 185
  FOCALCROS, 186
  FROS, 186
  HICROS, 156, 157, 159, 181–183
  IROS, 156, 186
  MINICROS, 186
  MULTICROS, 186
  power CROS, 154, 185
  unilateral loss, 170–178
Deafness management quotient, 214
Delivery systems, 253–259
  ASHA guidelines, 258–259
Digital processing, 261–264
Dynamic range, 108, 111, 112, 130, 131, 140, 160, 270
Ear level aids, 113, 122, 127, 132, 154–155, 158–159, 171, 174, 194
Earmolds, 42–43, 192, 195–196
  connectors, 46, 49, 192
  impression techniques, 43–44
  inserts, 47, 56
  instant earmolds, 44–45
  materials, 43, 45
  modification, 49–58
  open, 156, 159, 173, 178–181
  performance, 60
  standard, 57, 180
  stock earmolds, 45
  styles, 46, 48
  types, 46, 47
  vented, 54–58
Earphones, 31–34, 39, 40, 192
Electroacoustic measurements, 68–89
  automatic gain control, 85–86
  environmental tests, 86
  equivalent input noise level, 85
  freuency range, 82–83
  frequency response, 81–83
  gain, 72, 78–81
  harmonic distortion, 83–85
  humidity, 88
  induction coil, 85
  saturation sound pressure level, 78
  shock, 87
  temperature, 87
  vibration, 88–89
Environmental tests, 86–89
Feedback, 59, 196
FOCALCROS (see also CROS amplification), 186
Frequency range (see also Electroacoustic measurements), 82–83
Frequency response, 46–47, 50, 55, 57, 72, 106,

113, 114, 122, 125, 155, 227
measurement (*see also* Electroacoustic measurements), 81–83
Frequency transposition, 216
FROS (*see also* CROS amplification), 186
FTC, 15
Gain, 107–109, 139, 140
measurement, 72, 78–81
reference test gain (*see also* Electroacoustic measurements), 81
Gain control, 23, 35, 38, 107, 109, 193
HAIC, 16
electroacoustic measures, 73–89
Harmonic distortion, 62, 64, 71–73, 91, 109, 111, 113, 140
measurement (*see also* Electroacoustic measurements), 83–85
Head baffle, 171
Head shadow, 119, 120, 122, 123, 142, 171–172, 173, 181–184
Hearing aid evaluation (selection procedures), 127, 133–137, 143–144, 160–163, 211
Hearing aid industry, 14–16
Hearing aid orientation, 188–205
adults, 202–205
audiologist's role, 190–191
batteries, 194–195
care of hearing aids, 196–197
checking the aid, 198–199
children, 201–202
components, 192–193
earmolds, 195–196
inserting the aid, 193–194
introduction of hearing aid, 191–200
introduction to amplified sound, 200–205
repairs, 199–200
switches and controls, 193
telephone, use of, 197
HICROS (*see also* CROS amplification), 156, 157, 159, 181–183
High frequency emphasis, 114
High frequency hearing loss, 128–129, 133–134
Implanted hearing aids, 267–268, 270
Induction loop systems, 30, 39, 61, 198, 229, 233–235
Intensity of speech, 90–93
Intermodulation distortion, 89, 113
IROS (*see also* CROS amplification), 156, 186
Listening check, 198–199
Localization, 116, 117, 120
Low frequency emphasis aids, 104, 114, 155, 227
Master hearing aids, 138–139, 242
Maximum output (see SSPL)
Microphones, 26–29, 40, 192
carbon, 8–10, 12

crystal, 11
directional, 29, 123–125, 143, 261
electret, 13, 26–28, 36, 38
MINICROS (*see also* CROS amplification), 186
Most comfortable loudness level (MCL), 11, 108
MULTICROS (*see also* CROS amplification), 186
Peak clipping, 35, 73, 110–112, 140, 160
Performance intensity function, 92, 93
Power CROS (*see also* CROS amplification), 154, 185
Presbycusics, 93, 181, 204–205, 208, 271
Receivers (*see* Earphones)
Recruitment, 108, 133
Resistance and resistors, 22–23, 36, 38
Saturation sound pressure level (SSPL), 73, 109, 110, 112, 139, 160, 227
measurement (*see also* Electroacoustic measurements), 78
Signal-to-noise ratio, 91, 93, 118, 123, 124, 162, 171, 187, 223, 263
Soundproofing, 246–250
Speech discrimination measures, 92, 130, 141, 142, 149, 150–152, 161, 162, 171, 173, 184, 210, 215, 217–218
Speech intelligibility, 57–58, 90–106, 109–111, 113–115, 117–119, 123–125, 131, 155, 180, 184, 210, 211, 240
Speech sounds, 96–103
coarticulation, 96, 103–104
consonants, 101–103
diphthongs, 102
distinctive features, 98
formants, 99
semivowels, 102
suprasegmentals, 103–104
vowels, 99–100
Speech spectrum, 94–96
Surgical modification, 264–267
fenestration, 264–265
homograft, 265
of ear canal, 266
tympanoplasty, 265
Telecoil, 29–31, 39, 40, 60–61, 85, 125–126, 142, 197, 233, 250
adapters, 30, 31, 60, 197
Threshold of discomfort (*see* Uncomfortable loudness level)
Threshold shift, 216–217
Tone control, 34, 38, 156, 193
Transistors, 12–13, 24–26, 35, 38, 40
Uncomfortable loudness level (UCL), 108, 112, 139, 162
Vacuum tubes, 10–11
Y-cords, 121, 157